The American Disease

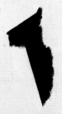

The American Disease

ORIGINS OF NARCOTIC CONTROL

EXPANDED EDITION

by David F. Musto, M.D.

NEW YORK   OXFORD
OXFORD UNIVERSITY PRESS

OXFORD UNIVERSITY PRESS

Oxford   New York   Toronto
Delhi   Bombay   Calcutta   Madras   Karachi
Petaling Jaya   Singapore   Hong Kong   Tokyo
Nairobi   Dar es Salaam   Cape Town
Melbourne   Auckland

and associated companies in
Beirut   Berlin   Ibadan   Nicosia

First published in 1973 by Yale University Press

Expanded edition first published in paperback in 1987
by Oxford University Press, Inc.,
200 Madison Avenue, New York, New York 10016

Oxford is a registered trademark of Oxford University Press

Library of Congress Cataloging-in-Publication Data
Musto, David F., 1936–
The American disease.
Includes index.
1. Narcotic habit—United States—History.   2. Narcotics, Control of—
United States—History.   3. Narcotic laws—United States—History.
4. Narcotic addicts—Rehabilitation—United States—History.
I. Title. [DNLM: 1. Drug and Narcotic Control—history—United States.
2. Legislation, Drug—history—United States.   3. Public Opinion.
4. Substance Dependence—history—United States. HV 5825 M991a]
HV5825.M84   1987   362.2'93'0973   87-14047
ISBN 0-19-505211-0 (pbk.)

10   9   8   7   6   5   4   3
Printed in the United States of America

This book is dedicated to
Dr. Albert J. Solnit

Contents

Abbreviations for Manuscript Sources

AP   Papers of Harry J. Anslinger. Deposited in the Pennsylvania Historical Collections of Pennsylvania State University.

BP   Papers of the Rt. Rev. Charles H. Brent. Deposited in the Manuscript Division of the Library of Congress.

BCR   Records of the Bureau of Chemistry, Department of Agriculture. Deposited in the National Archives; all references are to file no. 140 of Record Group 97.

BuP   Papers of Dr. Willis P. Butler, Shreveport, La.

JDR   Records of the Justice Department. Deposited in the National Archives; all references are to box 7 of Record Group 60.

PHSR   Records of the Public Health Service. Deposited in the National Archives; all references are to Record Group 90, file no. 2123.

RPU   Records of the Prohibition Unit, Bureau of Internal Revenue, Department of the Treasury. Now in the Justice Department, Bureau of Narcotics and Dangerous Drugs.

WP   Papers of Dr. Hamilton Wright. Deposited in the National Archives, Record Group 43, "Records of United States Delegations to the International Opium Commission and Conferences, 1909–1913" (entries 33 through 46), and "Records of Hamilton Wright" (entries 47 through 52).

Preface to the Expanded Edition

Drug use is linked to some of the most controversial issues we face today: drug testing at school and the workplace, controlling the spread of AIDS among and from those who use needles when taking drugs, attempts to stop the flow of drugs into the United States, and efforts to reduce the demand for drugs. We also face the menace of "crack," a smokable form of cocaine, which has frightened Americans with its seductive attractions and sad effects on users. We have gone through over two decades of widespread drug use, which has made us weary of the substances and their tragic consequences for so many users.

How can we understand this epidemic? It is important for us to know the history of drug abuse in America if we are to make wise decisions concerning drug abuse now and in the future. The United States has an extensive history in the use and abuse of drugs reaching far back into the nineteenth century. When we are in the middle of a drug crisis, however, we tend to forget this history and assume that we must face our drug onslaught with no guideposts. Unaware of how we have overcome past drug problems, we are liable to panic.

Almost fifteen years have passed since the publication of *The American Disease*—a period of intense concern about drug abuse. During this time billions of dollars have been spent fighting drug abuse through law enforcement, treatment, and research. We have witnessed more than one "war on drugs," and we have heard that our nation has "turned the corner" in this war. Proposals for a variety of solutions to the drug problem, ranging from much stricter laws—even quarantine for addicts—to the legalization of drugs, have raised expectations that our society will solve its drug problem, as one federal government slogan had it in the early 1970s, "once and for all."

The messages contained in *The American Disease* have not been a source of great optimism that the drug problem can be easily controlled or solved by some simple formula. What has most impressed me is that our use of drugs and the social damage that inevitably follows has so closely paralleled our earlier fascination with drugs, which peaked around the turn of the century. Our lack of public memory for the earlier waves of opiates and cocaine has unintentionally created an experiment with nature. The United States has been exposed a second time to the seduction of drugs

and has been particularly susceptible because the earlier generations that had learned a hard lesson about drugs were no longer
around. When cocaine reappeared in the 1970s, few people remembered the previous American experience with the drug: at first,
in the 1880s, it had been welcomed as an ideal tonic, but after a
decade or so its image had become more questionable, and by 1900
it was considered to be the most dangerous of all drugs. That process of learning slowly but deeply the lessons of prolonged drug
use led to cocaine's decline in the 1920s. Interdiction, crop substitu-
tions, and so forth were ultimately minor factors in the practical
disappearance of cocaine; what appeared to matter most was dis-
illusionment with the initial claims for a new drug and shock at
its effects on the lives of individuals and their families.

In this light, *The American Disease* remains at least as relevant
to contemporary drug issues as it was when first published. Perhaps
such lessons will be more sympathetically viewed in the 1980s and
1990s. In 1973 many hoped that the drug problem would be over
soon—possibly in a few years—or that we would at least come up
with a strategy that would rapidly contain the problem. Simple
solutions abounded. The myth that Britain had solved its heroin
problem by giving away heroin in the 1920s proved to be wishful
thinking. In fact, Britain had no heroin problem in the 1920s and
enacted its Dangerous Drugs Act of 1920 because such legislation
was required by the Versailles Treaty.[1]

Our first major national anti-narcotic law, the Harrison Act of
1914, was intended to curb recreational narcotics use and nonmedical addiction. It came after decades of increasing concern over
drug consumption in the United States, when we had little or no
legal controls over the sale and distribution of narcotics. Anyone
advocating that drugs should be legalized can look at a century
during which our nation was one of the few in the Western world
to allow unregulated drug use. The viewer will not see, however,
a happy equilibrium resulting from that open drug economy in the
nineteenth century, but rather an eventual demand by the public
that action be taken to curb availability. We thus oscillate from
periods of drug tolerance to drug intolerance. Equilibrium is a state
in which drugs, including alcohol, have rarely been found in the
United States.

A recent study of the American drug experience questions a
strongly held tenet of critics of the Harrison Act, that the law sim-

ply turned respectable drug users into criminals. If there had been no Harrison Act, this argument runs, addicts would have been free to obtain their drugs and pursue normal or relatively normal lives. Professor David Courtwright has argued in *Dark Paradise* that even had there not been a Harrison Act and an anti-maintenance interpretation by the Supreme Court in 1919, "the background of the typical opiate addict in 1940 would not have differed much from the one observed in historical reality."[2] Rather than merely creating criminals by forcing addicts to steal to buy drugs, the Harrison Act arrived as noncriminal addicts were already declining in numbers, partly because of the changing prescribing practices of physicians and a growing public intolerance of drug use. This trend left the less savory addicts more conspicuous. Analyses such as this suggest that ascribing simple causes to our drug problem—for example, the passage of the Harrison Act—is no more tenable than positing simple solutions.

And yet, as I see signs of a gradual decline in drug use and a growing intolerance reminiscent of the end stage of our previous drug wave, I cannot feel an unalloyed sense of relief that a difficult time for our nation may fade quietly away over the next decade or so. I have two worries. The first is that the intensity of intolerance may in itself cause trouble for Americans as the aim increasingly becomes eradication of drug use and drug users. *The American Disease* illustrates how the fear of cocaine was transferred to a fear of the Southern black and became mixed up with whites' anxiety about violence during a time of great racial tension in the United States. Evidence shows how Southern lawmakers, alarmed over the specter of black hostility, were maneuvered in an attempt to achieve passage of anti-drug laws. Emotions such as anger and intolerance can be easily manipulated as well as misdirected at inappropriate groups. If, by some law of American attitudinal change, we must again endure a reaction against drugs as fierce as that earlier in this century, then we must remain alert to the potentially harmful consequences.

The other worry arises from my belief that one of the signal reasons for a resurgence of drug excesses in the 1960s was the loss of public memory for the realities of drug effects, which were well known in the United States at the turn of the century. How can practical knowledge of drugs be transmitted across generations without—as in the 1930s and 1940s—becoming distilled into simple horror stories that collapse before the reality of drug use? The problem is more difficult if drug use does, in fact, decline again to the levels of the 1940s, for then there will appear to be little reason to put resources into educational programs and other efforts aimed at fighting drug abuse. If the stimulus is gone, the response will also fade. This is a question that deserves considerable thought, although at the moment such planning may seem to be premature and to reflect excessive optimism about a future decline in drug consumption.

This edition of *The American Disease* contains the original text with typographical and other minor errors corrected. I would be happy to learn of any additional errors. To the end of the first edition I have added a chapter covering the years from the mid-1960s to the mid-1980s. Within one chapter I have not been able to cover in detail equal to the earlier chapters the last 20 years, which have produced a mountain of documents and a multitude of professionals in the drug field. I must leave a more thorough examination to a later date, but I have tried to provide an account of the recent years that puts into perspective the swings in public attitude and governmental response to what remains an issue of great interest to us all.

I am grateful to Dr. Herbert D. Kleber for his advice on the trends of the last twenty years. I also wish to thank Ellen Zak Danforth for her unflagging efforts as my research assistant. Finally, I want to express my deep appreciation to Jeanne Musto, who has been my partner in this as well as other publications.

New Haven, Connecticut   D. F. M.
April 1987

1 Virginia Berridge and Griffith Edwards, *Opium and the People, Opiate Use in Nineteenth-Century England* (New York: St. Martin's Press, 1981), pp. 254–55, 268.

2 David T. Courtwright, *Dark Paradise, Opiate Addiction in America before 1940* (Cambridge, Mass.: Harvard Univ. Press, 1982), p. 142.

Preface

The word "narcotics" has usually connoted more than simply opium and its derivatives. In law and in custom "narcotics" has included the coca leaf and its active ingredient cocaine, and the cannabis plant, the source of marihuana and the powerful resin hashish. In this study several other drugs enter the history of narcotic controls. Chloral hydrate, a drug still used to induce sleep, was considered at the turn of the century to have serious potential for excessive use and as a result often found its way into antinarcotic laws. Alcohol, of course, cannot be easily separated, either in its effects or as a target for legal control, from the antinarcotic campaign which paralleled the drive for national liquor prohibition.

Crude opium is the dried juice of the opium poppy and contains many alkaloids with varying properties. About ten per cent of crude opium is extractable as morphine, the chief active ingredient. A simple chemical process discovered in the last quarter of the nineteenth century converts morphine into diacetylmorphine, more commonly known as heroin. Another alkaloid found in crude opium, codeine, is less addictive than morphine and is relatively accessible in cough medicines and analgesic preparations. Crude opium can also be prepared for smoking by dehydration and concentration.

The active alkaloid in the coca leaf is cocaine. Cocaine produces euphoria and hyperactivity and is similar in many respects to the amphetamines. Other drugs of current interest in addition to the amphetamines, barbiturates, LSD, etc., are not considered in detail in this history, although attitudes associated with older drug issues appear to have been transferred with little change to these more recent preparations.

While preparing this book, I have been constantly aware of how divisive and politically loaded the subject of drug abuse is—and has been for the past century. Nothing has reminded me more of the drug controversy than working with divided and troubled families in which each member insists that "fairness" consists in taking his side and condemning the others. Although this history will not provide an answer to the problem of drug use, perhaps it will lessen some of the distortions which interfere with public debate.

This research into narcotic controls began in 1968 while I was a member of the Public Health Service in Washington, D.C. In order to gather more information on long-standing issues in narcotics, Dr.

Stanley F. Yolles, then Director of the National Institute of Mental Health, requested an inquiry, particularly into the narcotic clinics which flourished in the United States in the early 1920s. Without any great difficulty a number of documents relating to American drug laws and attitudes toward drug users were located in such nearby institutions as the National Archives and the Library of Congress. It was soon apparent that these primary sources had been largely neglected in published accounts of American narcotic control. While studying the records I began to question both conflicting historical explanations with which proponents of the "medical" and "police" approaches justified their policies. These "histories" appeared to be more in the nature of political party platforms than accurate descriptions of the process of narcotic control in the United States.

Working within the Public Health Service while conducting such an investigation had distinct advantages, but also some understandable drawbacks. For example, it was not possible for me to examine the records of rival federal agencies. Therefore when I returned to New Haven in 1969, the study was only begun and would have ended there except for the support and opportunity for research offered at the Yale Child Study Center. Dr. Albert J. Solnit, the center's director, and the late Dr. Seymour L. Lustman, professor of pediatrics and psychiatry, encouraged the completion of this history and provided an environment in which a controversial issue could be freely pursued.

In resuming the study, access was sought to the early records of the federal narcotics agencies. Such a request to the Bureau of Narcotics and Dangerous Drugs received approval. The Bureau's director, John E. Ingersoll, and his then executive assistant, John Warner, made the clinic files and other relevant records available for unrestricted examination. I was impressed by the interest of both health and law enforcement officials in a thorough study of the origins of narcotic control.

Later I had the opportunity to discuss with Alfred R. Lindesmith of the University of Indiana his career as an investigator of narcotic policies, and he kindly provided me with a number of useful historical documents. I interviewed former narcotics commissioner Harry J. Anslinger and examined his papers which he had deposited in the Pennsylvania Historical Collections of Pennsylvania State University. Among others who generously gave of their time to assist this research are Dr. Walter Bromberg, Dr. Willis P. Butler, H. Emmett Corrick, Dr. Morris Fishbein, Robert P. Fischelis, George Griffenhagen, Malachi L. Harney, Dr. Victor G. Heiser, Jean Jones, Dr. Samuel Lambert, Jr., Helen Taft Manning, Dr. Peter Olch, Glenn Sonnedecker, Dr. Wilson T. Sowder, and Jeffrey Stewart.

I am especially grateful to James Harvey Young of Emory University, who gave the manuscript a close and constructive reading. The medical and scientific aspects of the manuscript received careful examination by Dr. Daniel X. Freedman of the University of Chicago. Various parts of the manuscript were reviewed by colleagues whose aid is deeply appreciated: Alan Trachtenberg, Jonathan Spence, Dr. Albert J. Solnit, G. Gaddis Smith, Howard R. Lamar, Dr. James P. Comer, and Alexander Bickel.

The investigation benefitted from the able and industrious efforts of my research assistant in Washington, Michael Adler. In New Haven I have been fortunate to have the aid of Barbara Granger, whose enthusiasm and perseverance never faltered. I also wish to thank two hard-working bursary students, Thomas Casserly and Joan E. Williams. Repeated typings were borne cheerfully by Carol Schlesinger, Barbara Granger, Mary Koines, and Grace Michele.

I am indebted for assistance from the staffs of the following institutions: Archives of the American Medical Association, Library of the American Pharmaceutical Association, Library of the American Psychiatric Association, Library of the Bureau of Narcotics and Dangerous Drugs, Georgia State Library, Louisiana State Board of Health, Library of Congress, National Archives, National Library of Medicine, Library of The National Institute of Mental Health, New York Academy of Medicine, New York State Archives, Medical Society of the County of New York, Municipal Archives and the Secretary of the Department of Health of the City of New York, Pennsylvania Historical Collections of the Pennsylvania State University, College of Physicians of Philadelphia, The Proprietary Association, Library of the University of Washington, Washington State Historical Society, Wellcome Institute of the History of Medicine, and the Yale Medical, Medical Historical, and Sterling Memorial Libraries.

At the Yale Press I have been most fortunate to have had the encouragement and editorial guidance of Jane Isay. I also wish to thank Robert Zangrando, now of Akron University, who urged me to undertake this book, and Anne Wilde for her valuable assistance.

To my wife Jeanne I owe the greatest debt for patiently enduring the book's preparation, critically reading each page, and maintaining our childrens' optimism that the task would eventually be concluded.

D.F.M.

New Haven, Connecticut
January 1973

The American Disease

NARCOTICS IN NINETEENTH-CENTURY AMERICA

Before 1800, opium was available in America in its crude form as an ingredient of multidrug prescriptions, or in such extracts as laudanum, containing alcohol, or "black drop," containing no alcohol. Valued for its calming and soporific effects, opium was also a specific against symptoms of gastrointestinal illnesses such as cholera, food poisoning, and parasites. Its relatively mild psychological effect when taken by mouth or as part of a more complex prescription was enhanced by frequent use, and the drug was supplied freely by physicians. In addition, self-dosing with patent medicines and the ministrations of quacks contributed to narcotic intake. The medical profession's need for something that worked in a world of mysterious mortal diseases and infections cannot be overlooked as a major stimulus for the growth of the opium market. A drug that calmed was especially appealing since physicians could at least treat the patient's anxiety.

Technological advances in organic chemistry during the early nineteenth century led to plentiful supplies of potent habit-forming drugs. Alkaloids in crude opium were separated and crystallized to isolate active principles that give opium its physiological and psychic effects. Analysis of the coca leaf occurred in mid-century, and cocaine was finally isolated.[1]

Opium and Its Derivatives

Morphine grew in popularity as its great power over pain became better appreciated. It was cheap, compact, and had a standard strength—unlike tinctures of other forms of opium extracted from the crude plant. When the hypodermic needle became popular in the middle of the century it permitted direct injection into the body of a powerful, purified substance. Of the many substances injected experimentally, morphine was found to be exceptionally effective as a pain-killer and calming agent, and it came into medical practice after the Civil War. Writers have remarked on the coincidence to explain the apparent frequency of addiction in the United States in the latter half of the century.[2] Of course, this line of reasoning does not explain the relatively few addicts proportionally or absolutely in such nations as France, Germany, Great Britain, Russia, and Italy, which also fought wars during the latter half of the nineteenth century and also used morphine as an analgesic.

Whatever the cause, a relatively high level of opium consumption was established in the United States during the nineteenth century. This appetite for narcotics calls for some examination if only because opiate addiction has been described in the United States as "un-American" and "non-Western." [3]

Because opium has not been commercially grown to any great extent in America, the national supply was imported. Before 1915 (1909 for smoking opium) no restriction other than a tariff was placed upon importation, and except for opium for smoking, these tariffs were modest. Tariff records reveal the demand for opium and opiates during most of the nineteenth and early twentieth centuries. It is reasonable to assume that smuggling did not severely modify the overall trends of opium importation, because the period of free entry (1890–96) did not dramatically alter the importation curve. The imported opium was mostly crude, although it did include opium prepared for smoking. The United States exported almost no manufactured opiates before World War I because European drugs undersold them on the world market. [4]

Crude opium contained an estimated 9 percent morphine content extractable by American pharmaceutical concerns. One of the largest morphine-producing firms in the nineteenth century, Rosengarten and Company of Philadelphia (later merged into what is now Merck, Sharpe and Dohme), began manufacturing morphine salts in 1832. The first statistics on the importation of opium date from 1840 and reveal a continual increase in consumption during the rest of the century. The per capita importation of crude opium reached its peak in 1896. The Civil War, far from initiating opiate use on a large scale in the United States, hardly makes a ripple in its constantly expanding consumption, but addicted Civil War veterans, a group of unknown size, may have spread addiction by recruiting other users. Although there is some reduction in crude opium imports during 1861–65, presumably due to the blockade of the South, the amounts imported within a few years before and after the war are very similar. The rapid rise in crude opium did not begin until the 1870s; then it quickly outstripped the annual increase in population. Morphine did not begin to be imported in great amounts until the late 1870s. [5] Another cause of increased consumption was the widespread use of opiates by physicians and manufacturers of patent medicines during a period when there was little fear of their use. The unregulated patent medicine craze in the United States hit its peak in the late nineteenth century—a time when the opiate content in these medicines was probably also at its highest.

The characteristics of opium and its derivatives were ideal for the patent medicine manufacturers. There was no requirement that patent medicines containing opiates be so labeled in interstate commerce until the Pure Food and Drug Act of 1906. Many proprietary medicines that could be bought at any store or by mail order contained morphine, cocaine, laudanum, or (after 1898) heroin. Attempts at state regulation of sales were not successful during the last century.[6] Even "cures" for the opium habit frequently contained large amounts of opiates. Hay fever remedies commonly contained cocaine as their active ingredient. Coca-Cola, until 1903, contained cocaine (and since then caffeine).[7] Opiates and cocaine became popular—if unrecognized—items in the everyday life of Americans. The manufacturers were remarkably effective during the nineteenth century in preventing any congressional action to require even the disclosure of dangerous drugs in commercial preparations.[8]

After 1896, the per capita importation of crude opium gradually began to decline and, just before prohibitive laws rendered the importation statistics valueless, had fallen to the level of the 1880s. That level was not low, but consumption did drop as agitation mounted for strict controls. One traditional opium import which did not decline after 1900 was smoking opium, in spite of its holding no special interest for prescribing physicians, patent medicine manufacturers, or wounded Civil War veterans. Smoking opium, solely a pastime, lacked any of the elaborate advertising campaigns which boosted morphine and cocaine preparations; it had had a slow but steady rise in per capita consumption since import statistics began in 1860.[9] Suddenly in 1909 smoking opium was excluded from the United States. Weighing heavily against it was its symbolic association since mid-century with the Chinese, who were actively persecuted, especially on the West Coast. By then they were almost totally excluded from immigrating into the United States.

The prohibition of smoking opium also served notice to other nations that America was determined to rid itself of the evils of addiction. In 1909 the United States convened the first international meeting to consider opium traffic between nations, specifically that traffic into China which was so unwelcome to the Chinese government. Although motivation for American initiative in the Chinese problem was a mixture of moral leadership, protection of U.S. domestic welfare, and a desire to soften up Chinese resistance to American financial investments, the United States was also led by the nature of the narcotic trade to seek control of international shipments of crude narcotics to manufacturing countries and thence to markets. But the United States, on the eve of entering an international conference it had called to help China with its opium problem, discovered it had no national opium restrictions. To save face, it quickly enacted one. American prejudice against the Chinese, and the association of smoking opium with aliens, was in effect an immense aid in securing legislation in the program to help China. Indeed, a prime reason for calling the International Opium Commission was to mollify China's resentment of treatment of Chinese in the United States.

What might explain the pattern of decline of opium importation for consumption in the United States before the Harrison Act in 1914? First would be a growing fear of opiates and especially of morphine addiction, which was marked by the quick spread of antimorphine laws in various states in the 1890s.[10] That opium addiction was undesirable had long been common opinion in the United States. Oliver Wendell Holmes, Sr., in an address delivered just before the Civil War, blamed its prevalence on the ignorance of physicians. Holmes, then dean of Harvard Medical School, reported that in the western United States "the constant prescription of opiates by certain physicians . . . has rendered the habitual use of that drug in that region very prevalent. . . . A frightful endemic demoralization betrays itself in the frequency with which the haggard features and drooping shoulders of the opium drunkards are met with in the street."

As the century progressed and the hypodermic injection of opiates increased their physiological effect, the danger of morphine addiction was more widely broadcast. For this reason patent medicine makers resisted attempts to require the listing of ingredients on labels. The knowledge that such substances were in baby soothing syrups and other compounds would hurt sales. Nevertheless growing publicity disclosing the contents of patent medicines, early regulatory laws in the states, and public opinion all worked together as forces to curb this use of opiates and cocaine.

Another possible explanation, although untestable, is that the opiates had nearly saturated the market for such drugs: that is, those who were environmentally or biochemically disposed to opiates had been fairly well located by the marketers and the consumption curve leveled off as the demand was met. Such reasoning could apply also to a product like cigarettes, the use of which grew at a fantastic rate with the beginning of World War I but eventually leveled off in per capita consumption: although they are easily available not everyone desires to smoke them.

The numbers of those overusing opiates must have increased during the nineteenth century as the per capita importation of crude opium increased from less than 12 grains annually in the 1840s to more than 52 grains in the 1890s.[11] Eventually the medical consensus was that morphine had been overused by the physician, addiction was a substantial possibility, and addition of narcotics to patent medicines should be minimized or stopped. There is reason to emphasize the gradual development of this medical opinion since physicians, as well as everyone else, had what now seems a very delayed realization that dangerously addicting substances were distributed with little worry for their effect. Cocaine and heroin were both introduced from excellent laboratories by men with considerable clinical experience who judged them to be relatively harmless, in fact, to be possible cures for morphine and alcohol addiction.[12]

By 1900, America had developed a comparatively large addict population, perhaps 250,000, along with a fear of addiction and addicting drugs.[13] This fear had certain elements which have been powerful enough to permit the most profoundly punitive methods to be employed in the fight against addicts and suppliers. For at least seventy years purveyors of these drugs for nonmedical uses have been branded "worse than murderers," in that destroying the personality is worse than simply killing the body. What is most human is what is destroyed in the drug habitués, the opponents of narcotics argued.

In the nineteenth century addicts were identified with foreign groups and internal minorities who were already actively feared and the objects of elaborate and massive social and legal restraints. Two repressed groups which were associated with the use of certain drugs were the Chinese and the Negroes. The Chinese and their custom of opium smoking were closely watched after their entry into the United States about 1870. At first, the Chinese represented only one more group brought in to help build railroads, but, particularly after economic depression made them a labor surplus and a threat to American citizens, many forms of antagonism arose to drive them out or at least to isolate them. Along with this prejudice came a fear of opium smoking as one of the ways in which the Chinese were supposed to undermine American society.[14]

Cocaine was especially feared in the South by 1900 because of its euphoric and stimulating properties. The South feared that Negro cocaine users might become oblivious of their prescribed bounds and attack white society.[15] Morphine did not become so closely associated with an ethnic minority, perhaps because from its inception it was considered a simple substitute for medicinal opium and suitable for all classes. When opiates began to be feared for their addictive properties, morphine was most closely attached to the "lower classes" or the "underworld," but without greater specificity.[16]

The crusade for alcohol prohibition which culminated in the adoption of the 18th Amendment started in the South and West early in this century. Intrastate Prohibition weighed most heavily on the poor since, until the Webb-Kenyon Act of 1913, it was quite legal to purchase liquor in bulk from wet states for shipment into dry states. When poor southerners, and particularly Negroes, were alleged to turn to cola drinks laced with cocaine or to cocaine itself for excitement as a result of liquor scarcity, more laws against cocaine quickly followed. Here, however, the South was at a loss for comprehensive legal control since the goal was to prohibit interstate as well as intrastate shipment. This could be done only with a federal statute which would threaten the states' police and commerce powers. Consequently, the story of the Harrison Act's passage contains many examples of the South's fear of the Negro as a ground for permitting a deviation from strict interpretation of the Constitution.

Cocaine

Cocaine is a good example of a drug whose dangers became widely accepted although at first it was immensely popular. It was pure, cheap, and widely distributed; its advocates distrusted not only the opinions of their opponents but also their motivation. Co-

caine users were so impressed by its euphoric properties that they
were unable to evaluate the drug objectively.

Cocaine achieved popularity in the United States as a general
tonic, for sinusitis and hay fever, and as a cure for the opium,
morphine, and alcohol habits. Learned journals published accounts
which just avoided advising unlimited intake of cocaine.[17] Medical
entrepreneurs such as the neurologist William Hammond, former
surgeon general of the army, swore by it and took a wineglass of
it with each meal. He was also proud to announce cocaine as the
official remedy of the Hay Fever Association, a solid endorsement
for anyone (see p. 252, n. 7). Sigmund Freud is perhaps the best-
remembered proponent of cocaine as a general tonic and an addiction cure. He wrote several articles in the European medical press
on the wonderful substance to which his attention had been drawn
by American medical journals.[18]

In the United States the exhilarating properties of cocaine made
it a favorite ingredient of medicine, soda pop, wines, and so on. The
Parke Davis Company, an exceptionally enthusiastic producer of
cocaine, even sold coca-leaf cigarettes and coca cheroots to accompany their other products, which provided cocaine in a variety
of media and routes such as a liqueurlike alcohol mixture called
Coca Cordial, tablets, hypodermic injections, ointments, and sprays.

If cocaine was a spur to violence against whites in the South, as
was generally believed by whites, then reaction against its users
made sense. The fear of the cocainized black coincided with the
peak of lynchings, legal segregation, and voting laws all designed to
remove political and social power from him. Fear of cocaine might
have contributed to the dread that the black would rise above "his
place," as well as reflecting the extent to which cocaine may have
released defiance and retribution. So far, evidence does not suggest
that cocaine caused a crime wave but rather that anticipation of
black rebellion inspired white alarm. Anecdotes often told of super-
human strength, cunning, and efficiency resulting from cocaine.
One of the most terrifying beliefs about cocaine was that it actually
improved pistol marksmanship. Another myth, that cocaine made
blacks almost unaffected by mere .32 caliber bullets, is said to have
caused southern police departments to switch to .38 caliber revolv-
ers. These fantasies characterized white fear, not the reality of cocaine's effects, and gave one more reason for the repression of
blacks.[19]

The claim of widespread use of cocaine by Negroes is called into question by the report in 1914 of 2,100 consecutive Negro admissions to a Georgia asylum over the previous five years. The medical director acknowledged the newspaper reports of "cocainomania" among Negroes but was surprised to discover that only two cocaine users—and these incidental to the admitting diagnosis—were hospitalized between 1909 and 1914. He offered an explanation for cocaine disuse among Negroes—that poverty prevented a drug problem equal to that among whites.[20]

The most accepted medical use of cocaine was as a surface anesthetic, for example, on the eye to permit surgery on a conscious patient, or as an injection near a nerve to stop conduction of pain stimuli. When sniffed, cocaine crystals shrink mucous membranes and drain sinuses. Along with sinus drainage, the patient gets a "high." Eventually such substitutes or modifications of cocaine were developed as benzocaine and procaine, which do not have such euphoric effects but are still capable of preventing nerve conduction.

Since cocaine was by no means limited to physicians' prescriptions, the "lower classes," particularly in "dry" states, found they could get a jolt which took the place of hard liquor. Bars began putting a pinch of cocaine in a shot of whiskey and cocaine was peddled door to door. By 1900, state laws and municipal ordinances were being rapidly enacted against these activities. But law-abiding middle and upper-class employers also found practical uses for cocaine; it was reportedly distributed to construction and mine workers to keep them going at a high pitch and with little food.[21] This value of cocaine had been first discovered by the Spanish in sixteenth-century Peru and was put to work among the native slaves who mined silver. Cocaine thus was economically valuable, but the fear of its overstimulating powers among social subgroups predominated, in the United States, and its provision to laborers waned.

STATE LAWS

State laws designed to curb the abuse of morphine and cocaine came mostly in the last decade of the nineteenth century. The realization of "abuse" and its seriousness gradually undermined confidence in simple regulatory laws and led to a determination that decisive action must be taken. Addiction became a challenge to medical and legal institutions. State and municipal laws generally required cocaine or morphine to be ordered on a physician's prescription, which then had to be retained for perhaps a year for inspection. The laws had one great loophole: the patent medicine manufacturers repeatedly obtained exemptions for certain quantities of narcotics in proprietary medicines. These loopholes permitted the narcotized patent medicines to be sold, but the laws lulled the public into believing that this abuse of narcotics was under control. To some extent these lacunary antinarcotic laws did alert the more wary, and manufacturers began to be cautious. But as curbs on the sale of narcotics for nonmedicinal use, the laws were not effective; they were not well enforced because, among other factors, the states did not have sufficient manpower to maintain surveillance.

Although a state might enact an antinarcotic law and even enforce it, bordering states without such laws often provided drugs for users and sellers. New York State reformers bitterly criticized New Jersey's lax narcotic regulations, which vitiated enforcement of New York's carefully framed legislation.[22] Furthermore, although the law-abiding physician had more paper work, unethical physicians could circumvent state and local laws and the consequent paper work in various ways. The "dope doctors" could simply purchase drugs by mail from another state and then dispense them to their "patients," thereby bypassing laws which relied on prescriptions and pharmacies to monitor drug use. Generally, physicians resented the legal advantage of patent medicines which, by means of statutory exemptions, contained narcotic dosages capable of producing addiction. These evasions were in painful contradiction to the intent of legislation and a distinct reminder of the political influence of those profiting from narcotic sales.

Federal control over narcotic use and the prescription practices of the medical profession were thought in 1900 to be unconstitutional. Gradually, federal commerce and tax powers were broadened by Supreme Court decisions, notably those upholding a federal tax on colored oleomargarine, federal prohibition against transportation of women across state lines for immoral purposes, the interstate transportation of lottery tickets, and carrying liquor into a state that prohibited liquor imports. But that congressional activity was still circumscribed by the Constitution was reflected in the Supreme Court ruling in *Hammer* v. *Dagenhart* (1918) wherein the court declared that congress could not regulate the interstate shipment of goods produced by child labor.[23] The ruling clearly indicated that federal police powers under the guise of tax or interstate commerce powers had narrow application.

As a result of constitutional uncertainty over legislation enabling federal law to prevail in an area of morals, there was little effort until after 1900 to enact a federal law to control the sale and prescription of narcotics. After the passage of the Pure Food and Drug Act (1906), some elements of the pharmacy trade supported a regulatory antinarcotic law based on the interstate commerce clause, a movement seconded by Dr. Harvey Wiley of the Agriculture Department.[24] Finally, by 1912, when the State Department's campaign for a federal antinarcotic law was making substantial progress, proponents opted for basing it on government's revenue powers. Thus the framing of an antinarcotic law paralleled the widening possibilities open to Congress in the area of policing morals. Even so, the Harrison Act of 1914 had to survive a number of unfavorable or close court decisions until its broad police powers were upheld in 1919. And as late as 1937 the Marihuana Tax Act was carefully kept separate from the Harrison Act in order to discourage more court attacks.[25] The Drug Abuse Act of 1970 scrapped the Harrison Act's foundation on revenue powers and rests on the interstate commerce powers of Congress, returning to the basis proposed more than sixty years before. In the last half century, the interstate commerce clause has been substantially broadened so that its powers can sustain strict regulation of drug use without the need to portray a police function as a revenue measure.[26]

REFORMERS

Lay reformers took a vigorous and uncomplicated stand on narcotics. In general, two problems enflamed them: corporate disregard of public welfare and individual immorality. This dichotomy is artificial but it helps to identify the objects of the reformers' zeal and it made a difference in the kinds of laws proposed. Reformers like Samuel Hopkins Adams, whose "Great American Fraud" series in *Collier's* in 1905–07 revealed the danger of patent medicines, were of course concerned over the damage done to unsuspecting victims of such medicines. Adams directed his attack against pharmaceutical manufacturers whose expensive and inaccurate advertising promotions sold harmful nostrums to the public. In keeping with his exposés of crooked politicians and corporations, Adams argued that regulatory laws should be aimed at the suppliers.[27] For other reformers, though, the addict evoked fears; their agitation resulted in legislation directed more at the user, who might be sent to jail for possession, than at the manufacturer who produced barrels of morphine and heroin. The Southerner's fear of the Negro and the Westerner's fear of the Chinese predominated in this approach to the drug problem. The origin of concern thus affected the aim and quality of the laws. Both classes of reformers looked to federal legislation as the most effective weapon, and both tended to measure progress in the reform campaign by the amount of legislation enacted.

The reformers can also be examined from another viewpoint. One group thought in moral abstractions while another was interested in a practical solution. The Right Reverend Charles Brent, who played an important role in the movement for narcotic control, was an abstract reformer who saw the narcotics problem, like any other social problem, to be a question which required first of all a moral approach to the decision.[28] Did narcotics have a value other than as a medicine? No: unlike alcohol they had no beverage or caloric value. Should such substances be permitted for casual use? No: there was no justification, since there was the possibility only of danger in narcotics for nonmedicinal uses. Therefore recreational use of narcotics should be prohibited, their traffic curtailed on a world scale, and a scourge eliminated from the earth. To compromise, to permit some (for instance the Chinese) to use narcotics would be inconsistent with morality, and therefore not permissible. Reformers like Brent were charitable but unwilling to compromise.

Other reformers sought a practical and partial solution which edged toward total narcotic restriction but was modified to allow for the cravings of addicts. These compromises often came from political divisions smaller than the federal government. In contrast to Bishop Brent's proposals, the compromise programs were based on the assumption that the supply of and the desire for narcotics could not be eliminated, and therefore any attempt at total prohibition would be a failure.[29]

Narcotics, however, constituted only a small part of the American reform movement at the turn of the century. In the last decade of the nineteenth century, rising public interest in protecting the environment and health was evident in exposés, public education and reform proposals in Congress for such things as a pure food law, but not until the presidential years of Theodore Roosevelt was this interest translated into substantial national legislation. Roosevelt's advocacy of ecology and conservation followed a popular revulsion against the excessive concentration of wealth and the manner in which it was amassed, and the disregard of general welfare by powerful private interest.

Upton Sinclair's bitterness led to *The Jungle,* in which the young Socialist portrayed the slaughterhouse owner's utter disregard for employee welfare. Often credited with giving the final push toward enactment of the Meat Inspection Act in 1906, Sinclair soon became disillusioned with his efforts at substantial reform through idealistic principles: the big meat packers benefited from the reforms enacted by Congress since small business firms could not afford the new inspection requirements nor meet the standards of foreign nations which had criticized the purity of American meat exports.

But if some reforms were actually an assistance to institutions reformers hated, other reforms were the nuisance or corrective their advocates desired. An aggressive administrator of the new regulations restricting environmental and physiological damage was Dr. Harvey Washington Wiley, who developed the Agriculture Department's Bureau of Chemistry into an avid detector of unsavory manufacturing practices.[30] He was condemned by industry because his criticisms and regulations often appeared to go beyond all reasonable limits. For example, he wanted to prohibit caffeine-containing drinks such as Coca-Cola as well as patent medicines containing narcotics. His particular attention to unlabeled additives resulted in an indictment of the Coca-Cola Company and the holding up of shipments of French wines not labeled to show sulfur dioxide as a preservative. These disputes required the attention of the President, the Supreme Court, or a Cabinet officer. Theodore Roosevelt's support of Wiley waned in 1908 as the criticisms grew, and he felt some personal evaluation was necessary. He called Wiley to the White House to confront industrial spokesmen. All went well until the conversation turned to the President's treasured sugar substitute, saccharin. Wiley at once declared saccharin a threat to health which should be prohibited in foods. Roosevelt angrily reacted: "Anybody who says saccharin is injurious is an idiot. Dr. Rixey gives it to me every day!" His doubt about Wiley strengthened by this encounter,

Roosevelt established the Referee Board of Consulting Scientific Experts. By 1912 Wiley had been forced out of government service because of his aggressive and, some thought, unreasonable antagonism to food and drug impurities and false claims.[31]

THE HEALTH PROFESSIONS AND NARCOTICS

Medicine and pharmacy were in active stages of professional organization when they became involved with the issue of narcotic control. The status of both pharmacists and physicians was less than desirable, and both suffered from weak licensing laws, meager training requirements, and a surplus of practitioners. Their intense battles for professional advancement and unification had an effect on the progress and final form of antinarcotic legislation.

Although the state of medicine in the nineteenth century was improving, its only tangible progress lay in some ability to contain a few communicable diseases. Yet, if the physician could not effect cure, he could assuage pain and apprehension: opiates were preeminent for these functions and were apparently used with great frequency. Drugs are still overused in this casual, convenient way— penicillin, the sulfas, tetracycline, barbiturates, and so on—they carry a message of effective treatment to the patient, fulfilling his emotional needs even if sometimes risky and superfluous from an objective viewpoint.

The American Medical Association (founded in 1847), which now appears monolithic and powerful, was a weak institution at the close of the last century. The vast majority of doctors refrained from membership. The AMA's battle for higher standards of training, licensure, and practice was threatening to many within the profession and seemed to the public to be but a covert plea for special preferment by one of several schools of medical practice.[32] While one may admit that the AMA reform program improved the political, economic, and social status of the medical profession, the public welfare was also to be improved. The Flexner Report, with its independent and corroborating analysis of the profession's weaknesses, was accepted by impartial critics.[33] Meanwhile, however, the low standards of the nineteenth century predominated and were consistent with the great reliance on such symptomatic relief agents as the opiates.

Although the drive to organize pharmacy was contemporary with the AMA's efforts, it was not so successful. However fragmented medicine might appear, pharmacy was far more fundamentally split into special-interest groups, often divided on questions of legislation, ethics, and professional standards. The druggist operated a competitive retail business to which his prescription service usually contributed only a fraction of his profits. He had some difficulty adhering to the strict professional standards enunciated by the American Pharmaceutical Association (1852)—stressing the ancient science of pharmacy—as the highest priority in his business. He found an ideal relationship with the physician was particularly difficult to attain since the oversupply of doctors led many of them to do their own dispensing. Similarly, pharmaceutical manufacturers, importers, exporters, and wholesalers were also engaged in businesses far removed from the archetypal pharmacist dispensing an intricate prescription. The various professional components often felt that their particular interests could not be adequately served by an association in which all elements of pharmacy had an equal voice. Dissatisfaction with the APhA led to many trade associations with specific membership criteria.[34]

Physicians and pharmacists were vocal and effective in their lobbying efforts. Each saw that in addition to aiding the public welfare, strict narcotic laws could be a distinct advantage for institutional development if great care was exercised in their framing. Knowledge of this rivalry and ambition clarifies legislative history; it also reminds us that in the competition to find a convenient law it was rather easy to lose sight of the victim of drug abuse. The public's fear of addicts and minority-group drug users might supply the powerful motive force for legislation, but the law's final form would await the approval of the institutional interests affected.

THE AMERICAN PHARMACEUTICAL ASSOCIATION

The pharmacists who were eager to proclaim themselves professionals, as opposed to mere retailers of prepared medicines and sundries, became members of the American Pharmaceutical Association. Retail druggists were divided over patent medicines, some making profits from the preparations, others embarrassed by such trade. Nevertheless, many druggists stocked proprietaries in self-defense. The APhA frowned on narcotic use for other than medical purposes, and the association's leaders fought proprietary medicines, as did the AMA, on both moral and self-interest grounds: they were dangerous, self-medication had inherent risks, and legitimate trade was taken from the pharmacists who prepared their own products.[35]

In September 1901, the American Pharmaceutical Association convened in St. Louis. The Section on Legislation and Education heard lawyer-pharmacist James H. Beal report that the model state pharmacy law which had been adopted at the previous convention was gaining popularity, and that a number of states had already enacted some of its provisions. Nevertheless, the desire of physicians to register as pharmacists without examinations continued. Beal also spoke of a new issue that merited the close attention of pharmacists. He called the section's attention to enactment in the previous year by Kansas and Tennessee of restrictions on habit-forming drugs, specifically cocaine and morphine. Beal warned: "If pharmacists do not take up and deal rigorously with these matters, they will be dealt with by the general public, and in a way not likely to be altogether agreeable to the pharmacists." Movements to restrict habit-forming drugs focused also on alcohol, chloral hydrate, other hypnotics, and a few other preparations. In Colorado, morphine and cocaine were tied together in proposed legislation with "malt, vinous, and spiritous liquors," which would be available only on a physician's prescription. Although the bill was defeated, it showed a trend toward drug and alcohol legislation which the pharmacists quickly realized must be dealt with before it went beyond their ability to influence.[36]

Atlanta's trouble with cocaine in its "Negro quarters" was brought to the attention of the association by its second vice-president, G. F. Payne. Several drugstores had been catering to the "extensive addiction" among Negroes and, although he doubted that stores were receiving most of their income from it, as was the rumor, he knew a lot of money was exchanging hands. A city ordinance had merely moved the "cocaine joints" out of town, whereas Georgia state restrictions appeared to have closed them completely. He noted that the cocaine was only 25 percent pure, but "the darkies seemed to be very well satisfied with that kind of cocaine." Another speaker spoke of increasingly popular sleeping medicines which also deserved study and restriction, and moved for the formation of a committee to look into the whole problem. An ad hoc committee

was approved and directed to "consider the question of acquirement of drug habits, and the best methods of legislative regulation
of the danger." [37]

This committee represented concern by a competent and broadly
based organization whose members had an important role in the
supply of drugs to the public. All members of the organization were
pharmacists and were in a good position to gather facts about the
prescription and purchase of morphine and cocaine, the chief
offenders at this time. At an early stage in the national movement for
narcotic laws the committee had an opportunity to report on attitudes toward habit-forming drugs and consider recommendations
for their control.

A year later the American Pharmaceutical Association met in
Philadelphia to celebrate its fiftieth anniversary. The Section on
Education and Legislation was assured by its chairman, E. G.
Eberle, that professionalization was still moving apace. Fewer
physicians were dispensing, and the enactment of salutary pharmacy
laws continued, but some activities needed closer watching. The
federal government gave away serum against infectious diseases
more liberally than seemed warranted, leading to competition with
private enterprise. Also the free medical dispensary, although laud-
able in its aims, was "another evil in disguise." A good solution to free-
loading was the scheme proposed by the medical and pharmaceutical professions of Pennsylvania to require dispensary patients to be
registered, under penalty of a considerable fine, so that only the
deserving received free care. As for habit-forming drugs, Eberle
hesitated to comment on the upcoming report of the ad hoc committee, but he believed the best law would not be one with many
penalties, or one based on fear, but one which simply required the
druggist to be of "moral character." [38]

The Committee on the Acquirement of the Drug Habit had
studied the statistics of narcotic importation over the previous five
years (1898–1902). Inspection of imports revealed the startling fact
that, although the population had increased by only 10 percent, importation of cocaine had risen 40 percent, opium 500 percent, and
morphine 600 percent.[39] The committee believed that the increasing
use of habit-forming drugs was not the fault of physicians, since
those with whom they had contact were generally prescribing less
than formerly as the danger of addiction became more widely appreciated.

Questionnaires had been sent to about a thousand physicians and pharmacists in New York, Brooklyn, Philadelphia, Baltimore, and a scattering of towns in Pennsylvania and New Jersey; about 30 percent replied. The questionnaire did not list alcohol among the drugs nor mention cannabis, but it did include preparations such as laudanum and chloral hydrate. On the estimate of five habitués reported per pharmacist, the committee concluded that there were about 200,000 habitués in the United States. This rough value is close to a later estimate for this period by the Public Health Service.[40] Two groups, the committee reported, Negroes and women, easily succumbed to cocaine:

> The use of cocaine by unfortunate women generally, and by Negroes in certain parts of the country, is simply appalling. No idea of this can be had unless personally investigated. The police officers of these questionable districts tell us that the habitués are made madly wild by cocaine, which they have no difficulty at all in buying, sometimes being peddled around from door to door, but always adulterated with acetanilid.

Several recommendations were offered. Smoking opium should be suppressed by the federal government by banning its importation. Since retail druggists rarely sold smoking opium and physicians were not known to prescribe it, such a recommendation was morally and economically sound. The only group that valued smoking opium, the Chinese, did not intimidate the committee: "If the Chinaman cannot get along without his 'dope', we can get along without him. The great increase in the quantity of this special kind of opium proves one of two things, or both: either our exclusion laws are being violated, or the smoking of opium is largely practiced by others than Chinese." [41] The last two recommendations were less specific: at the state level, uniform laws should be framed by state medical and pharmaceutical associations to protect citizens from habit-forming drugs. Finally, the association should refuse membership to traffickers in these drugs.

After a year of further study, and with the assistance of Beal, the committee recommended a model state law. This model of 1903 provides an insight into the status of habit-forming drugs before adoption of any federal controls. First, the proposal for regulation at the state level reflected the belief that the simplest way to control habit-forming drugs within the United States was through the states' police powers. Any intrusion by federal police power would meet resistance from strict constructionists and criticism as an enforcement task beyond the capacity of the small federal establishment. Moreover, the American Pharmaceutical Association's history of successful influence within state legislatures made lobbying on the state level a familiar operation. Therefore a state law would be customary and of assured validity.

Beal had conferred with various experts as to which drugs should be controlled. He included cocaine, opium and its derivatives (which would include heroin, morphine, and codeine), and chloral hydrate. These drugs should be given only under written order of a licensed practitioner, and prescriptions should not be refilled.

Beal then confronted an issue which is still actively debated: Should physicians be permitted to prescribe for habitués? Trying to take a middle course, he realized on the one hand that if this were permitted, unscrupulous physicians could prey on the victims of addiction and reap a harvest. On the other hand, a significant body of opinion in 1903 held that opium (and especially morphine) habitués could not be deprived of their drugs without "great danger to their lives." The use of opiates might even be part of the cure or treatment of the disease. Since this was the case, he argued, the goal of the law should be to restrict, rather than to prevent entirely, the sale of narcotics. Beal concluded: *"The principal object of the law must be to prevent the creation of drug habits,* rather than to reform those who are already enslaved, however desirable the latter might be, and the draft has accordingly been constructed upon this theory." [42]

Prescription of the forbidden drugs to a "habitual user" was outlawed provided "that the provisions . . . shall not be construed to prevent any lawfully authorized practitioner of medicine from prescribing in good faith for the use of any habitual user of narcotic drugs such substances as he may deem necessary for the treatment of such habit." Any prescription written by a licensed practitioner (physician, dentist, or veterinarian) was to be kept by the pharmacist for inspection for a period of two years. As one would expect in the pharmacists' model law, no provision was made for dispensing by physicians.

Preparations containing no more than specified amounts of a narcotic, such as less than ⅛ grain of morphine in one fluid ounce, were exempt from the law. Recognizing the seemingly invulnerable

popularity of narcotized patent medicines and their makers, the
restrictions would not apply in any way to "preparations recommended in good faith for diarrhea or cholera, properly packaged."
This exemption reflects the great prevalence of intestinal ailments
at the turn of the century and also touches on a complaint of
physicians: too many druggists "recommended" drugs for diseases,
and thereby encroached on the doctors' special province.[43]

Along with the submission of Beal's model law, the Committee
on the Acquirement of the Drug Habit presented its second and
final report.[44] Even more questionnaires had been sent out than
previously and the report represented (with a free admission that
it was fragmentary) conditions and fears from the whole nation.
Some of the findings are of interest. For example, of 150 drug
habitués reported in Alabama, 8 were heroin addicts. This indicates
a fairly rapid spread of heroin into the drug-abuse class since it first
became commercially available in 1898.[45] Georgia reported that almost every Negro prostitute was addicted to cocaine. Maryland,
Georgia, Ohio, and other states gave examples of disreputable
physicians and druggists who sold gigantic amounts of cocaine or
other drugs. Michigan reported an increase in sales to Negroes.
Pennsylvania also reported several heroin addiction cases and a
small retail dealer's purchase of ¼-grain morphine tablets in 100,000-
tablet lots. Virginia reported an enormous growth in the cocaine
habit among Negroes.

The committee did not want to imply, however, that the abuse
of drugs was confined to "the fallen and lower classes." Although
the lower and criminal classes were the most difficult to cure, had
frequent relapses, and stole in order to get their stimulants, the
higher classes, even those of intellect and with social prestige, were
not strangers to the overuse of habit-forming substances. The committee concluded, in the 1903 *Proceedings* of the APhA, with an
observation which suggested law enforcement as an adjunct to cure,
a presentiment of the federal narcotic policy of the 1920s: "those
who think they cannot break the results of the habit are those who
are free to obtain the drug by purchase or otherwise" (pp. 467–68,
471).

Acquiring the habit was related to many factors in American life,
the committee continued. Lawyers and preachers took cocaine in
order to be "bright." Even worse, "many of the leading lights of
the medical profession . . . become slaves to a vice which they

are supposed to combat." Patent medicines contained the drugs to produce quick relief regardless of the illness. Physicians believed they could build up a good practice by demonstrating to their patients the relaxing or pleasurable effect of one hypodermic shot. "Society's whirl demands late hours," the committee averred, believing that the need for immediate sleep led many to overuse sedatives. Headaches the next day could be cured by patent "headache powders" and so a vicious cycle started. Availability of drugs at a soda fountain diminished the wariness of the customer. With the use of narcotics increasing, "evil effects from it [will] come to succeeding generations" (p. 477).

Although the report made some serious allegations, there was no attempt to hide the incompleteness of the data or the uncertainty in various classes of response. Replies from prisons and asylums were particularly suspect because no accurate record was kept, although "we believe the state should exact it." It was recommended that in any later investigation one person in each locality should carefully gather and evaluate information, since questionnaires had limited value and comprehensiveness (pp. 467, 473). This frank and self-critical analysis became rarer as the debate over narcotics intensified in the next decades. From every trade group, regardless of the profit to be made from habit-forming drugs, the committee received the distinct impression that legislation was needed and expected. Smoking opium, a particularly indefensible vice, should be prohibited. Domestically, stringent state regulation of sellers with fines, imprisonment, and surrender of license would be required to stop the evil. Since illicit sales would naturally accompany drug restriction, the need for severe penalties was obvious (p. 477).

The criminal class posed a special problem. The "drug fiend" preying on society seemed unlikely to be cured. Even after a period of apparent respectability, he might begin stealing to obtain the drug. The chairman felt forced to conclude that perhaps certain classes of people, "the demi-monde, known criminals or those whose occupations are shady," should be totally prohibited from the drug. Information from the police that most drug abusers become so "after they had joined the ranks of the underworld, does not lessen the danger to society" (p. 475). How certain groups were to be kept from narcotics was not explained. Men in the army and navy were rapidly increasing their use of opium, perhaps due to their contact with the natives and Chinese in the Philippines during the insur-

rection there (1899–1902). No evidence pointed to the responsibility
of service physicians for the spread of the drug habit, but the great
increase in men separated from the armed services for addiction
during the previous year was evidence to the committee that their
companions—civilians and "lewd men and women"—had introduced
them to the habit.[46]

"Unless very stern and speedy action is taken *now,* the people
of the United States will pay dearly for the neglect in the not distant
future," warned the committee's chairman. He had little faith in an
appeal

> to the moral sense of the men who are today supplying retail
> drugstores with all the drugs they can sell, nor of the class of
> druggists who supply the "dope fiends." There is but one appeal to
> such men, and that is through fear—fear of their pocketbooks
> or fear of jail—and the only way to stop them from continuing
> their practice is to make the penalty severe enough to be adequate
> to the danger of their crime. Let it be administered in this spirit.
> The murderer who destroys a man's body is an angel beside one
> who destroys that man's soul and mind.[47]

DISTRICT OF COLUMBIA PHARMACY ACT, 1906

The pharmacists' early formulation of a national policy led to endorsement of state laws that would restrict to pharmacists and
physicians the supply of habit-forming drugs. A second and slightly
revised model law was adopted by the NWDA, NARD, APhA, and
the PAA in December 1905, formally extending the drug trades'
support of the 1903 APhA model. In May 1906 Congress adopted
for the District of Columbia a pharmacy act which druggists, particularly the American Pharmaceutical Association, considered exemplary.[48] It followed closely the language of the model state
pharmacy law promulgated by Beal in 1900 and included two sections adopting most of the association's model narcotic law of 1903.[49]

As a general pharmacy law, the Act protected registered pharmacists from those without a license, as well as from the sale of drugs
by hawkers and door-to-door peddlers. As usual, physicians were
exempt from the law with regard to their own patients, for whom
they could compound and dispense medicines.

Changes from the model narcotic statute reflected compromises reached in most attempts to restrict dangerous but popular medications. Minimal amounts of morphine, opium, cocaine, and chloral hydrate exempted in patent or proprietary medicines were doubled over Beal's earlier recommendation. The phrase "derivatives of opium" was omitted throughout the Act, thereby exempting any derivative that might be habit forming, such as heroin. The practice particularly offensive to physicians, "recommendation" of preparations for cholera and diarrhea by pharmacists, was rephrased to read "sold in good faith." Prescriptions for narcotics could be renewed only on the written order of the physician and were ordered kept three years for examination.

Congress appears to have strengthened provisions against addiction maintenance. Beal's model law seems somewhat more liberal in its provision that the physician could prescribe in good faith substances he might feel necessary for treatment of the habit. The District of Columbia law permitted the prescription of habit-forming drugs only when "necessary for the cure" of addiction. The physician must prove that he acted in good faith and believed the drug "necessary for the cure of drug addiction . . . or for the treatment of disease, injury, or deformity, and for no other purpose whatsoever." [50]

This law, although applicable only to the District of Columbia, assumed considerable importance later in relation to the question whether Congress had ever considered allowing drugs simply for the comfort of an addict. In the same spirit, Congress had mandated, a year earlier, nonmedical narcotic prohibition for the Philippine Islands.[51]

A month after passage of the District of Columbia Pharmacy Act, Congress approved the long-debated and controversial Pure Food and Drug Act. Administration of this Act was placed in the Bureau of Chemistry of the Department of Agriculture, headed by Dr. Harvey W. Wiley.

Although Wiley was not chiefly concerned with narcotics—most of his professional life had been devoted to the purity of food—the Act required the listing of narcotics, including cannabis, on the labels of patent medicines shipped in interstate commerce. Within a few years of the inclusion of this simple device, it was estimated that patent medicines containing such drugs dropped in sale by about a third.[52] Nevertheless, large sales did continue and pharmacists enlisted Wiley's aid in drafting an amendment to the Pure

Food and Drug Act which would eliminate any medicines containing habit-forming drugs from interstate commerce except under the prescription of a physician. In Wiley's opinion, through such an amendment "the whole commerce in so-called patent medicines containing these habit-forming drugs would be practically destroyed." [53] This would be an important trade victory for the retail and compounding pharmacists, for it would increase dispensing by pharmacists, decrease sales in grocery stores, and eliminate sales across state lines by mail-order houses. The amendment would also accomplish a reform which most impartial authorities agreed was desirable for the health of the nation.

Wiley recommended this change in the Pure Food and Drug Act to the State Department at the beginning of 1908, when some federal action was contemplated as a token of American concern about the international narcotic traffic.[54] Assistant Secretary of State Robert Bacon was interested in the Wiley amendment but claimed it came too late for submission to the current session of Congress.[55] By summer the situation had changed as far as the State Department was concerned. The department now felt that a simple amendment to an existing law would not suffice. A separate federal law was required, opposing in some respect nonmedical opium consumption.[56] The State Department now came into prominence as a leading proponent of narcotic legislation both nationally and internationally. The drug trades receded somewhat from public attention to work more quietly, but just as effectively, in the molding of restrictive legislation. The value of educating pharmaceutical groups as to their best interests in narcotic control was evident in the eventual legislation at the federal level. The drug trades were able to veto a number of schemes to control narcotics which violated, in their view, the legitimate interests and prerogatives of their industry.

2 Diplomats and Reformers

The State Department's unexpected leadership in the domestic antinarcotic movement originated with one of the peaks of American imperialism, the drive at the China market, and the seizure from Spain of the Philippine Islands.

THE CHINA MARKET

At the close of the nineteenth century, the Far East beckoned as a market for American investors. According to enthusiastic calculation, a pair of shoes sold to each Chinese would keep American shoe factories busy for years. American financial leaders coming out of the depression of 1893 believed that expanding markets were the key to future prosperity, blaming bad times on saturation of the home market.[1]

China may have needed almost everything manufactured, but China was also surrounded and intimidated by the great powers of Europe. America's penetration of China so far had been chiefly by missionaries. Perhaps the most promising investment market was railroads, an essential part of China's modernization plan and also a source of considerable income to the foreign syndicates which financed them. China's repayment was practically guaranteed by Western control of her maritime customs service, and her enforced acquiescence to the demands of foreign powers promised a good basis on which to loan hundreds of millions of dollars.[2]

Understandably, Russia, France, Great Britain, Germany, and Japan did not wish to include the United States in profits from their loan agreements. The weakness of diplomatic notes without military support was clear, but Theodore Roosevelt thought that American public opinion would not sanction the use of American troops in China to protect commercial interests.[3] The president therefore employed the power of words, like those framed in Secretary of State Hay's "open door" messages. Hay sought equal rights for all nations in the various treaty ports and spheres of interest and a guarantee of the territorial integrity of the Chinese Empire. After the Spanish-American War, the words of the United States were reinforced by the extensive territorial possessions it had gained in the Far East.

AMERICA ACQUIRES THE PHILIPPINES AND AN OPIUM PROBLEM

An expansionist mood, stories of Spanish atrocities against defense-less Cubans, and confidence in an American mission to bring democracy to the world led to the United States' declaration of war on Spain on 25 April 1898. The war's otiose character did not dim American enthusiasm, and its four-month duration made effective opposition impossible. It was difficult to criticize a war in which 341 battle casualties gave the nation Puerto Rico, Guam, and the Philippines as well as control of Cuba for some years. The Philippines, received, in the words of President McKinley, as a gift from the gods, intoxicated Americans who now saw indisputable proof of their new status as a world power and an opportunity to accept the eagerly sought burden of uplifting inferior peoples.[4] The financial and commercial implications of a solid foothold in the Far East were also kept in mind. The United States had in one stroke become a world power in the style of the European nations; an entrepreneur in the expanding market of the Far East. Magnificent responsibilities showered on the nation as it rushed to learn more of those faraway lands about which most Americans, Finley Peter Dunne claimed, did not know "whether they were islands or canned goods." [5]

American intentions toward the natives were honorable and characteristically altruistic. Meanwhile, the Filipinos, having fought side by side with the American troops to drive out the Spanish, thought that the United States was going to free the islands and turn the government over to them. It was difficult to convince them that the Islands were not yet ready for self-government. The Americans also feared that the Germans would seize the Islands if they were independent. America's refusal to grant independence led to a painfully prolonged war against the insurrectionists, which was finally declared crushed in April 1902.[6] In August the first Episcopal bishop of the Philippines, Charles Henry Brent, arrived, traveling with the returning civil governor William Howard Taft. The Right Reverend Mr. Brent, who had been an assistant minister in a poor Boston parish, functioned ably as a missionary bishop, developing schools, hospitals, and often providing a moral conscience for the Philippine Commission that had responsibility under the War Department for the management of the Islands.[7] His contact with the Philippine opium problem made Brent an international leader in the antiopium movement.

Annual trips home and the confidence placed in him by Presidents Roosevelt and Taft assured Bishop Brent of a prominent voice in Philippine affairs.[8] He had no doubt about the overall wisdom of the policy of McKinley and Roosevelt, being certain of the natives' inability to govern themselves. He saw America bringing to colonialism a new attitude and competence that would improve on English methods and on the laissez-faire style of the French administrators.

Opium provided the Islands' government with an early test of its moral intentions.[9] For more than half a century the Spanish had operated a government opium monopoly. Opium was contracted out to merchants who paid taxes on their sales to the Chinese, the only ethnic group permitted to purchase it. When Spanish control suddenly ended, opium imports increased. A cholera epidemic in 1902 reportedly made opium use widespread among the natives, because the constipating qualities of the alkaloids in opium were thought to be life-saving. A tradition of government monopoly of opium sales, supported by a sizable number of Chinese opium smokers and a growing number of natives smoking or eating opium, presented the federal government with an unprecedented problem and unprecedented latitude in the choice of a solution. The Supreme Court had decided in 1901 that doctrines of states' rights were inapplicable to the insular possessions; Congress and the Philippine Commission, therefore, had authority to take almost any action with regard to the opium question.[10]

The first solution proposed was pragmatic: reinstitution of the opium monopoly, restriction of sales to Chinese, and application of the revenue to the immense task of public education.[11] Commissioner of Public Instruction James Smith strongly favored this approach, and his recommendation was approved by Governor Taft. The bill started routinely through the machinery of the Philippine government, but between the second and final readings it was "electrocuted by Presidential lightning." [12] The Reverend Wilbur Crafts, leader of the International Reform Bureau in the United States, recalled that he heard almost casually of this moral outrage—a government pandering to opium craving by degenerate races. Quickly, by letter and by telegraph, he organized opposition: messages flowed into the White House asking President Roosevelt to veto the bill. To profit from such ignoble trade would involve the United States in the support of indefensible vices. Bishop Brent also opposed the scheme on grounds identical with those he gave when returning donations earned through gambling.[13] When the opposition first appeared, Secretary of War Root cabled Taft: "Hold opium monopoly bill. Further investigation. Many protests." [14] Soon opposition proved so strong that the bill was withdrawn.

The opium problem, however, remained. Taft appointed an investigating committee to examine how neighboring regions of the Far East dealt with the problem.[15] The committee, composed of Commissioner of Health Major Edward C. Carter, U.S. Army; Dr. José Albert, a prominent local physician; and Bishop Brent left Manila on 17 August 1903 to gather information in Japan, Formosa, Shanghai, Hong Kong, Saigon, Singapore, Burma, and Java.

A few months later Brent wrote at length to Secretary Taft to prepare him for the committee's report and to give a personal account of the investigation. Brent was disgusted that in Saigon "the French paid no attention whatever to the moral aspects of the question." But, more happily, "in the Straits Settlements we were met with that courtesy and interest that characterizes all the English officials with whom we have been brought into contact." Brent concluded, "the only effective laws we have met with are those enacted by Japan for the main part of the Empire, and for Formosa, and it is somewhat after the pattern of what she has done that we will mold our suggestions." [16] The final report was submitted to the Governor on 15 June 1904. Its conclusions were relatively simple. For three years opium sales should become a government monopoly with only males over the age of 21 licensed to smoke. After gradually reducing individual rations, opium and opiates would be totally prohibited except for medicinal purposes. The report rejected control by high tariffs or licenses, local option, registration of dealers, and immediate prohibition. Provision should be made for hospital cures and instruction in the schools on the evils of opium, to discourage the young from forming the habit. Opium dens were to be closed and poppy cultivation prohibited. The report's authors considered it in accord with contemporary medical opinion: the craving for opium is irrespressible and a habitué gradually increases his intake until systematic intoxication leads to moral and physical degeneration. Although crimes committed under the influence of the drug were thought to be less violent than those stemming from alcohol, extreme craving caused by lack of opiates was connected with crime. Immediate prohibition, therefore, would not be wise or effective. The ultimate goal, however, should be total prohibition, as well as free treatment for habitués who wished to rid themselves of the vice. Meanwhile, to keep the opium abuse from spreading, some form of registration was needed.[17]

American domestic reaction to opium use in the Philippines was more drastic than the committees' recommendations. In March 1905 Congress ordered immediate opium prohibition for Filipinos except for medicinal purposes.[18] In three years prohibition would apply to non-Filipinos. In the meantime, the Philippine Commission could make what provisions it wished to tide over the non-Filipino users until March 1908. Of course, the three-year legal use of opium would apply chiefly to the Chinese. Congress thereby reinstituted an ethnic distinction which the investigating committee had opposed in the "interests of equity and justice." [19]

The Philippine Commission decided on a program of expensive licenses for dealers and the registration of adult male Chinese habitual users. Beginning in October 1907, opium allotments to the registrants gradually decreased and sales ended completely in six months.[20] Effectiveness of Philippine opium prohibition continued to be debated, and as late as 1930 American investigators found that smoking opium was easily obtainable.[21]

OPIUM IN CHINA

Having resolved the opium question in the Philippines, Americans intent upon international control of narcotics now focused on the Sino-Indian opium trade. Since the late eighteenth century Indian opium had been shipped to China; from this trade India received considerable tax revenue. The moral implication of such commerce was often regretted in England as well as elsewhere. To reformers, opium smuggling was unfortunate, but to make the opium evil a revenue source was intolerable.

The British government feared that if the Indian opium trade were suspended, the great opium-producing nations of Persia and Turkey would quickly take it over or that China would merely grow more poppies. Such an event would make England moral, but the Indian government would have an unbalanced budget, and the Chinese would continue to smoke opium. Moreover, a British investigation into opium use in 1895 concluded that opium was more like the Westerner's liquor than a substance to be feared and abhorred.[22]

Britons who denounced the Sino-Indian traffic and Chinese who saw in opium a curse to their nation (and a reason why China accepted foreign domination) found support in the Philippine Commission's view of opium as one of the gravest evils in the Orient. Shortly after the commission's findings were published, several other events accelerated the fight against the Sino-Indian opium trade. The Liberal Party won an overwhelming victory in the parliamentary elections of January 1906. The Liberals' reform program included a long-standing recommendation to eliminate the Indian opium exports to China.[23] As a result of parliamentary pressure, the British Foreign Office approached China, offering to abolish that trade to the extent that China decreased cultivation of poppies and use of opium. By the close of 1906 agreement had been reached to reduce, under inspection, both the Chinese consumption and Indian shipments of opium by 10 percent annually, so that the whole trade could end in 1916.[24] Chinese hatred of foreign domination spurred her to unexpected fulfillment of this agreement. These forces for modernization were equally antiforeign and anti-imperialist.[25]

The Boxer movement, which culminated in the Rebellion of 1900, was the most violent expression of China's growing nationalistic and anti-imperialistic sentiment. The Boxers revered traditional values and reviled the new technologies, but other Chinese, many students, and some officials who coveted the scientific and military power of the West and Japan sought avenues in which China could move forward and surpass her enemies.

Simple hatred of foreign domination and yearning for technological progress united in opposition to opium addiction. Opium was accused of sapping the strength and initiative of the nation so that it lagged in education, science, technology, and military effectiveness. Students and other youth joined the antiopium campaign which had always been the official (albeit never effectively enforced) position of the government. So many groups now combined to fight opium that a vigorous and sustained eradication program was possible for the first time.[26] In 1906, strict regulations for reducing opium use were promulgated by the Dowager Empress. This popular action was in accord with the British-Chinese agreement. Although previously only the antiopium zealots had any optimism for the campaign, within a few years China's most severe critics agreed that the crusade had begun to succeed. The methods employed by the Chinese government were ruthless and could not have been carried out unless the government and Chinese society agreed that opium was an unmitigated evil. Fervent nationalism, which nominated opium as the scapegoat for a multitude of humiliations, was an effective weapon against the narcotic.

THE AMERICAN RESPONSE TO CHINESE ADDICTION

Chinese in the United States received some of their worst treatment during America's period of expansion in 1904 in the Far East. Tension between China and the United States reached a climax over the determination of Congress to exclude Chinese laborers. Brutality in the United States against Chinese travelers and immigrants of all kinds furnished ammunition to the anti-imperialists in China.[27] With an inadequate army, and knowing that burning the American Embassy would only bring back the marines, Chinese merchants protested by organizing a voluntary embargo against American goods in 1905.[28] Although formally disavowed by the Chinese government, the embargo was popular and in certain trading areas effective. The growth of the embargo, and a fear of what total cessation of trade would mean to those who thirsted after the endless Chinese market, agitated American traders. President Roosevelt privately admitted the justice of the Chinese protest but felt it unmanly to allow America to be pushed around: he asked Congress for $100,000 to send troops to the Far East.[29]

On 24 July 1906, after the embargo had begun to take effect and while British and Chinese opposition to opium accelerated, Bishop Brent wrote to Roosevelt urging an international meeting of the United States, other great powers with interests in the Far East, and Japan to help China with its opium struggle. Only such concerted action, he pleaded, could shut off the flood of opium into China and make effective the forthcoming opiate prohibition in the Philippines.[30]

Roosevelt's initial response was favorable. The proposal was well timed to ameliorate the tension between China and the United States, and an international meeting was one of Roosevelt's favored methods to promote the United States into the ranks of the foremost powers. Soon the Roosevelt-inspired Second Hague Peace

Conference was to convene; Roosevelt had just completed negotiations at Portsmouth, New Hampshire, to bring an end to the Russo-Japanese War. A humanitarian movement to ease the burden of opium in China would help his long-range goals: to mollify Chinese resentment against America, put the British in a less favorable light, and support Chinese antagonism against European entrenchment.[31] A less sanguine Secretary of State Elihu Root went along with the plan.

After most nations with possessions in the Far East had accepted the American invitation, the State Department requested of Congress $20,000 for appointment of three commissioners to investigate the international opium evil and prepare for the conference.[32] Who would take charge of this work for the State Department? Ideally the man should be familiar with the region and also with the problem of opium from a scientific point of view. Such a person lived in Washington, the dashing, ebullient Dr. Hamilton Wright.[33] Dr. Wright had previously worked in the Far East, setting up a laboratory in the Straits Settlements to study tropical diseases. He had gained some fame by discovering (erroneously) that beriberi was an infectious ailment. Even more than research, Wright had always enjoyed the political side of medical work. In 1899 his marriage to Elizabeth Washburn, member of a politically prominent family, opened many doors and advanced his hopes for a career.[34] Wright became enthusiastically involved with opium and was dubbed the father of American narcotic laws. He later recalled that his appointment seemed casual good luck:

My first intimation that there was to be an American Opium Commission came to me from O'Loughlen [*Chicago Tribune* correspondent Cal O'Laughlin]. I met him on Scott Circle on the morning of May 1st [1908]. We passed the time of day and he then asked me in his usual direct way if I would like to be a member of an opium commission about to be appointed by President Roosevelt. I inquired about it, could not get much information as O'L did not have much. But I saw at a glance that it was bound to be a large and extensive bit of work and I said that certainly I would like to be a member. O'L said that he thought that Roosevelt wanted me to serve and that I could see [presidential secretary] Loeb about it. I did so shortly thereafter at the White House offices.[35]

As another delegate to the commission, the President appointed Dr. Charles C. Tenney, secretary to the American Legation at Peking, a former missionary who had helped the Chinese to achieve educational reforms. Tenney strongly supported the Chinese anti-opium campaign and condemned the British for their immoral trade with China.[36]

The chairmanship was tendered to Judge Thomas Burke, one of Seattle's most prominent citizens, but for unknown reasons he declined it. Then the State Department turned to the originator of the conference proposal. Bishop Brent, who was also being urged by Roosevelt and Taft to transfer to the bishopric of Washington, D.C., accepted the chairmanship in July 1908, two years after his recommendation to the President. The three delegates, although residing in Washington, Manila, and Peking, began coordinating efforts for the conference scheduled for the first day of 1909 in Shanghai.

In a short time Dr. Wright devoured what information the State Department and the Library of Congress held on the subject of opium. But his debut with the Federal bureaucracy was a grave portent of his future diplomatic career. Hearing that Bishop Brent on a midyear trip to the United States might visit the White House to discuss delegation matters, Wright sent the President a memorandum on the general opium situation. This direct communication to the President reflected Wright's view of his role in government: a subordinate in the State Department because of technicalities, he was in reality independent of formalities—a distinguished scientist trying to accomplish quickly and efficiently an important political assignment.

Secretary of State Root, to whom Roosevelt turned over Wright's memorandum for comment, did not share Wright's perception. To Root, this attempt to attract the attention of the President would only confuse consideration of the subject and was a nuisance. "Dr. Wright should report to the State Department under which he is serving," admonished Root. "If Wright would go on and attend to his business the information he acquires will be used in the proper place."[37]

Soon Wright launched a national survey to collect information on the use of opium and its derivatives in the United States. He sent hundreds of questionnaires to prisons, police departments, boards of health and pharmacy, and morphine manufacturers, and he visited a number of cities to examine for himself the use and control of opiates. Wright's frenetic activity was evoked by the State Department's request to other nations for such information. He thought the Americans should lead the way.[38]

Another responsibility of the convening nation was to have exemplary opium laws. Here there was a more serious difficulty, for while calling on other nations to aid in eliminating the opium problem, the United States had no national laws limiting or prohibiting importation, use, sale, or manufacture of opium or coca leaves and their derivatives. This situation simply reflected the traditional constitutional reservation of police powers to the states. Nevertheless, the lack of a federal law embarrassed the commission officials, who believed that other nations would not understand the intricacies of the American Federal system.[39] Wright and Root wanted federal anti-narcotic legislation before the Shanghai meeting, only a few months away.

Wright may have believed it necessary to stress the evil of opium in America in order to secure passage of domestic legislation. His statistics were usually interpreted to maximize the danger of addiction, dramatize a supposed crisis in opiate consumption, mobilize fear of minorities, and yet never waver from the exuberant patriotism which colored the crusade for the Shanghai Conference.[40] An example of Wright's patriotic interpretation of evidence is found in a letter to Brent announcing that an enormous amount of opium and its derivates and cocaine was supplied to the army and navy, but that he had been assured that the drugs had been stolen by unscrupulous persons in the medical department and sold surreptitiously in our larger cities.[41]

In New England, particularly in his adopted Maine, Wright saw a close relationship between Prohibition and the use of opiates: in teetotaling states morphine sales over the previous ten years had increased 150 percent.[42] Nationally, patent medicines containing opiates had decreased in sales between 25 and 50 percent since the pure food laws went into effect.[43] His study also uncovered the existence "ten or fifteen years ago" of opium joints in Boston and New York operated by "Harvard students and students of our larger universities." [44]

Except for a brief contretemps between Wright and Root over travel expenses, all seemed to be going well for the American delegation. The commission continued to grow into a representative group. Persia and Turkey, which produced most of the opium introduced

into the Far East, were invited (Persia accepted) and at the last
moment Italy and Austria-Hungary asked to be included.

Enactment of a federal law regulating opiates was the only problem that remained after the survey. But Wright and others were
soon caught in a bind as they considered legislative programs: to
close all loopholes meant offending pharmacists, manufacturers, and
physicians by a multitude of detailed controls; easing up on the
controls would provide ways for the unscrupulous dealer to continue
his evil trade. And then, of course, a perennial problem continued
to complicate the matter—the federal government had limited police
powers. The State Department thought the most likely prohibition to
gain quick congressional approval would be a ban on imported
smoking opium. With smoking opium as the target, planning moved
quickly forward.

Secretary of State Root, one of the ablest legal minds of his
period, tried to make the prohibition as simple as possible. He
proposed to Congress in 1908 a combination of the legislation per-
taining to the import of opiates into the Philippines (of March 1905)
and the standard statute used in the prevention of illegal imports.
He modified the Philippine legislation to make it possible for
citizens to import opiates other than smoking opium.[45]

Root made no claim that he was proposing a definitive law to
deal with the opium problem in the United States. No new methods
of enforcement were proposed, and only the importation of opium
for smoking was actually outlawed. A simple and broadly acceptable
approach was mandatory if the United States was "to have legislation on this subject in time to save our face in the conference at
Shanghai."[46] When the Act was approved (9 February 1909), the
American delegation proudly and with dramatic flourish announced
the victory to the commission, then in session.[47]

That this first federal antinarcotic legislation was largely a matter
of face-saving is demonstrated in an exchange between the head of
the Agriculture Department's Bureau of Chemistry, Dr. Harvey
Wiley, and the State Department in the fall of 1908. Dr. Wiley over-
saw the enforcement of the Pure Food and Drug Act of 1906 and was
widely considered the chief architect of that progressive legislation.
The State Department requested that Wiley examine a bill proposed to outlaw smoking opium imports.[48] Not realizing the propaganda purposes of the legislation, Dr. Wiley replied that a new law
was unnecessary since Section 11 of the Pure Food and Drug Act

made provision for the banning of any imported drug that was
dangerous to the health of the people of the United States.[49] A quick
response from Assistant Secretary Robert Bacon informed him that
banning itself was not so essential as the enactment of specific antiopium legislation to prove the nations' sincerity in Shanghai.[50]

As the State Department maneuvered the legislation through
Congress before the Shanghai meeting convened, Brent and Wright
made their separate ways to Manila where they were to confer on
plans for the meeting. After stopping in San Francisco to investigate
the narcotic problem there, Wright again reminded the State Department of the importance of a bill to abolish smoking opium, although he knew the more serious problem was domestic abuse of
narcotics in all forms.[51] With reference to the larger issue, he asserted that manufacturers were ready to agree to the recording of
drug sales by Internal Revenue Bureau tax stamps. Pharmacists
would likewise be required to account for all drug dispensing. Such
records would enable state officials with police powers to locate
trends and areas of abuse so that current state laws could be effectively enforced or stronger ones enacted. Curiously, he made no
mention of the physician's role in providing narcotics or creating
addiction, although this was a concern to other reformers.

Wright spent December in the Philippines with Bishop Brent. A
small problem, but typical of the situations he created, arose when
he desired to confer with the Philippine government's Secretary of
the Interior Department, Dean Worcester. Wright maintained his
rank was equal to that of a minister and that Worcester should visit
him; Worcester countered that a secretary of the Philippine Department had the rank of ambassador, and so Wright should come to
him.[52] It is unclear whether these men ever met. Wright and Brent
moved on to Shanghai and the opening of the Shanghai Commission.

The Shanghai Opium Commission

The commission convened on the first of February, having been
postponed for a month out of respect for the death of the Dowager
Empress. Originally Brent had hoped for a conference, a diplomatic
meeting that could lead to official action by represented governments. At the request of Great Britain and the Netherlands, however, the meeting was ranked as a commission, a fact-finding body
which could make only recommendations and not commitments.[53]
Brent was chosen chairman and conducted the meeting in a con-

ciliatory spirit, seeking to obtain unanimous support for the final resolutions. Attempting to please all nations led to less dogmatic stands than Brent desired, but this plan had the advantage of creating at least a moral commitment, so the Americans thought, to a set of resolutions. Accordingly, the resolutions were later used in the United States to pressure Congress and other groups to fulfill "America's pledges" to the rest of the world. The commission and the resolutions also helped inaugurate an American tradition in narcotic control—enactment of strict domestic legislation in the United States as an example to other nations.

Problems that still plague international control of narcotic traffic appeared at the 1909 meeting. Although thirteen nations were represented, Turkey did not attend and Persia appointed a mere local merchant to represent its interests. Most nations were mildly interested in the subject but unwilling to exert much effort for non-medical prohibition as proposed by the United States; it was impossible to get general agreement that the use of opium for other than medicinal purposes was evil and immoral.[54] The cautious attitude of most nations increased the American delegates' determination to prove their sincerity with solid legislation and dramatic action to control narcotics. Their assumption was that if other nations controlled their internal growth, manufacture, and export of narcotics, the United States would be freed from its burdens, since the poppy and the coca leaf had never been grown in significant commercial quantities in America. Later Wright told influential congressmen that when other nations took the strong stand he advocated for American domestic control of narcotics, our customs service would be cheaper, since fewer agents would be required to protect the nation from smuggling.[55] The desire to show the others, to prove America's good intentions, and to provide an example all supported the new campaign for strict federal narcotic laws.

The Shanghai Opium Commission met for almost four weeks. Although initially wary, the Chinese delegates eventually expressed their country's appreciation at being treated as an equal in a conference dealing with a Chinese question. Apparently this was the first such meeting in which China was afforded equal status.[56] Delegates who had prepared reports of conditions in their own countries presented them. Resolutions were debated. The British were unwilling to open discussion on the Sino-Indian opium agreements, since India strongly objected to any changes in the profitable trade and Britain felt that it was a matter between London and Peking. Persia, whose commercial representative contributed little to the discussion, had accepted the invitation at a late date and had not had time to prepare a national report.

The resolutions were merely recommendations; they would never be submitted for ratification to the governments represented. Given this limitation, they did articulate some of the American sentiment, though they were usually qualified. For example, Resolution Two called on each government to take measures for the gradual suppression of opium smoking with due regard to the varying circumstances of each country concerned. In the light of near unanimous agreement that opium for other than medicinal uses should be prohibited "or carefully regulated," each nation was called upon by Resolution Three to "reexamine" its own laws. Resolution Four, which Wright later boasted to Congress was the delegation's prime achievement (although there was no significant opposition), stated that nations could not export opium to other nations whose laws prohibit the importation. It would have been difficult to vote against this resolution but, on the other hand, no international system was established by which close control could be maintained.[57]

Particularly appealing to the Americans was the unanimous agreement that drastic measures should be taken by each government to control morphine and other opium derivatives. Originally a British resolution, amended slightly by the American delegation, it provided U.S. delegations and those involved in interim domestic maneuvers with ammunition for pursuing strict federal legislation: it would be humiliating for the United States to demand controls by other nations but have no exemplary laws of its own.[58]

UNITED STATES APPEAL FOR AN INTERNATIONAL CONFERENCE

The United States delegates had challenged themselves to prove America's sincerity. They hoped that another meeting would soon be called to design formal international cooperation to eliminate the narcotic menace; but the American proposal for a post-Shanghai conference was not accepted as one of the resolutions.[59] Most other nations were not interested. Great Britain did not wish to enter a conference until trade between India and China could be brought into a more popular and defensible form. Turkey had not sent a

representative to the Shanghai meeting and gave no promise of appearing at any later conference. Eventually other nations equally
essential to international control, for example France and Germany,
proved to have little interest in such a meeting. The prospect for
quick agreement by any nation other than China to meet again on
the subject of opium did not seem good.

Within a week of the Shanghai Commission's adjournment, the
United States inaugurated a new president, William Howard Taft,
who had strongly supported Brent's activities against opium and
whose foreign policy goals were congenial to a plan for international
control of narcotics.[60] Taft had heartily encouraged the initial steps
to call the Shanghai Commission, was familiar with the Orient, and
had full confidence in Brent.

But within the State Department the wisdom of America's carrying the crusade beyond Shanghai was questioned, particularly by
Huntington Wilson, chief of the newly created Far East Division
and Wright's immediate superior. Another meeting had not been
announced in the original planning for the commission, and it was
beyond the department's purview to suggest to Congress domestic
laws on drug control. Furthermore, in such a meeting America's
own trade agreements with China might be brought up, and this
possibility was no more attractive to the United States than discussion of the Sino-Indian trade agreement was to the British.[61] Wright,
angrily aware of Wilson's opposition to the United States delegation's moral commitment, believed that Wilson was jealous of his
sudden prominence in Chinese affairs and frightened by the support
given Wright's bid to be appointed minister to China the previous
spring.[62] Brent had written Theodore Roosevelt on Wright's behalf
but was relieved when Wright lost out. His message to Wright was
amicably blunt: the doctor should stick to medicine; he was not a
diplomat and in a sensitive situation he was bound to "kick over
the traces." "I would hate to see you enter diplomacy," concluded
Brent, "without a pretty sure chance of success, which I doubt."
Continuing in this vein later that year, Brent wrote to Wright, "A
man who has the scientific ability that you have might continue along
the lines in which he has already distinguished himself." [63] Wright
chose not to take this advice.

Meanwhile, Taft's Secretary of State, Philander C. Knox, adopted
a European custom and initiated aggressive diplomatic efforts to
obtain financial concessions in such areas of market expansion as

China and Latin America. But this period of renewed American determination to penetrate the China market coincided with Chinese nationalism and resistance to new foreign investments, even though American offers promised the "methods and improvements of Western civilization." [64] Other nations that had hopes for large investments continued to oppose American interests.

Memories of the Chinese embargo and more recent demonstrations of resistance to foreign investment gave Wright hope that an American call for another international meeting to assist China would be approved by the State Department. For this approval he had to go over Wilson's head and confer directly with the Secretary of State. To Wright's relief, Knox "realized in two minutes the importance of the affair and its bearing on his determined efforts to make the United States felt in the commercial life of China." Wright recalled telling the Secretary:

> Our move to help China in her opium reform gave us more prestige in China than any of our recent friendly acts toward her. If we continue and press steadily for the Conference, China will recognize that we are sincere in her behalf, and the whole business may be used as oil to smooth the troubled water of our aggressive commercial policy there.
>
> "Go ahead," replied the Secretary. [65]

During the next two years Wright rode to the high point of his diplomatic career. He carried on negotiations with Congress, drafted proposals for domestic antinarcotic laws, threatened and cajoled foreign ambassadors, and planned in intricate detail just what economic concessions to require of China in return for all the good that was being done for her.

The first step in calling the international conference, letters of invitation to the powers represented at Shanghai, were to be sent on 1 September 1909. In the middle of August Wright rushed back to Washington from a brief vacation in Maine because he was uneasy. His concern was warranted, for Wilson, his bête noire, had mislaid the official documents. They were then found in Wilson's motorcar and sent. [66] In the letters over the signature of Assistant Secretary A. A. Adee, Wright asked for a reply by 30 November. Privately he admitted he didn't see why the conference could not meet at least by the following May (1910). Anticipating quick results at home and abroad, he belittled the fainthearted Wilson, who thought it would take two years to bring the conference into reality. Wright worked feverishly at drafting domestic legislation, kept the zealous reformers from getting too impatient, and thoroughly enjoyed himself.[67] But Wilson had correctly estimated that two years would pass before the conference opened.

The program for the conference was patterned on the Brussels Convention of 1890 concerning the slave and liquor traffic in Africa. The provisions of that convention had been enforced by a permanent commission, just as Wright expected that an international board would oversee adherence to the agreements reached at the opium conference. Britain, he believed, having insisted in its treaties with China upon monitoring the diminishing Sino-Indian opium trade and China's elimination of domestic poppy growth, would make a similar demand of any other international agreement.[68] Since without British cooperation no solid results would be possible, every whisper from Whitehall was carefully examined for the divination of Great Britain's real intentions.

Dr. Wright considered American demands for currency reform in China, as well as a number of other financial improvements to strengthen the Chinese economy, as only fair requests considering what the United States was trying to do for China.[69] Economic reforms were desired by American investors and had been a prime goal of the State Department.

DOMESTIC LEGISLATION: THE FOSTER ANTINARCOTIC BILL

Wright believed that the Shanghai meeting gave the United States a moral obligation to appear with a clean slate before asking other nations to enact drastic legislation. He was quite ready to frame such laws, but he faced strong opposition even within the State Department. He had spent most of the summer of 1909 in Washington trying to formulate a bill and gathering the data for a strong report to Congress when "he of the eolithic mind [Huntington Wilson] cried halt." [70] Wilson, having lost on the question of another conference, now argued that proposing domestic legislation was an unwarranted action by the State Department.

Frustrated by this block to his ambitious project, Wright saw no recourse but once again to take the question to Secretary of State Knox. The Secretary asked him to put in writing "not only its bearings on the home problem, but as it affected our foreign relations especially with China." In a week or so Knox gave his approval and Wright was back on the rails.[71]

By late 1909, Wright had a plan for domestic legislation. He decided to seek the control of drug traffic through federal powers of taxation. His bill would require every drug dealer to register, pay a small tax, and record all transactions. The drug container would be required to carry a revenue stamp; interstate traffic would be prohibited between individuals who had not paid the tax. Wright's bill spelled out heavy penal provisions, and possession of drugs other than those specified in the bill would constitute evidence for conviction. State boards of pharmacy and local and municipal authorities would have access to information about the transactions so that they might enforce "the proper relations that should exist between the physician, the dispensing druggist, [and] those who have some real need of the drugs." Significantly, in view of future trends in narcotic control, Wright believed in 1909 that it was impossible for the federal government to regulate such a relationship.[72]

Wright submitted a draft to Representative James R. Mann of Illinois, chairman of the House Committee on Interstate and Foreign Commerce. Mann had shown interest in legislation to preserve or regain morality: the Supreme Court would in 1913 uphold legislation associated with his name to prevent the transporation of women across state lines for immoral purposes. Mann doubted that Wright's tax approach, with its burdensome details falling on the retail druggist, was likely to succeed, so he recommended alternative legislation based on the regulation of interstate commerce.[73]

The bill which Mann preferred to Wright's had been introduced by Mann in the House in May 1908, at the request of retail druggists in cooperation with the Agriculture Department, and had failed to pass.

Wright's proposed legislation was eventually introduced on 30 April 1910 by Representative David Foster of Vermont, chairman of the House Committee on Foreign Affairs.[74] The direct antecedent of the Harrison Act, the Foster bill was designed to uncover all traffic in opiates, cocaine, chloral hydrate, and cannabis regardless of the minute quantities that might be involved. Records would be scrupulously kept, bonds given, and reports rendered as required. Violations were to be punished by not less than $500 or more than $5,000 and for no less than one year's imprisonment or more than five. Nothing in the law stipulated any such restriction on the retail distribution of habit-forming drugs as limiting sales or prescriptions to medical needs. Nor did the bill allow any exemption for patent medicines or household remedies containing relatively small amounts of the controlled drugs. Therefore any purchase of a narcotic would require tax stamps and record keeping under very severe penalties for error or omission. Perhaps the ulterior goal was to make such retail sales more troublesome than profitable and thereby eliminate the trade.[75]

On 31 May 1910, when Wright had once thought that the International Conference would convene, he appeared before the House Committee on Ways and Means to support the Foster bill.[76] Most of the arguments presented orally were contained in the Shanghai Commission report, which had been recently sent to Congress with a message from the President recommending appropriate domestic legislation.[77] The report was designed to impress Congress with the need for legislation and for an appropriation of $25,000 to finance federal "efforts to mitigate if not entirely stamp out the opium evil." [78] The Shanghai meeting was portrayed as extremely hopeful and much to the credit of the United States, but incomplete and looking to Congress for the legislation that would permit the United States "to see the thorough solution of not only China's oppressive opium problem, but that of other countries not so heavily burdened" (*Report,* p. 75). As proof that the country had a serious narcotic problem the report claimed that since 1860 importation of crude opium had risen more rapidly than the American population (p. 38). State legislation was unable to stem the importation of narcotics.[79]

The severity of the bill's penalties as compared with, for example, the District of Columbia Pharmacy Act, was explained by the fear that even such seemingly harmless opium preparations as laudanum and paregoric, sold to minors in many states, could lead to addiction (p. 59). The report depicted the pharmacy and medical professions as untrustworthy: many pharmacists sold addictive drugs indiscriminately and many unscrupulous physicians dispensed habit-forming drugs in large quantities from their offices (p. 59). "It would be wise," the report recommended, "for state laws to make possession of drugs except for medicinal purposes, evidence for conviction." [80] Information gathered in Wright's national survey indicated that among physicians about 2 percent and among nurses about 1 percent were habitués of some form of opium. Only 0.7 percent of other professional classes and 0.2 percent of the general population were addicted (p. 47). Such drugs were practically unknown in colleges and universities; opium smoking had not affected servicemen who had been in the Far East during the previous ten years.[81] Wright expressed embarrassment at the United States' consumption of opium as compared with European nations; the abstinence of the latter was due, he felt, to their strict national laws and their "good sense" (p. 46).

In regard to opium smoking in the United States, Wright reported that the Chinese were the primary source of infection, but that it had then spread from white to white and from black to black. He did not want to engage in scare tactics about the spread of this habit from the Chinese to the American population, but he did observe that "one of the most unfortunate phases of the habit of smoking opium in this country [was] the large number of women who have become involved and were living as common-law wives or cohabiting with Chinese in the Chinatowns of our various cities." [82]

Wright did not stress the dangers of opium smoking since Congress had obligingly enacted the recent law in time for the Shanghai meeting. The menace of cocaine was more serious, however, although it had been a national problem for only about twenty years. Wright assured Congress that cocaine was more appalling in its effects than any other drug (*Report*, p. 48). Most citizens knew of its general harmful effects, but its identification with the Negro had not received due attention. Why Wright thought this identification had not been sufficiently publicized is unclear, but he warned of cocaine's "encouragement . . . among the humbler ranks of the Negro population in the South." In the South the cocaine problem among Negroes greatly troubled law enforcement officers, he stated. The "lower order of working Negro [being] not willing, as a rule, to go to much trouble or send to any distance for anything," intoxication by the drug made "it certain that it was brought directly to him from New York and other northern states where it [was] manufactured." Wright also reported that contractors gave the drug to their Negro employees to get more work out of them.[83]

Criminal classes everywhere were starting to use cocaine, especially those concerned in the white slave traffic. Cocaine use threatened to creep into the higher social ranks of the country. Should anyone doubt the need for stricter control of this substance, the report concluded, "it has been authoritatively stated that cocaine is often the direct incentive to the crime of rape by the Negroes of the South and other sections of the country" (pp. 48–49).

The purpose of Wright's strong statements in regard to cocaine and Negroes was, of course, to encourage the legislation he sought, partly by motivating hesitant southern Democrats who feared any precedent of federal involvement in the police powers reserved to the states. But the fear of Negro cocaine users could as easily be found reported in northern and southern newspapers and in medical journals as in State Department reports and congressional hearings.[84]

The Foster bill's goal was to bring the "whole traffic and the use of [habit-forming] drugs into the light of day and thereby create a public opinion against the use of them." [85] The traffic was deemed so serious that "quite 10 percent of the retail drug stores of the United States would be put out of business if the illicit sales of the drugs were stopped." [86] Therefore, because the nation was being debauched by habit-forming drugs, and also because the Shanghai declarations resulted from American initiative, it was "the bounden duty of our government to be the first to enact [drug-control] legislation." [87] In spite of the report and the obligations Wright enumerated, no action was taken by the committee before summer adjournment.

In the elections of November 1910 the Democrats gained control of the House for the first time in eighteen years. A substantial interval would pass before the newly elected members took office on 4 March, but ranking Democrats, mostly from the South, quickly assumed a greater importance in the future of any legislation. Perhaps that accounts for Wright's even more open fear-mongering on the dangers of the Negro cocaine addict when hearings on the Foster bill reopened.

DEFEAT OF THE FOSTER BILL

The December sessions heard arguments in support of strict control of habit-forming drugs, and several members of the drug trades favorably inclined toward the Foster bill appeared at the hearings. After the Christmas recess the opposition was heard. A week before hearings were resumed, Wright came to New York to conciliate doubtful medical and pharmaceutical interests. The drug-trade leaders gathered at the home of Dr. William J. Schieffelin, president of the National Wholesale Druggists Association (NWDA) and a prominent member of various national reform movements.[88] After this meeting, trade representatives hoped that modifications would be made in the bill. Druggists, however, continued their attacks. The Drug Trade Section of the New York Board of Trade came out in opposition to the Foster bill, which it now described as pleasing no one except Dr. Wright. The section also correctly predicted that no action would be taken during the last session of the 61st Congress.[89]

Attitudes toward narcotic control varied considerably within the drug industry. Restrictions on small amounts of narcotics that could make a best seller out of an otherwise slow item (mainly proprietary medicines) were opposed by retail drug interests. Legislation that would permit sales of narcotics only to pharmacists was opposed by manufacturers of medicine exclusively for dispensing physicians.

On the final day of hearings, 11 January 1911, a message from the President was transmitted to Congress reiterating the obligation of the United States "to see that its house is in order before the International Opium Conference meets in The Hague in 1911." Drafted principally by Wright, this Message on the Opium Traffic declared that enactment of the Foster bill was a "pressing necessity" as a consequence of drug abuse in the United States as well as American moral responsibilities undertaken before other nations.[90]

The House Committee on Ways and Means devoted the day to the Foster bill, providing the opportunity for the first extended debate before Congress between interests concerned with narcotic control. Opponents spoke first, then supporters. A representative of the NWDA, Dr. Charles West, began the attack. He opposed the inclusion of any drugs other than opium, morphine, cocaine, and their derivatives. Cannabis, he said, was not what might be called a habit-forming drug. He attacked the use of stamps and labels at every turn, arguing that additional help would be needed to separate orders, check inventories, and keep records; a tremendous financial burden would be placed on the jobbers and wholesalers. Proprietaries should be exempted as provided in many state laws. The word "knowingly" should be added for protection against an unintentional violation of the act. Dr. West felt the penalties were excessively severe. After a few other criticisms he endorsed the goal of the law, "but what we want is a simple law, one that can be enforced and will not inflict too much hardship on the trade." [91] At the hearings of 11 January, Dr. West was questioned by Representative Francis Burton Harrison (future sponsor of the Harrison Narcotic Act), Harrison focused on cola soda pop. "What about this material they call Coca-Cola?" he asked the NWDA representative, "Isn't it a habit-forming drink?" Dr. West agreed that it was a habit-forming drink and that perhaps Pepsi-Cola was in the same class. Rep. Harrison then stated that coca leaves should be included in the bill, since from them were made "Coca-Cola and Pepsi-Cola and all those things that are sold to Negroes all over the South."

Representative Henry Boutell suspected that a strict law would create bootleggers and not solve the addiction problem. Harrison countered that if less were sold, the public would develop less of a craving and thus not have much need for the bootlegger. The chairman, Representative Sereno Payne, suggested one good result of elaborate and stringent provisions: "regulation . . . would . . . make it so unprofitable to sell the stuff [proprietaries] that wholesale druggists might go out of that line of business." Dr. Schieffelin took a more positive view of the legislation. He wanted legitimate druggists to handle drugs with clean hands; bootleggers could have the other traffic. He made a sharp distinction between alcohol on the one hand and opiates and cocaine on the other; he considered the latter substances a great danger, leading probably to death and almost certainly to insanity. Agreeing with the critics who had spoken, he suggested that labeling requirements be replaced by a system of registry numbers which each transactor could place on the containers. He also supported some provision exempting proprietaries containing limited amounts of narcotics.

Charles Woodruff, a lawyer representing six large drug manufacturers, denied that the industry was thoughtless about public welfare: his firms had for years worked to keep morphine and later cocaine out of the hands of dope fiends and disreputable persons. Multiple regulations would just make "a goat out of the manufacturer. The welfare of this country depends on the welfare of the manufacturer." Dr. William Muir of Brooklyn, speaking for the New York Pharmaceutical Association, showed the plight of the honest retailer. Cannabis, for example, was an ingredient of corn cures. Every time a corn cure was sold, the druggist would have to make a record of it. The druggists weren't interested in helping collect statistics for future legislation, a goal suggested for the law.

Dr. Muir warned the committee that retail druggists were now up in arms against the bill: only the day before five hundred druggists in Brooklyn had met and opposed the measure. He disputed estimates on prevalence of drug abuse. Declaring that education could control the problem, Muir pointed to a decline in the sale of cocaine, which he attributed to public enlightenment. Just because opium causes some harm, he argued, is no reason to stamp it out; one should think of the good it does in relieving pain. "A good many people are killed by automobiles: but there is [also] a good deal of pleasure gotten out of them," he said. Representative Payne, in response to Muir, summarized the goal of federal legislation: not to limit opium's pain-relieving uses but to eliminate the use of drugs "prepared to satisfy a habit."

The American Pharmaceutical Association was represented by the chairman of its Committee on National Legislation, Henry B. Hynson. Amendments recommended by the association clearly illustrated its willingness to go beyond most drug-interest groups in the search for effective reforms. The association criticized the list of uncontrolled drugs as too short; it wanted synthetic drugs to be listed and heroin to receive specific mention. Hynson pinpointed some ambiguities in the bill's definitions and further emphasized the association's desire to have a strong law by warning the committee that if they added the word "knowingly" it would "envalidate the whole matter." Yet, as regards the possible police powers of such an act, he added, the several states should retain control of the writers of prescriptions within their borders.

Charles B. Towns, operator of a drug and alcohol hospital in New York, also defended the Foster bill. Towns attacked the veracity of the witnesses representing the wholesalers, saying he could name names and cite instances of habitués' purchases from the wholesalers. Towns opposed almost all stimulants. He greatly feared opium's effects on the mind and body. Anyone could get addicted to morphine by taking ¼ grain daily for three weeks, no matter what his character. Codeine was especially dangerous, and as for cannabis, "there is no drug in the *Pharmacopoeia* today that would produce the pleasurable sensations you would get from cannabis . . . and of all the drugs on earth I would certainly put that on the list." Moreover, experience had convinced him that it was a habit-forming drug. He believed that federal and state laws must cooperate and complement each other in the control of habit-forming drugs. Although he had noted a decline in the use and sale of cocaine, he figured the legitimate need for the drug to be very small compared to the amount being sold in the United States. He agreed with pharmaceutical representatives that 50 percent of the addictions resulted from overzealous physicians who prescribed habit-forming drugs.

From the Bureau of Chemistry came Dr. Wiley and his assistant Dr. L. F. Kebler, who appeared with samples of narcotic-containing proprietary medicines including addiction remedies and infants' soothing syrups. Some preparations were from physicians who operated opium-cure sanitaria or who sold bottled opium cures through the mail. Since these "cures" contained large amounts of narcotics, Dr. Kebler contested the wisdom of the druggists who wanted to exempt proprietaries from the general law.[92]

Dr. Wiley wanted a prohibitory law, but he would accept less. Caffeine should be added to the list, as well as acetanilid, antipyrene, and phenacetin. He belittled the contention that large firms could not keep accurate records of habit-forming drugs (p. 87).

The drug trade's chief requirements—provisions for exempt proprietaries, simple record keeping, and softer penalties—had to be met if federal laws controlling or monitoring the traffic in dangerous drugs were to be passed. Two weeks after the hearings, Representative Payne wrote to Huntington Wilson hinting that the Foster bill might not be acted upon in this last session of the 61st Congress because of the time pressure. He chided the delay caused by trying to decide who would be honored by introducing the bill—Mr. Mann or Mr. Foster.[93]

Wright remained optimistic, but the drug trades had won. The *American Druggist and Pharmaceutical Record* of February 1911 headlined the decision simply "Foster Bill Killed." In his enthusiasm and political naïveté, Wright had not taken into consideration the great threat his bill posed to everyday routine and sales in the drug trades. The Foster bill's uncompromising provisions were impressive; not a milligram of a habit-forming drug would have been lost in the legitimate trade had this bill been passed and enforced. But such an altruistic bill could not be accepted by manufacturers and local druggists. Smoking opium could be denied to the Chinese, but babies were not to be protected from narcotized "Mrs. Winslow's Soothing Syrup" or "Hooper's Anodyne, the Infant's Friend."

THE HAGUE CONFERENCE

Congress had failed Wright, and now prospects for the great international conference were filled with uncertainty. Delay after delay marked planning for its opening session. Wright and some of the State Department staff began to suspect a conspiracy against the American crusade. He was tempted to push a little harder, but from the American Embassy in Paris came the warning that the other nations were tired of American insistence. Now as Ambassador to France, Robert Bacon reminded the anxious planners that "everyone else has so much more at stake than we, they cannot be driven too hard." [94]

The doctor turned to publicity for support of the American proposals. He told his brother-in-law Frank Baldwin of the *Outlook* that he was willing to write an article on the economic aspects of the opium question, but the *Outlook* editors preferred something more "picturesque" on opium; for example, "selling girl babies into slavery." [95] Wright rejected that idea. Dr. Lambert's aid was enlisted to get Theodore Roosevelt, the *Outlook*'s contributing editor, to write an article on opium.[96] Nothing ever came of this, although Wright tried constantly to get at least a stirring editorial paragraph out of Roosevelt.

Even more disheartening delays by Germany, Great Britain, and the Netherlands suggested that these essential nations did not want an early conference if any at all. In August 1911, Wright sought out the Dutch minister to the United States, then vacationing in Maine, and threatened (with Knox's approval) that if the Netherlands continued to procrastinate, the United States might convene the conference in Washington. This forceful action seemed to increase the rate of note-exchanging among the powers. In early September Wright was back in Maine telling the vacationing British ambassador James Bryce that the United States had received a great deal of information indicating a conspiracy to delay the conference. Bryce agreed to urge London to inform the Netherlands that Great Britain was now ready to attend the conference. Wright's pressure tactics proved to be unnecessary in this instance because one day prior to his meeting with Bryce Great Britain had informed the Netherlands of its readiness. The German Empire was spared one of Wright's persuasive visits, for on the day he was to embark for

Berlin, Germany agreed to attend. Perhaps these experiences encouraged Dr. Wright's style of blunt diplomacy.[97]

On the first day of December 1911 the International Conference on Opium convened at The Hague. America sent two of its former Shanghai delegates, Bishop Brent and Dr. Wright, and added Henry J. Finger, a prominent California pharmacist who had been recommended by Knox's physician brother. Wright was mortified by this choice. He had hoped for an expert on international law if he could not have Professor Jeremiah Jenks (whose economic plans Wright so admired).

Bishop Brent, through his acquaintance with the Archbishop of Canterbury and other leaders of the antiopium movement, had smoothed British acceptance of the American-inspired conference. At one time he was so persuaded by his British friends, who thought that Wright antagonized other nations with his emphasis on American righteousness and implications of foreign duplicity, that he advised Wright to quit the antinarcotic campaign for the sake of the international movement. Wright refused.[98]

Chosen to chair the conference, Bishop Brent again symbolized the American moral stewardship that brought twelve nations to The Hague to consider ways to regulate international narcotic traffic. Turkey still declined to attend, and Austria–Hungary, although present in Shanghai, chose not to return. Those assembled at The Hague had individual concerns that influenced their actions. England, proud that a new agreement with China made provision for rapid termination of the odious opium traffic with India, now pressed the conference for action against cocaine and morphine.[99] Germany sought to protect its giant chemical industry from an agreement to limit production if that agreement was less than unanimous among the manufacturing nations—there was no reason to curtail a profitable business if another nation, perhaps Switzerland, were to take up the slack.

Portugal defended the opium industry in Macao, and Persia its own thriving poppy cultivation. The conference host, the Netherlands, was involved in the narcotic traffic in the Dutch East Indies. France was ambivalent; she received revenue from opium smoking in French Indochina but feared the reported increased use of potent opium derivatives in her colonial possessions. Japan assumed a position of ignorance with regard to charges of her illegal introduction of morphine and hypodermic syringes into China. Russia had a poppy-farming industry, but not of great size. Siam, on the other hand, processed a considerable amount of opium, and the problem and profits of opium were familiar.

Curiously, Italy insisted that the conference include the subject of Indian hemp as the price for her participation, but her delegation came only to the first day's session.[100] Since nations other than the United States did not want to include hemp as a menacing drug, it was not thoroughly discussed. The most the American delegation was able to secure was an addendum to the Opium Convention, the "Protocol of Cloture," which read in regard to Indian hemp:

> The Conference is of the unanimous opinion that it is advisable to study the question of Indian hemp from the statistical and scientific point of view, with a view to regulating its abuses, if the necessity of such a course makes itself felt, by internal legislation or by an international agreement.[101]

The United States delegation was disappointed that the Convention could not be put into effect upon ratification by the dozen contracting nations. The Americans were counseled to wait for adherence from the world's forty-six powers, particularly those deeply involved in the opium and cocaine traffic, such as the absent Turkey, Switzerland, Bolivia, and Peru. The Germans protested that it was an unusual practice to frame a world convention with only twelve powers represented, that some procedure must be made for the signatures of other states: until those states took unanimous action there was no point in any one nation's acting against its own industrial or agricultural interests.

Germany then attacked the American delegation in a rather weak spot. What assurances could be given that, having signed and ratified the Convention, the United States would enact implementing legislation? Wright loftily replied that the good faith of the United States was a sufficient guarantee that Congress would pass the necessary legislation to enforce the Convention if Germany would sign and ratify it; but he knew by then that meaningful federal control would be very difficult to obtain.[102] Yet here was one more instance in which enactment of exemplary domestic laws became necessary in order to avoid international embarrassment. Other nations already had more stringent domestic legislation than the United States. Even the notorious opium traffic in French Indochina was theoretically controlled by an elaborate set of rules and regulations. In Shanghai the United States delegation had accepted an obligation to enact federal narcotic control. The pressure to live up to this standard of morality would be felt most heavily by the State Department and the President.

Chapter 3 of The Hague Opium Convention had a bearing on the movement for American narcotic legislation. It called for control of all phases of the preparation and distribution of medicinal opium, morphine, heroin, cocaine, and any new derivative that could be scientifically shown to offer similar dangers. Exempted from proposed control were preparations containing less than 0.2 percent morphine and less than 0.1 percent heroin or cocaine. The contracting powers agreed to "endeavor" to control their own traffic in the above substances. The Convention placed the major burden of narcotic control on domestic legislation, and the apparent failure of this approach led in ten years to the Geneva Opium Conference, which shifted the locus of control to international restraints.[103]

China had a difficult role at The Hague. She wanted to protect her territorial integrity against other powers who argued that if China allowed importation of British opium she could not exclude that of other nations. They failed in this attempt to keep their opium traffic with China. Several articles of the final Convention embodied measures to aid China in her program against opium, such as closing opium divans in Chinese areas under extraterritorial control.

A mechanism was conceived for the signature and ratification of the Convention. It was agreed that all powers, not just those at the conference, must sign and ratify it before it could come into effect. The Netherlands would notify signatories of progress. If the signatures of all powers were not obtained by the last day of 1912, a second conference would be called for July 1913, and the Convention was signed by the participating powers on 23 January 1912, and the first Hague Opium Conference ended. Efforts now were made to obtain signatures of the unrepresented nations. The United States had little difficulty in persuading the Latin American republics to sign the Convention. Even Peru with its considerable interest in coca production eventually adhered.

The Second Opium Conference met on 31 July 1913 to consider the report that thirty-four nations had signed, leaving twelve, including Turkey and Switzerland, still to be persuaded. The meeting lasted only eight days. At its close each nation that wished to deposit its ratification of the Convention before all nations had signed was permitted to do so. If at the end of 1913 the Convention remained incompletely signed, a third conference would be held at The Hague in 1914 to consider putting it into effect among those who had signed.

Since Bishop Brent did not choose to participate in the Second Conference in 1913, Hamilton Wright was chosen to head the American delegation. While the conference met, the second Balkan War, involving Bulgaria, Serbia, Greece, Romania, and Turkey, was being fought. All of these nations, incidentally, were among the twelve which still had not signed the Convention. The United States' Senate ratification was formally deposited at The Hague on 10 December 1913, but when the year closed the Convention remained less than unanimously subscribed.

The United States requested and obtained postponement of the Third Conference, proposed for May 1914, in an attempt to get its own domestic legislation enacted before this perhaps final meeting. Yet, when the conference convened on 15 June, the United States still lacked domestic legislation, for the Harrison bill, having passed the House in the summer of 1913, was deadlocked in the Senate. Hamilton Wright was not selected even to attend the Third Conference for reasons that will become apparent in the next chapter.

Endeavoring to salvage something tangible in spite of Germany's unwillingness to ratify unless other powers, especially Turkey, did so, the final Protocol of Cloture provided that the Convention might go into effect on 31 December 1914 among those signatory powers which had deposited ratifications. The conference closed on 25 June 1914, three days before the assassination of Archduke Ferdinand. Forty-four governments had signed the Convention: only Serbia and Turkey refused to do so. Less than half the signatories, however, had ratified it, and in the next five years only seven nations would put it into effect.[104]

3 The Harrison Act

In January 1912 Wright returned to the United States with two goals: increasing the number of signatories to the Convention and dispelling any doubt that this nation would pass the necessary domestic legislation. Southern resistance to any invasion of states' rights made Democratic control of the House especially significant for the narcotic reformers. Representative Francis Burton Harrison, a well-born Tammany Democrat, agreed to shepherd the antinarcotic legislation through the House. Harrison's task was to assure his colleagues that the various trade interests and concerned parties had achieved a generally acceptable narcotic bill or at least one that would engender no unyielding hostility. He did not display as much interest in the specific form or philosophy of the legislation as in its political viability.

Strongly backed by such adamant reformers as Drs. Harvey Wiley, Alexander Lambert, and William Schieffelin, Dr. Wright believed that the legislative goal should be elimination of narcotics except for medical purposes. As a result, the first Harrison bill in the 62nd Congress did not differ greatly from the ill-fated Foster bill of 1910.[1] It contained no provision for exempting small amounts of narcotics in patent medicines. Revenue stamps, record keeping and various details such as bonds, license fees, and severe penalties were retained, although still strongly opposed by the retail druggists. Wright could not easily bring himself to compromise. Weakening the bill would have made him susceptible to the same criticisms he heaped on the foreign governments that did not rigorously and heroically stamp out the evil of narcotics.

THE NATIONAL DRUG TRADE CONFERENCE

Believing that the movement to control narcotics was gaining strength and that some legislation was likely to be enacted, the American Pharmaceutical Association sought to give the various components of the drug trades a united voice, or at least a forum, in which the interests of each would receive the maximum possible support of the others. Meeting in Denver during October 1912, the association called for a convocation. As a result, the National Drug Trade Conference (NDTC) was created and met in Washington, D.C., on 15 January 1913, with its chief business the proposed antinarcotic bill. Each major trade association was permitted three representatives, and no resolution could be passed unless it was unanimous.[2] This set of rules worked relatively well for the problem at hand because pressure from outside forces was considerable. During the three-day meeting, constituent members were able to compromise on a common position. In later years, however, and on other subjects, the NDTC reached unanimity less often.

All groups opposed the Harrison bill as it then stood. The American Association of Pharmaceutical Chemists and the National Association of Medicinal Products (NAMP), both makers of prescription drugs, were against the legislation on grounds of its "too complex procedure." The National Association of Retail Druggists (NARD) found inconsistencies, especially in the keeping of records. The National Wholesale Druggists' Association would abide by the law if enacted but also found it inconsistent in various respects. The principle of the law was endorsed by the APhA although the details appeared to be a burden on the retail drug trade, especially the record-keeping provisions. In a familiar jousting for superiority, Wright invited the NDTC to meet with him at the State Department, but the NDTC, as its first unanimous resolution responded by inviting Wright to meet with them at the Hotel Willard.

He accepted, and Wright and Representative Harrison heard the druggists' criticism. The NDTC members found that evening session an irritating encounter with the federal bureaucracy for they had worked at great length to prepare a detailed and unanimously approved criticism of the bill. For Representative Harrison, who had to meet his wife at the theater, "or she would fear I had taken an overdose of narcotics," it was a rushed evening. Wright got so angry with the proposed changes to his bill that he walked out of the meeting declaring that any further discussion would take place at the State Department. This hectic encounter strengthened the NDTC's resolve to approve no bill until its views were taken into consideration. Wright's angry action had helped unify opposition to the Harrison bill.[3]

A few days after the confrontation, Harrison decided that Wright would have to work out a bill suitable to the NDTC; he would then see to its passage through the House. Several revisions suggested by the NDTC were accepted into the bill.[4]

The NDTC established an Executive Committee based primarily in Washington and able to meet quickly to discuss the sometimes rapidly changing status of legislation.[5] The American Medical Association, which also had been consulted about the Foster bill, was always represented in the NDTC conferences, either by Martin I. Wilbert, a pharmacist in the Public Health Service and a member of the AMA's Council on Pharmacy and Chemistry, or by a leading legislative adviser to the AMA, the able lawyer-physician Dr. William C. Woodward, Health Director of Washington, D.C. Both men had had prominent roles in health legislation.

Dr. Woodward participated in legislative conflict from about 1910 to 1940. He fought in the initial Harrison bill battles, against federal health insurance and for uniform state narcotic laws. One of his last appearances before Congress in regard to drug abuse was to oppose on behalf of the AMA the Marijuana Tax Act of 1937. Although in 1913 he was concerned with framing and passing a satisfactory federal narcotic law, later enforcement activities caused him to fight the Harrison Act during the 1920s.

Both Wilbert and Woodward favored restrictive legislation and were opposed to narcotic-containing proprietary and patent drugs, but both also favored legislation with a maximum chance of actual passage. Through one or the other representative the AMA was constantly apprised of the actions of the NDTC and was able to cooperate in influencing Congress.

THE AMA AND NARCOTIC LEGISLATION

The AMA's role in narcotic legislation reflected its stage of institutional development. By 1913 the American Medical Association, from a relatively small group centered mostly in the eastern states, was well on its way to consolidation of American medical practitioners. Like the American Pharmaceutical Association, it represented a group desire to strengthen the education and raise the status of physicians. Although founded in 1847, it did not begin its period of rapid growth and powerful influence until this century. Membership increased from 8,500 in 1900 to 36,000 in 1913, and to more than 44,000 by 1920. The AMA realized the need to enter into political activity in order to achieve its professional goals. It maintained surveillance on laws affecting its interest at each political level. The battle for the Pure Food and Drug Act in the first decade of the century whetted the AMA's legislative weapons, and from then on it knew when, how, and whom to contact in the state, local, or federal echelon involved. The Council on Health and Public Instruction, created in 1910, contained within it the Bureau of Legislation, headed by Dr. Woodward. This bureau was permitted to use its discretion in legislative matters not specifically covered by resolutions passed at general business sessions. Further impetus to the collection of laws and decisions, formulation of model laws, and improvement of communication with the public occurred at the beginning of 1913 with the establishment of the Medicolegal Bureau, also within the council.[6]

Prior to World War I, the AMA was guided by a rather small coterie of physicians who were strongly influenced by the reform enthusiasm of the Progressive Era. The AMA supported uniform licensing procedures, a federal department of health, the Pure Food and Drug Act, and federal support of worthy medical schools. In 1916 Wright's comrade, Dr. Lambert, as the head of the AMA Judicial Council, submitted a favorable report of the European experience with social insurance.[7] Lambert, as well as the English-born Dr. George H. Simmons,[8] editor of the *Journal of the American Medical Association* (*JAMA*), admired the British health insurance scheme for the poor that resulted in better health care for millions of the needy as well as in higher incomes for physicians. During this stage of its development, the AMA welcomed the federal government as a valued collaborator in achieving its professional goals.

By 1918, with a vastly enlarged membership drawn from the nation's general practitioners, a different attitude arose within the AMA—a fear of federal control leading, perhaps, to "state medicine," rejection of state-supported health insurance schemes, opposition to widespread building of Veterans Administration hospitals and federal funding of state maternal and child care programs, and antagonism to almost any other government-sponsored action in the health field that would limit the prerogatives of the independent practitioner.[9] After Prohibition, the AMA opposed the Willis–Campbell Act's limit on each physician of one hundred prescriptions in every ninety days for medicinal wine or whiskey as another example of governmental interference in what was clearly a health issue.[10]

The Harrison antinarcotic legislation, enacted in December 1914, came during the AMA's transition from favoring federal assistance to an antipathy toward Washington's entry into the health field. By the 1920s the AMA felt medical standards could be most effectively maintained by the profession itself, without federal help. Therefore it is not surprising that the Harrison Act received strong opposition from the AMA in the early 1920s, when fear of federal domination affected all political issues involving the medical profession. If the government could establish control over one part of the practice of medicine, even if the goal was admirable, what could the government not do? [11]

Before the watershed of World War I and during the controversy over the Pure Food and Drug Act, Dr. Simmons had taken a very strong stand with regard to habit-forming drugs. In an editorial,[12] the *JAMA* declared unalterable opposition to any provision in the Act that would permit manufacture of medicines containing small amounts of opium, morphine, heroin, chloral hydrate, and other narcotics. Such an exemption was "as vicious as [it was] . . . stupid." The insidious small dose carried the great danger of gradual increase leading to addiction. In words similar to those of Bishop Brent a few years earlier concerning the Philippine opium monopoly, Simmons said there should be no compromise with crime. Opponents of the doctor's stand suggested the profession wanted a monopoly on all narcotic sales to the public and wanted a fee for every citizen's head cold.

THE PHARMACISTS AND NARCOTIC LEGISLATION

Although sensing the value of cooperation, one point at which the doctors and pharmacists diverged was on the extent to which each profession should dispense narcotics. The druggists insisted that a physician prescribe only after examination and diagnosis. Without such a provision, they feared physicians could set up narcotic dispensaries in their offices and "prescribe" for all who came in. Pharmacists conceded that the physician could dispense to his patients, but to them only.[13] Establishing this distinction was not specifically linked to narcotics but had been a long-standing goal of druggists. The dispensing physician, a rarity now, was then the target of pharmacists' ire. But as competition among physicians decreased and they became more prosperous, their need for a sideline declined and with it, dispensing.

Similarly, friction was caused by any suggestion that physicians need keep fewer records than pharmacists, as provided by some of the early narcotic bills.[14] Druggists felt that such a requirement reflected on the pharmacist's honesty and was a consequence of the growing prestige and influence of the medical profession. Also, druggists suspected that physicians, by not having to keep records of all transactions, would continue to sell huge amounts of drugs.[15] Eventually a compromise permitted the physician to abstain from record keeping when out of his office, say at the bedside of an ill patient; or, as the law finally read, when "in personal attendance" on his patient. Neither the retail druggist nor the practicing physician welcomed the record-keeping duties that were anticipated from the antinarcotic legislation, but any requirement that would rest more heavily or more effectively on the druggist than on the physician was opposed by the NDTC.

PASSAGE OF THE HARRISON ACT

The presidency of Woodrow Wilson began in March 1913, with Democrats now in control of both Houses. Initially Wright was delighted with this change. Wilson and Secretary of State William Jennings Bryan supported strict regulation of narcotics and seemed to have nothing but admiration for America's initiative in international control. Wright gave a glowing report of his first meetings with Bryan. According to Wright, his account of the fight for worldwide narcotic control was repeatedly punctuated by Bryan's amazed exclamation: "How did you manage it?" [16]

A joint committee set up by the State and Treasury Departments attempted to write a bill acceptable to the drug trades, the medical profession, and the Internal Revenue Bureau, which would have enforcement responsibility. Wright felt he was close to the end of a three-year fight with trade interests. At last, on 10 June 1913, the chairman of the NDTC signed a draft of the bill, which was then introduced into the first session of the 63rd Congress by Harrison as HR 6282, destined for eventual passage as the Harrison Act.[17]

The descendant of the stricter Foster bill, the Harrison bill of 1913 had incorporated numerous compromises. Records were simplified; standard order blanks would be filled in by any purchaser of narcotics and kept for two years so that the revenue agents could inspect them at will. Copies of the orders were to be kept by district internal revenue offices on permanent file. Physicians could dispense drugs without keeping records if in actual attendance on their patients. Numerous patent medicines containing no more than the permitted amounts of morphine, cocaine, opium, and heroin could continue to be sold by mail order and in general stores. Everyone

dealing in narcotics except the consumer would have to be registered. Retail dealers or practicing physicians could obtain a tax
stamp for one dollar a year. No bond was required, the drugs were
not taxed by weight, and chloral hydrate and cannabis were omitted
in the final version.

The Harrison subcommittee of the House Ways and Means Committee assured the full committee that the bill now had approval
of both the medical and trade interests. On 26 June 1913, only six-
teen days after the NDTC had accepted the draft, the House passed
HR 6282 with only minor changes in the phraseology.[18] When the
bill went to the Senate, however, progress slowed, for efforts to give
special interests an advantage started over again. Not until 18
February 1914 did the bill come out of the Senate Finance Committee. One change by this committee particularly aroused the
anger of the American Pharmaceutical Association: physicians were
to be permitted to provide narcotics when they "shall have been
specifically employed to prescribe for the patient receiving such
drug or article." [19] This change permitted anyone to apply by mail
for a drug from a physician. The amendment was inserted, the
Journal of the APhA believed, to accommodate a physician-owned
business that sold asthma cures by mail after having the patient
fill out a form describing his illness and asking for treatment.[20]
Other amendments of an unpalatable nature to one group or
another were now being offered. One proposed amendment to
the committee version simply exempted physicians and their aides
from the provisions of the Act.[21] The response to this change can
be well imagined. Dr. Woodward thought it possible that these
amendments were intended not to revise but to defeat the bill
arduously worked out the previous summer.

On 15 August 1914 the Senate passed HR 6282 but with amendments unsatisfactory to the House Conference Committee. Professional and trade organizations put pressure on the House and Senate
Conference Committee to achieve a workable compromise. These
efforts in the autumn of 1914 by the NDTC, the medical profession,
Wright, and the administration were successful; in October agreement was reached.[22]

The Senate had increased the heroin exempted in one ounce of
proprietary medicine from 1/12 grain, which the NDTC and the
House had approved, to ¼ grain, but this was reduced to ⅛ grain in
the compromise. The reduction was opposed by some makers of

proprietary medicines, but their opposition was not fatal. A few minor changes were made, such as lessening the effect of the bill's impact on our insular possessions, which already had stringent laws and were not part of the internal revenue system of the United States. Final action was delayed until the December 1914 session of the 63rd Congress, when the Conference Report was accepted without opposition.

On 14 December the bill passed and was signed by the President on the 17th. Finally the American government had redeemed its international pledges; a federal law brought some control to the traffic in opiates and cocaine. The practical significance of the Harrison Act, however, was still debated among the groups affected. There was no general agreement on what would be the desirable or actual enforcement of the law.

Wright had been gravely concerned by the impasse that had threatened the Harrison bill, but he had been removed from his prominent position in the State Department for the second time in June 1914. During the Democratic administration, antagonism to Wright had been a significant cause—at least in Secretary Bryan's view—of repeated refusals by the Appropriations Committee of the department's request for funds to participate in the Second Hague Conference.[23] After House passage of HR 6282, Wright had asked for a ministerial appointment, anywhere, on the basis of his good work on the opium matter. He was refused, allegedly because both the Secretary and the President had more Democratic applicants than they could satisfy.[24] Wright's influence had declined since 1911, and he found himself increasingly isolated from congressional and trade leaders.

In early 1914 some Democratic members of the House Appropriations Committee criticized Wright's proposed appointment to the Third Hague Conference. Secretary Bryan, increasingly uncertain about Wright's value and having occasionally detected liquor on Wright's breath, called him and demanded that he take the pledge of abstinence, at least for the duration of the Hague Conference. Humiliated, Wright refused and was thereupon dismissed from the State Department and from the Hague delegation.[25]

In the autumn of 1914, while the nation followed reports from a disintegrating Europe, Wright was totally absorbed in his private political career. Desperately he had sought support from medical authorities and the drug trade to influence the Conference Com-

mittee to reconsider the House and Senate versions of the Harrison
bill, to include nothing unsatisfactory to any of the interested parties.
He also wrote and telegraphed the President. After the antinarcotic
bill passed, he began searching for "some large task" to take up. His
correspondence is a pathetic series of rejections from prominent
individuals and institutions.[26] Although having denied that he was
an office-seeker or wanted any personal connection with the new
legislation, Wright asked the Treasury Department in January 1915
whether he might be needed for three months or so to get the whole
apparatus set up and coordinated, or perhaps to write the regulations enforcing the Act. The Treasury, however, did not need
him.[27] He maintained an interest in the Harrison Act, but after
1914 his antinarcotic activities diminished. He still cultivated Theodore Roosevelt as well as regular Republican politicians, but nothing came of his efforts. Casting about for activity, he went to
France in 1915 to help the Allied cause. While there he was injured
in an automobile accident from which he never fully recovered.
Wright died in Washington, D.C., in January 1917 at the age of 49.

Wright had recognized defects in the law. He especially regretted Section 6, which permitted exempt narcotic preparations,
but he agreed with Representative Harrison that without such a
provision the proprietary interests would have scuttled the bill.[28]
He also regretted that the provisions for record keeping were less
strict than originally proposed, but here he accepted the opinion of
Representative Mann, who believed more strenuous requirements
would result in the retail druggists' blocking the law.

Wright believed he had a powerful remedy for these defects. Since
the statute was the outcome of an international agreement, he assumed it could employ police powers within a state in addition to
the traditional powers associated with a federal revenue measure.
This would give great importance to the words "prescribed in good
faith," enabling the federal government to argue, as it did, that
this phrase prevented addiction maintenance. Without some legal
sanction for federal police powers in the states, the Act would be
limited to record keeping. Wright based his optimistic expectation
on the principle that a treaty to which the United States had become
a signatory and which had been ratified by the Senate, would take
precedence over state law. On this reasoning, if the Act did employ
police powers within a state, such extension of federal activity would
not be unconstitutional because the Act carried out a treaty, the

Hague Convention. This issue was later considered by the Supreme Court in the case of *Jin Fuey Moy* (1916). Wright's view was not sustained, the court majority holding with Justice Holmes that the specific form of the Harrison Act was not required by the Hague Convention. Charles Evans Hughes and Mahlon Pitney dissented, prompting Wright to express his appreciation and to assert that he had had Hughes' own teachings on the subject in mind when the law was drafted.[29]

The Federal Position

A position similar to Wright's on the extension of federal police powers was uneasily anticipated by Frank Freericks, although not on grounds of treaty-making powers of the federal government. The prominent lawyer–pharmacist maintained in the *Journal* of the APhA that the Harrison Act did involve police powers and would attempt to regulate the selling and mode of selling of narcotics to consumers. Freericks strongly disagreed with those who maintained that the Act was merely an information-gathering device that relegated the policing of drug traffic to the states. Those who had proposed it, he maintained, understood that the states were not successfully curbing the abuse of drugs and that the Act's purpose was to accomplish by federal powers what the states were unwilling or unable to do.[30]

Strong objection to Freerick's view was expressed by the *Journal*'s editor James H. Beal, one of the key NDTC negotiators with the federal government.[31] Also a lawyer and pharmacist, he disputed Freericks on the crucial question of police powers in the Harrison Act. In Beal's opinion there were no police powers whatsoever. If police powers were implied in the Act, or if anyone tried to develop such powers under its authority, the Act would be quickly declared unconstitutional. Beal had only loathing for any "physician [who] has so far lost his sense of professional responsibility as to be willing to sell habit-forming drugs to habitués." But the sole purpose of the Act was to gather information, which could then be conveyed to the state and local authorities. The states would continue to regulate the relationship between professionals and their clients. If the states failed in this task, then the Harrison law would be a failure: it could in no way remedy the states' inability to enforce, or refusal to enact, drug-abuse laws. Freericks had argued that should the Act lack police powers to regulate the physician's prescription of narcotics to his patients, then the law would merely transfer widespread selling of narcotics into a profitable monopoly for unscrupulous physicians. Beal answered that the phrase "in the pursuit of his professional practice only" would enable conviction of any unscrupulous physicians who simply sold drugs and prescriptions to satisfy the cravings of addicts.[32]

The Public Health Service shared Beal's view of HR 6282. In a revealing letter to a woman who had taken morphine for many years and now complained that her supply would be cut off because of the Harrison Act, the Surgeon General replied in March 1915 that the Act was intended simply to gather information, and she could continue to receive morphine from her physician.[33]

The Bureau of Internal Revenue, on the other hand, took a somewhat more stringent view. It prepared to bring actions against druggists and physicians as well as addicts who were violating the bureau's understanding of the Harrison Act's moral principle—that taking narcotics for other than medicinal purposes was harmful and should be prevented.[34]

The American Medical Association, in the person of Dr. Simmons, opposed the selling of narcotics to users without medical reasons. Whether or not the majority of physicians agreed that the habit was harmful is uncertain. But economics was only one factor complicating the physician's relationship to narcotics. The number of physician-addicts was high. Medicine was (and is) the leading profession in rate of addiction, about 2 percent according to Wright's survey. The profession was commonly believed to be one of the causes of most of the other addicts in the nation, and evidence, nowhere contradicted before Congress, revealed that physicians were the principal offenders.[35] Perhaps the attitude of the public was not unreasonable, for a small percentage of physicians could maintain a considerable number of addicts if no restrictions were placed on their prescription powers. In contrast to such high-minded spokesmen for the AMA as Drs. Lambert and Simmons, a minority of physicians made substantial profits by prescribing narcotics to addicts and intended to continue this practice until forced to stop. Others devoted only a small portion of their practice to addicts. Although some physicians continued to feel no discomfort in maintaining habitués, medical experts as well as laymen commonly believed that addiction promoted criminal appetites and inclination, ruined the reproductive organs, and caused insanity.

Some of the public believed the Harrison Act prohibited simple maintenance, and, in fact, the Internal Revenue agents would begin enforcement on the premise that maintenance violated "good faith" in the practice of medicine. Detailed records would now be available to indicate the number of prescriptions and the amount of narcotics sold by doctors. If the "nonmedical" consumption of narcotics did not decrease substantially, the licensed professional was an obvious and relatively easy target for legal action.

DRUGS, ALCOHOL, AND THE PUBLIC

Passage of the Harrison Act came after consultation with the trade and professional interests concerned, from the obligation of America to other nations, and with the support of reform groups, but it was not a question of primary national interest. Although drugs later became a great popular issue, the passage of the Harrison Act in 1914 seemed a routine slap at a moral evil, something like the Mann Act or the Anti-Lottery Acts. It went largely unnoticed because the question of controlling narcotics had none of the controversy associated with the prohibition of liquor. Perhaps half the nation saw nothing evil in moderate drinking. Most Americans described themselves as in favor of temperance, which could be interpreted as being opposed to public drunkenness. But almost no one ever used the term temperance in discussing the use of opiates or cocaine after 1900; by the teens of this century both classes of drugs were deemed in public debate to have no value except as medicine. The closest a public spokesman would come to defending such drugs would be to say that they were not especially harmful as compared say, with alcohol, and with a vigorous effort in progress to outlaw alcohol, the description did not protect narcotics from criticism.[36] By 1914 prominent newspapers, physicians, pharmacists, and congressmen believed opiates and cocaine predisposed habitués toward insanity and crime. They were widely seen as substances associated with foreigners or alien subgroups. Cocaine raised the specter of the wild Negro, opium the devious Chinese, morphine the tramps in the slums; it was feared that use of all these drugs was spreading into the "higher classes."[37]

The only question publicly debated with reference to narcotics was *how* to control, not (as in the case of liquor) *whether* to control. Addiction and liquor prohibition were linked only in an indirect way in congressional consideration of the Harrison and related acts. First some congressmen were concerned that the prohibition of interstate commerce in drugs might be extended by teetotaling zealots to liquor, which had a brisk and legal interstate traffic flowing from wet to dry states. This question was settled in early 1913 with the passage of the Webb-Kenyon Act, forbidding shipments of liquor to states that prohibited its sale. The fact that Congress passed this Act over President Taft's veto indicates the prohibitionists' growing strength in both houses.[38]

Some congressmen feared that strict prohibition would only drive liquor and drug traffic underground. This reasonable concern was apparently overcome by the conviction that compromise should not be made with unquestioned evils. Liquor prohibitionists argued effectively that some illicit traffic would be better than national over-indulgence in alcohol. The image of the ubiquitous saloon was a powerful propaganda weapon, for the saloon tempted not only the native American but especially the immigrant, whose moral qualities were under continuous attack by such groups as the Anti-Immigration League. Prohibitionists believed that their reform could be made to work, perhaps not perfectly but well enough to rid the nation of such glaring evils as the saloon. The movement was supported by the characteristic Progressive assumption that government could change or neutralize the habits of large groups by well-written legislation and honest enforcement.

Public and congressional distinction between narcotic control and liquor prohibition was clearly shown during the middle weeks of December 1914. Part of a rush of legislation, the Harrison Act was approved in a few minutes, a fact not even noted that week in the New York *Times* summary of that session's work.[39] On the other hand the House set aside the entire day of 22 December for debate on a resolution introduced by Alabama Congressman Richmond Hobson to submit to the states a constitutional amendment mandating prohibition of alcohol. Parades and speeches marked the entry of thousands of supporters into the Capitol. The visitors' sections of the House were packed with prohibitionists, and from the gallery was draped a petition with six million signatures calling upon Congress to submit the amendment to the states: the petition was the largest ever sent to Congress. At the Speaker's dais charts depicted the progress of Prohibition across the nation, and between the side columns, until removed for violating House rules, large cartoons attacked liquor.[40] Hobson, a hero of the Spanish-American War and in the 1920s and 1930s leader of a national lay movement against narcotics, delivered the day's longest and most impassioned appeal for Prohibition. Hobson's speech was modeled on his platform address "The Great Destroyer," which he was to deliver many more times in the future as the Anti-Saloon League's highest-paid publicist.[41]

Supporting the Prohibition resolution, Representative Charles A. Lindbergh, Sr., of Minnesota spoke for the opportunity to "record our votes in favor of our race—to save the boys and girls who will become the future citizens and rulers of our country." [42]

The attack against Hobson's resolution was led by Speaker of the House Oscar W. Underwood, also of Alabama.[43] Underwood, who had shepherded the Harrison Act through the House the previous week, described the Prohibition Amendment as a "tyrannous scheme to establish virtue and morality by law." [44] Congressman Mann, who had joined Harrison in arguing for the antinarcotic act the previous year, proposed that the Prohibition Amendment be submitted to conventions in the several states, an obstacle quickly rejected by the dry forces.

When the vote was taken the drys outnumbered the wets by 197 to 190, although they fell short of the two-thirds majority needed for adoption of the resolution. But it was a strong warning of what was to come; three years later almost to the day, the House passed a Prohibition resolution (282 to 128) differing little from the one submitted by Hobson. It outlawed the manufacture, sale, and transportation of liquor within, into, and out of the United States. The amendment was to become effective one year after three-quarters of the states had ratified. The Senate passed the proposed amendment on 18 December 1917, by 47 to 8, and within thirteen months it was part of the Constitution.

The funds spent annually by the liquor lobbyists, the Anti-Saloon League, the Women's Christian Temperance Union, and other organizations went into the millions of dollars. National Prohibition, even though twenty-seven of the forty-eight states were prohibitionist already, was bitterly debated. If the vote on the resolution to submit the amendment to the states had been secret it is unlikely it would have been passed. Since the vote was by roll call, the well-organized strategists for Prohibition were able to use political threats effectively. Many congressmen feared for their political careers should they vote nay. The United States had been at war since April 1917, and the hysteria that gripped the nation in its crusade against the Kaiser extended to a firm belief that liquor sapped the nation's strength and will power, and even depleted the cereal grains that could be used in bread for the troops and starving Europeans. Prohibition was not, however, merely the result of wartime excitement and fears: it had been steadily gaining ground since before 1900, beginning in the South and West and extending eventually over most of the country.[45] Prohibitionists, who favored the "pledge" against all liquor and would profess such a standard in their own lives, favored narcotic prohibition; the combatants in the fight against narcotics, however, were often divided on the liquor question. Bishop Brent had early distinguished between narcotic and liquor prohibition. He believed that liquor had a "beverage value" and therefore was in the class of nutrients; but narcotics, unless taken for medical reasons, had no value whatsoever. Wright's views on liquor seemed to go at least as far as Brent's; Representative Harrison was never accused of abstemiousness.[46]

During the four years between Hobson's resolution and ratification of the Prohibition Amendment, the control of addiction moved toward a more prohibitory style of enforcement. The required tightening of restraints on narcotics came from an amendment and Supreme Court rulings in early 1919, a few months after the national victory of the temperance forces. Occasionally breaking into newsprint, the evolution of the Harrison Act's enforcement policies, after initial setbacks, ended in the triumph of those who believed the law had a moral effect and was designed to prohibit the use of narcotics for the maintenance of "mere" addiction.

The Search for Cures

Opium use was extensive before the modern era.[1] By the Middle Ages opium was used in standard antidotes such as theriac, mithradatium, and philonium, which combined an elaborate array of substances with large amounts of opium. In the mid-sixteenth century opium was particularly associated with the Swiss firebrand Paracelsus, and it is likely that his followers began to use the word laudanum for the alcoholic tincture of opium. The laudanum that bemused DeQuincey and Coleridge, however, was the recipe of one of the greatest seventeenth-century English physicians, Thomas Sydenham: the opium was dissolved in sherry flavored with cinnamon, cloves, and saffron—an early cocktail. Sydenham considered opium "one of the most valued medicines in the world [which] does more honor to medicine than any remedy whatsoever." [2] The use of such concoctions as laudanum led to medical warnings of the hazards of opium. John Jones in his tract *The Mysteries of Opium Revealed* (1700) warned that the "effects of sudden leaving off the uses of opium after a long and lavish use thereof [were] great and even intolerable distresses, anxieties and depressions of spirit, which commonly end in a most miserable death, attended with strange agonies, unless men return to the use of opium; which soon raises them again, and certainly restores them." [3] This rather good description of the withdrawal syndrome included an early statement of a durable belief among physicians that death could easily result from a termination of habitual opium intake.

Jones's warning was only one reason that other eighteenth-century writers cautioned against frequent use of opium. Some physicians considered that opium addiction was dangerous not as a disease but that opium's pain-relieving powers might simply mask a disease that required other treatment for cure. To the question of who is susceptible to opium habituation, one also finds a comment by Samuel Crumpe (1793) suggesting that only in certain persons could opium take hold, depending on their constitution.[4] Jones and Crumpe state both sides of a dialogue on opium addiction that is still debated after two centuries: Can anyone become addicted or are only certain persons, psychopaths or biochemical misfits, likely to succumb? A modification of Crumpe's theme was the assertion that Orientals were much more resistant or susceptible to opium than Occidentals.[5] In

Victorian England the view was expressed in medical periodicals that the lower classes had a worse reaction to the use of opium than middle or upper classes, leading in the former to degeneracy and in the latter to no noticeable behavioral changes. As for the withdrawal syndrome, the eighteenth-century also inaugurated a long tradition of pharmacological manipulation during withdrawal to either replace the opium with another drug or to counteract its effects in order to make withdrawal safe.[6]

Opium preparations were remarkably popular in these centuries in the western world, although one could not be certain of their potency, which depended on the crude opium from which they were prepared. Dr. Pereira's standard British text of therapeutics (1854), also widely used in America, echoed Sydenham's description of opium as "undoubtedly the most important and valuable remedy in the whole Materia Medica." The effects of opium are "immediate, direct, and obvious; and its operation is not attended with pain or discomfort." Opium could be used for the "relief of maladies of everyday occurrence" with great success. Dr. Pereira recommended opium for almost every ailment for which a physician might be consulted:

> to mitigate pain, to allay spasm, to promote sleep, to relieve nervous restlessness, to produce perspiration and to check profuse mucous discharges from the bronchial tubes and gastro-intestinal canal. But experience has proved its value in relieving some diseases in which not one of these indications can be at all times distinctly traced.[7]

Some of the other remedies available to physicians were bloodletting, large doses of laxatives, mercurials, and other harmful (and in many cases very uncomfortable) applications, including various forms of skin irritation or denudation such as blistering. The sweet effect of opium in fevers, inflammatory diseases, delirium tremens, insanity, depression, convulsions, poisoning, hemorrhages, and venereal diseases must thus have appeared in many cases superior to an alternative regimen.

As to the dangers of opium use, medical opinion in Great Britain in the first half of the nineteenth century was divided. Perhaps the recent "opium wars" with China had encouraged moderate statements about the danger of the habit. The poor and destitute in China and Great Britain who took up opium smoking were generally agreed to suffer from it. Pereira (p. 1039) considered that continued opium smoking damaged the physical and moral character of the individual, "especially among the lower classes." He warned, in an earlier tradition, that "if the poison be withheld, death terminates the victim's existence." Yet there were respected contrary opinions that many years of opium smoking were not incompatible with longevity, a vigorous physical constitution, and a praiseworthy morality.[8] The difficulty of stopping opium smoking was recognized, and the withdrawal syndrome was described fairly accurately. In keeping with the concept of inheritance of acquired characteristics and damage to germ cells by disease or excesses, the offspring of opium smokers were understandably declared by Pereira to be "weak, stunted, and decrepit." Widespread use of opium in Great Britain was feared; Pereira believed that addiction was increasing, and import statistics were known to be rising, but no numerical estimate of habitués was offered (pp. 1040, 1025).

In contrast to Pereira's ambivalence, a leading American text, *Treatise on Therapeutics* (1868), by Dr. George Wood, professor of the theory and practice of medicine at the University of Pennsylvania and president of the American Philosophical Society, extolled opium uncritically:

A sensation of fullness is felt in the head, soon followed by a universal feeling of delicious ease and comfort, with an elevation and expansion of the whole moral and intellectual nature, which is, I think, the most characteristic of its effects. There is not the same uncontrollable excitement as from alcohol, but an exaltation of our better mental qualities, a warmer glow of benevolence, a disposition to do great things, but nobly and beneficently, a higher devotional spirit, and withal a stronger self-reliance, and consciousness of power. Nor is this consciousness altogether mistaken. For the intellectual and imaginative faculties are raised to the highest point compatible with individual capacity. The poet has never had brighter fancies, or deeper feelings, or greater felicity of expression, nor the philosopher a more penetrating or profounder insight than when under the influence of opium in this stage of its action. It seems to make the individual, for the time, a better and greater man. Sometimes there may be delusion; but it is not so much in relation to the due succession or dependence of thought, as in the elevation of the imagination and the soul above the level of reality. The hallucinations, the wildness, the delirious imaginations of alcoholic intoxication, are, in general, quite wanting. Along with this emotional and intellectual elevation, there is also increased muscular energy; and the capacity to act, and to bear fatigue, is greatly augmented.

After a length of time . . . this exaltation sinks into a corporal and mental calmness, which is scarcely less delicious than the previous excitement, and in a short time ends in sleep.[9]

A physician reading this description of opium would, in all likelihood, consider the substance to be a most efficacious and therapeutic device, or worth giving to a healthy friend.

Dr. Wood recognized the possibility of becoming a slave to opium, although he considered its effects less dangerous to the individual and society than those of alcohol. Nonetheless, overindulgence in opium, he wrote, could lead to the "lowest stage of degradation" when the user experiences a "total loss of self-respect, and indifference to the opinions of the community; and everything is sacrificed to the insatiable demands of the vice." But the cause of this fall from respectability could be found in the user's weak character. Since opium, unlike alcohol, did not destroy body tissue, the functions might be deranged but, "It is satisfactory to know that this evil habit may be corrected, without great difficulty, if the patient is in earnest." Sudden deprivation of opium, however, might lead to death. "The proper method of correcting the evil is by gradually withdrawing the cause; a diminution of the dose being made every day, so small as to be quite imperceptible in its effects . . . leading to a cure in somewhat more than a year" or even less (pp. 725–28).

By 1868 morphine had become a useful and common medicine. Dr. Wood considered it even more advantageous and safe than opium preparations, which had to be compounded from "parcels of opium [with a] diversity of strength." Generally, morphine was more agreeable to the patient and "less liable to provoke irregularities of mental action, and, with an equal excitant influence on the faculties and feelings, to derange them less frequently, and in less degree." Pain, insomnia, and nervous irritation were the chief indications of morphia.[10]

One of the greatest advantages of morphia over opium is the ease with which it can be injected by the hypodermic method into the subcutaneous tissue. To Dr. Wood it was remarkable that morphia, when injected, "even though applied at a distance from the seat of the disease, removes the pain quite as effectually as if injected into its immediate vicinity." As a consequence, "There are few affections in which opium is indicated, in which the salts of morphia have not been advantageously given in this way" (p. 762). Dr. Wood did not include in his description of morphine any warning about its habit-forming properties; perhaps his earlier discussion of opium habituation would apply to morphia also.

The writings of Pereira and Wood indicate that at the midpoint of the last century and well thereafter the danger of opium was balanced by its effective treatment of the symptoms of disease. The authors were skeptical about claims that opium was a serious danger to those classes of society above the lowest, to those who had will power, and even to those who were not Orientals. In fact, Pereira quotes some medical reports that opium users in the Orient were healthier than the average workers (p. 1039). Wood's praises for opium read very much like encomia over cocaine in the 1880s.[11] If opium was an actual assistance to the strong-willed, those who abused it were denigrated as weak-willed; enslavement to opium was real degradation but not cause for too much worry. Medical proponents of opium did not claim it was harmless, but that it was, like any powerful and effective medicine, capable of being abused.

RECOGNITION OF ADDICTION

Within a few years, warnings about the habit-forming propensities of morphia taken hypodermically began to accumulate in the medical literature. Dr. Clifford Allbutt, one of Great Britain's most eminent clinicians, stated in 1870 that he had not read any warnings against frequent and regular morphia injections; he feared the prevalence of practitioners "of whom the syringe and phial are as constant companions as was the lancet to their fathers." Nine of his patients with neuralgias appeared to have developed a morphia habit, yet he was uncertain whether this was really the case. Allbutt typifies the hesitancy among the best clinicians to assert the addictive properties of morphia:

Injected morphia seemed so different to swallowed morphia, no one had any experience of ill effects from it, and we all had the daily experience of it as a means of peace and comfort, while pain on the other hand was certainly the forerunner of wretchedness and exhaustion. Gradually, however, the conviction began to force itself upon my notice, that injections of morphia, though free from the ordinary evils of opium-eating, might, nevertheless, create the same artificial want and gain credit for assuaging a restlessness and depression of which it was itself the cause. . . . If this be so, we are incurring a grave risk in bidding people to inject whenever they need it, and in telling them that the morphia can have no ill effects upon them so long as it brings with it tranquillity and well being.[12]

This was not the first warning; a little earlier one had appeared in the German medical literature,[13] but Allbutt's was among the first in an English periodical, and it was published simultaneously on both sides of the Atlantic.

In Germany, mid-nineteenth-century publications came from two schools of thought, each with its own explanation for the addiction of certain persons. One school held that morphine craving was a psychological hunger related to the personality or constitution of the addict, while the opposition, represented by Eduard Levinstein of Berlin, argued that regular doses of morphine would make anyone an addict since the cause lay in a physiological reaction to opiates.[14] Dr. Levinstein was rather pessimistic about the cure of morphine addiction. In 1875 he reported that his own limited follow-up of patients weaned from opiates had a relapse rate of about 75 percent.[15] For withdrawal he suggested that in most cases the patients should agree to total seclusion and management by hospital staff, since voluntary outpatient treatment simply would not work. He did not favor gradual reduction, comparing it to cutting off a dog's tail one slice at a time. He recommended abrupt cessation of opiates along with medical management during the two to three days of extreme discomfort. He felt this was preferable to prolonging withdrawal over many weeks and exhausting the patient as well as his funds and confidence.[16]

Levinstein accurately described the withdrawal syndrome. Since the basis of addiction is the normal human physiological reaction, all classes of people could, and did, succumb. Moreover, he averred, morphine addiction affected an upstanding victim's moral sense and turned him into a hopeless liar, especially with regard to drugs. This meant that addiction could not be controlled in a setting where the patient could in any way get his own drug supply.[17] Levinstein, Wood, and Pereira agreed independently that decline of moral character is associated with chronic opiate use in either some or almost all instances.

Addiction had a long way to go before it was widely recognized as an unmitigated evil, a danger to society, and deserving of the most severe penalties, but the belief grew that prolonged use of opiates endangered anyone who indulged and could lead to immoral and criminal actions and social ineffectiveness. Any intellectual or social value in opium, even for the higher classes, was eventually discounted, and the ease of becoming an addict began to be accepted as an extreme hazard.

The notion of a vice-disease easily acquired, progressively damaging, and difficult to cure was a triad familiar to the public: opiate addiction easily fit this category. In the late nineteenth century there were two other common social afflictions, syphilis and alcoholism, that shared these characteristics. Both were largely associated with the lower classes and with gradual deterioration of the mind and body. The public probably came to consider opiate addiction a similar vice.[18] As the more direct causes of disease were discovered in the decades after Allbutt's warning, more sophisticated treatments arose—and the number of illnesses treated by alcohol and opiates diminished.

In the last decades of the nineteenth century bacteriology became the model for the medical profession. The bacteria causing tuberculosis, diphtheria, and cholera were located and studied. None of these diseases could be cured by administration of opiates. As a result, opiates had fewer and fewer specific uses other than subduing pain. Opium's use as a soothe-all, so useful to medicine in past centuries, began to appear unscientific, unprofessional, and an indulgence fraught with danger.

The microscope and the research laboratory led to great discoveries that began to change the practice of medicine and its theoretical foundations. Many old problems were reexamined by enthusiastic investigators. Even the cautious and brilliant bacteriologist Robert Koch announced in 1890 that he had discovered a cure for tuberculosis, and several years passed before it was realized that "tuberculin" was useless in treatment and actually could innoculate an individual with the disease. If Koch's zeal could carry him beyond his evidence, there were many other investigators who also believed that they had come upon the answer to mysterious problems.

Opiate addiction provided, then as now, one of the most baffling problems in medicine, and extensive research was conducted from the 1870s on. The two elements of opiate addiction that led to the most extensive investigation were tolerance and the withdrawal syndrome. In 1883 Marmé claimed to have discovered a breakdown product of morphine, oxydimorphine, which had effects the opposite of morphine. Increasing doses of morphine were required to neutralize its effect, and when morphine was stopped, the breakdown product caused the withdrawal syndrome.[19] This explanation attempted to explain both tolerance and withdrawal, but unfortunately oxydimorphine could not be located in the blood of addicts by other investigators, nor could it, prepared in vitro, cause any symptoms when injected into an addicted animal.[20]

Immunological theory provided the basis for Gioffredi's work in 1897 which appeared to demonstrate that an antitoxic substance was produced in the bodies of addicted dogs, which, when injected as a serum into kittens, protected against large doses of morphine.[21] Several other investigators also reported the production of an antitoxin to opiates.[22] If true, this would have been unusual since all other known antitoxins were stimulated by the complex proteins of viruses and bacteria. Later this antibody or antitoxin theory of addiction was espoused vigorously in the United States by Dr. Ernest S. Bishop of New York, a national leader among those physicians and laymen who believed that indefinite maintenance of some addicts was rational and humane.[23] Dr. Bishop collided head on with federal enforcement policies after 1919 and lost. One element in his defeat was the disproval of the antibody hypothesis, which led some of his opponents to conclude that there was no organic basis for withdrawal phenomena.

A somewhat similar theory, and one based on another popular medical belief, was the "autotoxin" theory of Dr. George E. Pettey.[24] Some laboratory evidence for this theory existed as well as that hypothesizing antibodies, but its immediate plausibility came from the invocation of intestinal autotoxins, a widely accepted cause for a multitude of ailments, and one advocated by Nobel Laureate Ellie Metchnikoff (1908).[25] According to Pettey, opiates stimulated the production of toxins in the intestines, which had the physiological effect associated with withdrawal phenomena. Morphine in increasing doses was necessary to counteract the toxin production; if it was stopped, the toxins would be unchecked. Therefore treatment would consist of purging the body of toxins and any lurking morphine that might remain to stimulate toxin production in the future.[26] In 1914, Valenti reported that serum of dogs taken during signs of abstinence and injected into normal dogs produced similar abstinence phenomena.[27]

Other explanations for addiction, often with voluminous laboratory data, included shedding of endothelial cells of endocrine glands leading to blocked secretions (Sollier 1898); an increased ability of the body to destroy morphine (Faust 1900); changes in cell protoplasm (Cloetta 1903); degenerative changes in brain cells (Willcox 1923); and changes in cell membrane permeability (Fauser and Ottenstein 1924).[28]

TREATMENT OF ADDICTION

There have been dozens of different theories for the treatment of addicts. A myriad of details as to timing, size of dose, and prognostic signs fill journal pages, but the fundamental treatment categories were few. Patients could be purged to eliminate toxins or morphine; or sedated during withdrawal by innumerable substances—bromides, barbiturates, trional, etc.; or put into a state of confusion or forgetfulness with hyoscine or atropine. A drug similar to the addicting opiate might be substituted, perhaps codeine or, for a while, heroin or even cocaine. An antagonist to some withdrawal symptoms, e.g., sweating or diarrhea, might be prescribed—perhaps one of the atropine-like drugs such as belladonna. Theory might determine how long the treatment was given, for a few days or a few weeks, or whether one element in the treatment was essential and one of the other standard treatments totally contraindicated. All treatment sought to make withdrawal as pleasant as possible, and some writers claimed that it could be quite comfortable. This goal might lead the therapists to employ slow or abrupt withdrawal. Of course at any one time there were some therapists who believed withdrawal was psychological and did not require medicines, and some who believed that withdrawal was life-threatening and therefore recommended indefinite maintenance. But from the mid-nineteenth century until about 1920, physicians continued to tell one another that withdrawal and perhaps a few weeks of aftercare would lead to the cure of addiction in most cases. Levinstein's prediction in 1875 of 75 percent relapse, and a United States Public Health Service study in 1942 that more than 75 percent of the addicts treated at Lexington Narcotic Hospital relapsed, bracket a period of therapeutic enthusiasm in the midst of which American narcotic laws were enacted and the enforcement style established.[29]

In the first decade of this century there was confidence that an addict was eminently curable. In 1900, dozens of sanitaria for alcohol and drug habits were scattered across the United States. Naturally, as private operations they catered to those who could pay, middle- and upper-class unfortunates who wanted to be cured or at least dried out for a while. The sanitarium operators wrote extensively on the drug and alcohol evils, proudly spreading their successful treatments. Two physician-proprietors, Dr. C. B. Pearson of Maryland and Dr. T. D. Crothers of Connecticut, took opposing views on how to treat the addict, each condemning the other's mode of operation, and each claiming remarkable effectiveness for his own.

Dr. Crothers, superintendent of Walnut Lodge Hospital in Hartford, maintained in *Morphinism and Narcomania* (1902) that the first prerequisite to treatment was "control of the patient" for his will must be subservient to the physician's.[30] An opposite view was expressed by Dr. Pearson, who preached an optimism about voluntary reduction of opiates. Among his many patients he said he had had great success, and his description of success where others failed should have been persuasive. All he asked was a sincere willingness to be cured:

> A prominent woman took treatment eleven times and failed each time. At last her finances became reduced to a sum just sufficient for her twelfth treatment. On this occasion she was entirely successful and remained free from morphinism until her death several years later. Everyone knows that morphinism does not improve with age, therefore it is evident that this lady could have succeeded at any of her previous attempts had she wished to.[31]

Dr. Pearson condemned physical restraint and believed that cures resulted from slow reduction, good food, and an understanding physician. This of course was sweet music to the ears of most general practitioners as well as to most patients. Less pleasing aspects were explained away by calling concern with the length of treatment a "puerile objection." And with voluntary gradual reduction and friendly treatment Dr. Pearson claimed success: "I look for 75% of permanent cures in straight cases of morphine addiction, who have never taken treatment and who are up and about at work, regardless of the amount used and length of addiction and a lower percentage of cures in the other types, according to circumstances." [32]

Perhaps it is harsh to attribute an obvious form of advertising to these or any other entrepreneurs, for if they thought they had a valid message they were entitled to communicate it in the medical and lay literature. Our knowledge that these treatments were worthless, that they made fortunes for their proprietors, and that their "scientific" pronouncements seemed so under the control of their investments, make it tempting to call them charlatans—but all this knowledge is after the fact. Their financial success elicited enmity from their less fortunate colleagues, just as Treasury Department agents who later investigated physicians seemed influenced by evidence of personal gain accruing from clinics or private practice, although there is no necessary connection between financial reward and charlatanism.

Charles B. Towns and His Treatment for Addiction

Of all the cure proclaimers there was an undisputed king, or perhaps emperor, so magnificent were his accomplishments and so influential his lobbying: Mr. Charles B. Towns. He worked at such a high level of national and international efforts to control narcotism that he appeared to many to be above mercenary considerations.

New York City has long held the distinction of harboring the largest number of narcotic addicts in this country. It is natural that sanitaria and specialists in the treatment of addiction and similar ailments would congregate there, but the leading addiction specialist came for unrelated reasons. At the turn of the century Towns arrived from Georgia, casting about for new fields to conquer. He. had no interest in addiction or even medicine, although he was destined to dominate much of the addiction controversy for the next twenty years. In Georgia, Towns had risen by his own efforts from farm boy to a supersalesman who had written "more life insurance than any other man south of Mason and Dixon's line up to that time." When he came to New York in 1901 he sought a larger arena for his talents as an insurance salesman but found something that excited him even more by its possibilities—the stock market. From 1901 to 1904 he was a partner in a brokerage firm that even-

tually failed. While discouraged over his first failure, Towns later
related that he was approached by a fellow who whispered, "I
have got a cure for the drug habit, morphine, opium, heroin, codeine
—any of 'em. We can make a lot of money out of it." Towns was
skeptical and sought the advice of his personal physician, who said
that the claim was ridiculous. With this opinion challenging him,
Towns began investigating the cure by putting advertisements in
the paper to locate drug fiends who wanted to be helped. Trying
the formula out on such persons and restraining them when they
wanted to get out of the hotel rooms Towns used for his experiments, he perfected the treatment so as to "eliminate all the suffering." [33]

As he gained patients for his treatment, Towns was shunned by
the regular medical profession. But in a few years he was somehow
able to interest Dr. Alexander Lambert of Cornell in his methods.
Although Towns would still not reveal the secret formula, he was
able to convince Lambert that he had an effective treatment for
addiction. Eventually Lambert, Theodore Roosevelt's close friend
and personal physician, introduced Towns to government officials
as a "straightforward, honest man—no 'faker,' " who had a most
useful treatment for drug addiction. When Towns wanted to find
a market for his "cure" in China, Lambert wrote Assistant Secretary
of State Robert Bacon, asking him to smooth Towns' way in China
so that he could use his treatment there; he reported it had been
investigated by the War Department and "really cures morphine
and opium addictures." [34]

Towns impressed the American delegation to the Shanghai Opium
Commission by his apparent success in China when, in 1908, he
claimed to have cured about 4,000 opium addicts there by his
method. By that time the Americans believed they had ready a historic announcement: "An everyday American fighter" had located
an effective treatment for addiction. The delegation wanted Towns
to announce to the assembled members of the commission the treatment that he had now decided to give to the world. It bothered
the Americans to have the commission declare itself incompetent
to evaluate such a message of hope; consequently, the Towns treatment was relegated to the delegation's official report to the Secretary of State. Nevertheless, the unique prominence given the Towns
treatment by the delegation was almost an official endorsement.
The attitude of the American delegates toward the possibility of a

simple cure complemented their repeated declarations at the commission meetings that a world prohibition of habit-forming drugs should be enacted, excepting only obvious medical uses in the alleviation of pain. The Towns treatment answered the problem of what to do with addicts, and so a possible dilemma was avoided by accepting Towns' claims at face value. If a cure indeed existed, the prohibition of narcotics for simple addiction maintenance or pleasure was no more cruel than the requirement for smallpox vaccination: the prohibition of nonmedical narcotic uses could be classified as a routine public health measure.

In transmitting Towns' regimen to the State Department, the delegation called attention to the fact that the "cure" had "already been favorably reported on by Drs. Lambert and Thomas at the instance of the Philippine Government." It was recommended that it be used under the supervision of Mr. Towns as far as practicable and that "he should be given full credit for the treatment." Towns was described as a man who had eschewed pecuniary exploitation, and his treatment, "properly carried out, is the most successful on record for the cure of the victim of the opiate habit in any of its forms." [35]

What was this generous gift to the afflicted? The formula follows.

fluid extract of prickly ash bark	1 part
fluid extract of hyoscyamus	1 part
15% tincture of belladonna	2 parts

It was given in ½ cc doses at half-hour intervals to an addict until signs of atropine effect were noted: dilatation of the pupil, slight dryness of the throat, and redness of the skin. But before beginning with the specific, a "complete evacuation of the bowels" must have been accomplished, and half an hour before beginning formula administration, the largest tolerable dose of the addicting substance was given "to bridge the patient over as long a period as possible without having to use the drug again." [36]

About 24 hours later, after a second cathartic had worked its effect, another dose of the addicting drug, but this time only one-half or one-third of the previous amount, was given. Allegedly this left the patient as comfortable as the previous maximum dose. Twelve hours later a third cathartic was given, and 6 to 8 hours later this was followed by 1 to 2 ounces of castor oil. Secretary Root was informed that this last cathartic, the third during treatment by the specific, should produce "a stool that consists of green mucous matter." When Dr. Lambert announced the treatment to the medical profession in September 1909, he wrote that "when this stool occurs, or shortly afterward, the patients often will feel suddenly relaxed and comfortable, and their previous discomfort ceases," thereby bringing the entire treatment to an end.[37]

This outline is drastically condensed from the original elaboration. Not mentioned, for example, is strychnine in small doses, which was necessary to combat the patient's exhaustion after the first day or so. Towns conceded, "In some cases and in those using large amounts of drugs a patient may have some discomfort during the treatment," but this was not much trouble. The patient "does not remain on the average more than five days." [38] One of the cure's detractors later labeled it "diarrhea, delirium and damnation," but it seemed very neat and scientific when presented in 1909 under the auspices of the federal government, Dr. Lambert, and the *Journal of the American Medical Association*.

Towns rose in the esteem of the medical profession's elite and in the opinion of the political powerwielders who were under pressure to do something about opium addiction in the Philippines, China, and the United States. Towns achieved a national and even an international role. His techniques as a salesman and his imposing personality took him far, and he was eventually accepted as one of the most knowledgeable and altruistic addiction experts in the United States. By 1920 the belief of Towns' physician that the cure was ridiculous began to be widely held also among the profession and the public, but while confidence in him lasted, Mr. Charles B. Towns was an active figure on the American drug stage.

WHAT IS ADDICTION?

The question of whether addiction is a disease became crucial during 1919 and 1920 in the United States and followed the Supreme Court declaration that maintenance of addiction without a cause such as intractable pain was illegal. But if addiction was a bona fide disease, perhaps addicts could be legally maintained after all. Leading physicians, who in the past had sought stringent antinarcotic laws and had also declared addiction a disease, now averred that it was not a disease at all, at least not an *organic* disease requiring doses of narcotics. Withdrawal symptoms and signs for which they had once recommended intricate physiological therapies were now said to be "purely functional manifestations and have no physical basis." [39] This conclusion came while the medical profession was split and each side bitterly accused the other of a conspiracy to either foster dope fiends or to jail sick patients. The battle was so intense that disproval in 1920 of the antibody theory, the favored hypothesis of addiction-disease advocates, was taken to mean that addiction and the withdrawal phenomena had no organic basis at all.[40]

Just as the belief that addiction was a disease drew upon the new studies in immunology in the late nineteenth century, so the decision in 1920 that addiction was functional came when the new psychology—psychoanalysis—could be invoked as an explanation of dysfunction and as a source of effective therapy. Psychoanalysis, an AMA report explained in 1920, had shown how the subconscious life had a strong hold on our conscious behavior. If the problems within the subconscious have caused regression, then psychoanalysis might be able to locate the "sore spot" and release the libido for "higher thought and emotional levels." The goal of treatment must be to "teach this otherwise normal drug addict to irradiate and sublimate this libido which he is so wantonly wasting on the fetish of drug addiction." If the addict was not normal, but a social misfit, he should be rehabilitated along the lines of vocational training and probation. Without correction he might become "organized and vocal," and "society may awaken to the fact that he is an IWW, a bolshevik, or what not." [41]

The assertion that the withdrawal syndrome is functional was a position taken by leading figures in national medicine in 1920, apparently to protect the gains made, in their view, toward outlawing addiction. They associated the argument that addiction is a disease with men whose motives they suspected, since leaders like Dr. Lambert had lost faith in medicine's power to cure addiction.[42] "Addiction-disease" seemed a handy cover for "dope doctors" who made enormous profits selling prescriptions or habit-forming drugs. Most physicians shied away from addicts as too troublesome, unsavory, and frustrating to warrant any therapeutic attempt; those physicians who would provide addicts with drugs seemed either an uninformed or a mercenary minority.[43] Since by 1920 faith in cure had already begun to fade, one had to choose between indefinitely maintaining what was thought to be an enormous number of addicts, over a million by federal estimate, or trying to stop all "non-medical" drug supplies. In this situation the question of whether addiction was a disease was paramount. It was difficult to advocate elimination of addicts and their drugs if addiction was a true disease, a permanent physiological disorder; in that case opiates could no more be withheld than digitalis from the chronic heart patient. It would appear that a desire to stop the dope doctors led prominent and able clinicians into believing that addiction withdrawal was functional and without an organic basis.

Later in the 1920s the belief in the organic reality of withdrawal, even if not understood, was again asserted by many in the medical profession, but it was still linked to psychological disorder. Dr. Lawrence Kolb, Sr. of the United States Public Health Service represents the highest level of medical research in addiction from the 1920s into the 1940s. In the 1920s he believed that "normal" persons did not choose to become addicted; therefore the addict by choice was a "psychopath." Addiction was only one aspect of the psychopath's life, which included other criminal activity and social ineptness. Dr. Kolb stated that the joy of a morphine injection would be felt only by the psychopath; a normal person would feel little or nothing. In his opinion the accidental case, whether addicted from patent medicine or a physician's malpractice, had been greatly reduced as a result of the Harrison Act, so that in the 1920s only psychopaths were seeking the pleasure of opiates. In 1925 he summarized some of his research:

> Opiates apparently do not produce mental pleasure in stable persons except a slight pleasure brought about in some cases by the reflex from relief of acute pain.
>
> In most unstable persons opiates produce mental pleasure during the early period of addiction. The degree of pleasure seems to depend upon the degree of instability.[44]

As for the pain and suffering of the withdrawal syndrome, the 1920s silenced the claims for specific treatments and cures of addiction by a series of careful and controlled studies in Philadelphia and New York.[45] The work of the Mayor's Committee on Drug Addiction (New York) has a finality about it because it was chaired by Dr. Alexander Lambert, one of the most respected clinicians in the nation and an advocate of a specific withdrawal method since 1909. Although Dr. Lambert had, in the hectic year of 1920, apparently abandoned the physiological basis of the withdrawal syndrome, a few years later he was again actively investigating various specific treatments.[46] In 1927 the Mayor's Committee, composed of Health Department physicians and other experts, was given financial support by the city and the use of a ward in Bellevue Hospital with a full medical staff. In 1928 and 1929, 318 addicts were studied at Bellevue with physical and psychological tests, and the various treatments suggested for addiction were applied to subgroups of the addicts. Controls were maintained for each test of an addiction treatment. The committee's report was published in 1930. Some of its conclusions were:

That the patients be given as rapid a reduction treatment as the age and physical condition and response to morphine dosage would permit.

Younger addicts in good physical condition could often be given abrupt withdrawal without danger.

A small number of well-adjusted drug addicts should be permitted to continue daily dosage under proper supervision.

There was no evidence to confirm claims of "cure" or a "specific" which would miraculously rid habitués of addiction. Withdrawal of narcotics does not constitute a "cure." [47]

The year 1930 may be taken as the close of the era of therapeutic optimism with regard to opiate addiction. It had been increasingly difficult since World War I to rouse enthusiasm for an addiction cure, and within a decade the full weight of clinical medicine was against any such claims. Everything had been tried and everything failed; the relapse rate was appalling. When Congress established narcotic institutions in 1929 the primary reason for federal aid to addiction was not to provide treatment; the Lexington and Fort Worth narcotic "farms" were unmistakably built for the large numbers of jailed addicts who had crowded federal penitentiaries. Yet in the debate over authorization, the warm hope was expressed that through these hospitals effective treatment or a new discovery would begin to wipe out the addiction menace.[48]

The search for an effective medical cure for addiction has so far failed. The occasional cure that has gained brief professional endorsement and popularity has later proved to be the result of wishful thinking, financial investment, or poorly designed evaluative methods. A not uncommon occurrence in the history of medicine, the powerful desire for a cure has produced a succession of them: eventually the patience and credulity of the medical profession and the public have become resistant to new claims.

A recent review of the opiates concluded that probably no other group of drugs has been so extensively studied with such uncertain results,[49] but this dismal information was not available to dampen the enthusiasm of earlier American reformers. Professional and public confidence that addiction could be successfully treated must be recollected in order to understand the history of narcotic control, particularly in the United States, where belief in medicine's ultimate triumph was never stronger than in the early decades of this century.

At present, the reasons for the initial nonmedical use of opium and similar substances is in dispute, the physiological basis for addiction is unknown, and a treatment with even a quarter the effectiveness of penicillin in pneumonia is lacking. The regular user's reaction to sudden deprivation of an opiate is generally well validated. According to a contemporary authority this phenomenon has the following characteristics in morphine addiction and is similar for other opiate-like drugs.

> The abstinence syndrome that develops when repeated injections of morphine are suddenly terminated is quite stereotyped. Although the patient may complain much earlier, frequent yawning, nasal discharge, tears, widening of the pupils, sweating, erection of the hair, and restlessness are usually observed 12 to 16 hours after the last dose. Later, muscular aches and twitches, abdominal cramps, vomiting, diarrhea, hypertension, insomnia, loss of appetite, agitation, profuse sweating and weight loss develop. . . . In addition, spontaneous ejaculations may occur in the male and profuse menstrual bleeding in the female.
>
> The constellation of signs, together with more variable behavior changes, reaches peak intensity on the second or third day after the last dose of morphine, and then subsides rapidly over the next week, but . . . a stable state may not be reached for six months or longer. If, at any time during this abstinence period, a single dose of morphine is administered, all the abstinence phenomena subside dramatically, only to reappear again within 4 to 6 hours at a level comparable to that had morphine not been administered. The untreated morphine abstinence syndrome is

rarely fatal except in patients with cardiac disease, active tuberculosis, or other debilitating illness.[50]

Mild abstinence symptoms can be produced in man by abruptly withdrawing morphine after two weeks' administration four times daily in doses of 15 or 20 milligrams (¼ to ⅓ grain). A yearning for a sense of well-being, or relief from pain, either of which may have led to the first use of an opiate, diminishes as the same amount of drug is readministered; more drug is required for the same effect. Apparently in many instances of opiate addiction, euphoria cannot be regained and the drug is then taken simply to prevent the onset of the abstinence phenomena. Other effects which decline as the same dose is repeated are depression of respiration, nausea, and vomiting. Pupil constriction and muscle spasms of the kind that cause constipation seem to respond indefinitely to the same dose. Adrenocorticotrophic hormone (ACTH) production is suppressed, with the result that the male becomes impotent and the female ceases to menstruate.

The mode of administration seems to affect the ease with which addiction develops and has been claimed to affect the ease of withdrawal from the drug. Smoking opium apparently has a rather mild effect, eating opium a stronger one; taking by mouth the purified principle morphine, or its derivative heroin, produces a more powerful result; the greatest impact results from intradermal, intramuscular or intravenous injection. If this appraisal is correct, the ingestion of crude opium before the nineteenth century would have had milder effects than hypodermic injections of purified opium derivatives. Still, the phenomenon of large numbers of people finding opiates to be irresistible and addictive was described before the last century. There is now little doubt that organic factors are an integral part of the addiction syndrome.

MORE ABOUT MR. TOWNS

After 1920 Towns continued work at the Charles B. Towns Hospital, using apparently the same treatment he had popularized in the first decade of the century. As his standing in the medical world fell, his claims became more and more extravagant and the substances he inveighed against multiplied to include tobacco, coffee, tea, bromides, marihuana, paraldehyde, etc., as well as opiates and

alcohol. He recounted his days of fame and acceptance in little
books; for example in this passage in a 44-page volume published in
1932:

> We have *never had a negative result* in any case, free from dis-
> ability, or from an incurable painful condition which enforced
> the continued use of an opiate—such as gall stones, cancer, etc.[51]

In the bright days of the Towns Hospital and its support by leading physicians the cure rate was usually set as high as 75 to 90
percent. This was based on the reasoning that if you never heard
from a patient again, he no longer needed your services. Or as a
brochure put the issue of successful treatment in 1914 after several
thousand patients had taken the five-day course:

> A little less than ten percent returned to us for a second treat-
> ment, a reasonable presumption being that the ninety percent
> from whom we have never heard further that left our care had
> no need to consult with us a second time.[52]

While the treatment had credibility, even Dr. Lambert did not
closely question this logic and in fact employed it himself, but when
evidence accumulated that the Towns treatment was ineffective,
the weakness of such claims for cure seemed evident to all.[53] Eleven
years after his initial research on the Towns treatment, Dr. Lambert
had lost his faith in merely withdrawing the drug. "I tried it," he
said, "in about 200 patients at Bellevue . . . and I had looked them
up afterwards. I found that about four or five percent really stayed
off." [54] Towns, however, still clung to his illusions about the patients
who did not return. When his medical friends asked him what percentage of his alcoholics were cured, by 1931 Mr. Towns would
reply that he had not the slightest idea:

> I tell these doctors that when a patient leaves this hospital, we
> are through with him. We never communicate with a patient,
> either directly or indirectly. . . . Our psychology in this particu-
> lar line, I believe, is sound. You can hardly expect to establish
> confidence in a drinker by constantly communicating with him,
> or by having him report regularly to you.[55]

Prevailing concepts of control of addiction in the United States
abandoned the medical approach, which Towns sold as avidly as
life insurance or stocks, and he faded from the national scene to

become the proprietor of just one more sanitarium in New York City. Towns did not change his medical theories, his treatment, or his style of presentation, but the nation discarded specific treatments and was soured on the fantastic claims from their proponents. At the beginning of his career in combating "habits that handicap," Towns' story reveals the deep belief among many leading Americans that a cure existed for addiction and that Towns had it. The flaws in his statistics were overlooked as both physicians and statesmen persuaded themselves that a simple cure existed for this difficult social problem. Towns' own confidence and his bearing must have been part of his triumph; Dr. Richard C. Cabot of Boston knew him as "one of the most persuasive and dominating personalities in the world." [56] But the chief factor of his success was the confidence Americans had in the progress of medicine and its ability to solve by such therapeutic inventions a complex social and personal ailment.

Perhaps it would be worthwhile to consider the cure as a type of medical cure in general. The physiological basis for the treatment was quite reasonable: Opiate withdrawal usually produces sweating, diarrhea, and vomiting. The atropine-like action of the formula was thought pharmacologically to counteract these symptoms, thereby aiding the patient in lasting out the withdrawal. Atropine also had the effect of causing a delirium confusion, a kind of twilight sleep which erased memory of the withdrawal. In an age of belief in various potent intestinal autotoxins and antitoxins, the wisdom of complete evacuation of the intestinal tract before treatment was quite understandable, as was the continued evacuation of the bowels during therapy. Cathartics rid the body of the poisons that might be causing withdrawal symptoms as well as of any opiates lurking in the intestinal tract that might stimulate antitoxins later on. Therefore, what might now seem a bizarre treatment without rationale was in reality a harmful regimen within an accepted set of beliefs.

The way in which the cure was presented by leading medical authorities also conveys a sense of the science as well as the art of medicine. There were endpoints to be looked for—atropine toxicity in the administration of the specific, and the characteristic "green, mucous stool" which meant the treatment was completed. In addition to these guidelines, the treatment was repeatedly characterized as one requiring great care, "for the success of this treatment," Dr.

Lambert admonished, "depends on the conscientious adherence to its many details." [57]

Now forgotten, the Towns cure is an example of some of the classic medical "cures" of the past that have combined arcane scientific knowledge, elaborate detail, and professional expertise. Benjamin Rush's purging and phlebotomy to cure yellow fever in the 1790s, and lobotomy in the twentieth century are two more examples. It will suffice to note that the Towns method had so many social and political pressures favoring it that refutation was difficult for a decade after its publication. It seemed to succeed because the alternatives—no effective medical cure for addiction, and the inaccuracy of some medical theories of the time—were unacceptable.

State and Local Narcotic Control

Early local and state narcotic controls in the United States grew out of the danger perceived by those American communities that were directly affected. Pennsylvania, the home of leading morphine manufacturers, enacted an antimorphine law as early as 1860. Two decades later Ohio passed a law against smoking opium, and in 1897, twelve years after the way had been prepared by pharmaceutical research for massive production of the compound, Illinois enacted a law against cocaine.[1] Soon thereafter, as the activity of the American Pharmaceutical Association between 1901 and 1903 suggests, efforts within the states to control opiates and cocaine rapidly reached across the nation. Cocaine's euphoric and stimulant qualities, as well as its association with crime and with a feared and repressed minority put it at the top of any list of outlawed substances. These characteristics of cocaine are similar to the description in the mid-1930s of marihuana's effects.

Local laws varied in their severity. Some were so complicated or all-inclusive that it was practically impossible to fulfill their requirements. Others were expressions of concern over narcotics, but with loopholes to protect the sale of patent medicines and other domestic remedies that contained narcotics.[2] The sale of drugs and patent medicines across state lines was affected little, if at all, by local measures. A typical law would provide for the sale of narcotized proprietaries without restriction, but would confine provision of pure drugs to pharmacists and physicians, requiring a prescription that would be retained by the pharmacist for inspection for a period of time, perhaps two or three years. Naturally, there were many ways around this modest regulation. A physician might dispense narcotics directly to his patients or to anyone coming to his office. Inspection of pharmacists' prescriptions was notoriously rare; in some drugstores one could simply purchase a dime or a quarter's worth of cocaine or morphine.

Some laws prohibited refilling of narcotic prescriptions in the attempt to cut off an unlimited supply of narcotics to anyone who had a tattered prescription. These laws generated arguments which became wearyingly familiar as the antinarcotic crusade progressed. On the one hand the wholesale and retail drug trades expressed concern for the poor who would be forced to visit a doctor every time a prescription for morphine or heroin had to be refilled. It was on behalf of unfortunates in the cities and in isolated rural communities that prescription refilling at the patient's request was sought. Complaints that a prescription which could be indefinitely refilled was in effect a dangerous and uncontrollable opportunity to obtain habit-forming drugs was met with avowals that no self-respecting druggist would lower himself to be a mere purveyor of such substances.

Physicians, on the other hand, could accept the wisdom of such prohibitions; they did not plan to overcharge just because the patient had to return for prescription renewal. The effect of prohibiting prescription refills was to create steady customers who came back daily or weekly for brief visits to some physicians to get new prescriptions. A small percentage of physicians devoted themselves to this "specialty." Their encounters with their numerous "patients" were short—some saw hundreds daily—but the fact that there was an encounter at all gave the public the satisfaction of knowing that addicts were "under the care of a physician."

Let's not confuse the nefarious with the respectable, the maintaining physicians argued, and treat patients with chronic diseases like addiction, dropsy, liver cirrhosis, and constipation as if they were criminals.[3]

Other physicians, the vast majority even according to advocates of addiction disease, shied away from treating, maintaining, or encouraging addicts. These doctors shared an attitude common in America: patient habitués were troublesome and untrustworthy. The rare physician who before 1919 publicly favored maintenance of addicts pleaded with his colleagues to cooperate, but the practitioners' interest in doing so, either initially or as antinarcotic legislation gained ground, appeared to be rather small.[4]

The health professions occupied a prominent position in the antinarcotic crusade. No one questioned the medical need of opiates in some medical situations, and so initially the profession had a generally free hand. Lawmakers relied on professional ethics to control use of narcotics, but in the day-to-day practice of medicine, legal definitions could not easily distinguish between well-meaning overuse, use in error, and indiscriminate dispensing that led to addiction. Legally, restriction of narcotic transactions to licensed health practitioners was fairly simple, and the thought that this regulatory approach would fail because of the professionals' own culpability was painful to contemplate, for the result would be an enforcement nightmare.

In the Harrison Act an attempt was made to distinguish legitimate from illegitimate prescription of narcotics by physicians. The Treasury and Justice Departments would argue in 1915 that supply of drugs for mere comfort or maintenance of addiction was illegitimate, but this interpretation was not supported by the Supreme Court until 1919. One can conceive the difficulty of framing legal rules for the practice of medicine, and it was this difficulty which earlier legislators believed could be avoided by trusting doctors to police themselves. When fear of narcotics grew, the health professions were high on the list of culprits.

Loopholes in various state narcotic laws also received criticism when alarm over addiction did not decline after legislation had been enacted. The patent-medicine makers, however, had some unusual weapons that protected their commercial well-being. Beyond the usual art of lobbying, proprietary manufacturers had clever contracts with newspapers that provided for cancellation of their large advertising contracts should any state law be enacted restricting the sales, labeling, or claims that the medicine makers chose to employ. This provision generally resulted in silencing the news media with regard to restrictions on patent medicines and revelations of their dangers. But by 1905 the criticism of narcotized proprietaries became so outspoken that the Proprietary Association of America, comprised of the leading manufacturers, favored strict limits on the amount of narcotics in across-the-counter remedies.[5]

Furthermore, until labeling requirements were mandated by the federal Pure Food and Drug Act (1906), not only did manufacturers not list the narcotic or alcohol contents, they often positively denied its presence when it was plentiful in the substance.[6] Apparently the remoteness of mail-order houses clouded their special role. By default, then, the health professions had a prominence greater than they deserved.

If the fear of drug abuse had diminished in the new century, the health professions would have had no worry. Fear accelerated, however, in spite of a leveling off in per capita narcotic importation. Record-keeping regulations made it possible for jurisdictions to examine the prescribing and dispensing habits of physicians and druggists. It was discovered, particularly after the Harrison Act made national narcotic record-keeping uniform, that a small percentage of the profession was simply selling narcotics, having received, as it were, a license from the state to do just that. Yet when the doctors were questioned or brought into court, they claimed they were merely practicing medicine and that they had every right to prescribe as they thought wise. Pharmacists were similarly brought under legal scrutiny. The law as applied to the health professions was difficult to enforce but could be made more stringent if the public so demanded. Professionals could be made to conform to law much more effectively than unlicensed peddlers or pushers. One cannot but wonder what would have been the public's response if it knew how many preparations handled by the health professions were completely inert or ineffective.

Reformers attacked the patent medicine problem in several ways. Some labeling requirements were achieved in 1906, and an unexpected loophole in labeling claims was corrected by the Sherley amendment in 1912.[7] Pressure mounted in state legislatures to force disclosure of all active ingredients in patent medicines. Surveys made by the American Pharmaceutical Association in 1915 and 1916 monitored the decline in narcotized patent medicines. In 1915, the first year the Harrison Act was in effect, 92 of the 1,108 packaged remedies available in retail stores contained opiates, cannabis, or chloral hydrate. Significantly, none contained cocaine. By 1916, only 61 of 1,078 remedies had any opiate, cannabis, or chloral hydrate. Of the five with cannabis, three were remedies for corns and two were cough preparations. Of the four with chloral hydrate one was a hair tonic, one an antiseptic lotion, one a toothache remedy, and one an ointment for eczema.[8]

As the number of narcotic proprietaries diminished, so did the narcotic content in many that remained. Pe-ru-na, a cheerful standby for generations, decreased its alcoholic content (required, the makers said, simply to retard spoilage) from 28 percent at the turn of the century to 17 percent, and by 1918 to nothing. Similarly, the morphine content of Mrs. Winslow's Soothing Syrup decreased from 0.4 grain in an ounce in 1908 to 0.16 grain in 1911, and then to no morphine by 1915. These changes were apparently undertaken because disclosure of narcotics or alcohol content decreased the popularity of proprietary remedies.[9]

The great furor over narcotic proprietaries represented the public's awareness of insidious drugging by unscrupulous interests. Relief that this menace was receding under the impact of hard-won federal legislation left the self-regulated health professions in an even more exposed position. They were becoming the last legitimate enterprises that could be legally constrained from endangering society with narcotics.

The peddler had been present from an early day; he was not considered an extremely difficult enforcement problem until the most restrictive legislation and court interpretation cracked down on licensed purveyors of narcotics. Once maximum legislative control was applied to the peddler or pusher, it became evident that narcotics would remain available in the largest American cities. Before the peddlers' durability became evident, though, the legal channels of narcotic traffic would have to be attacked.

THE USPHS AND MARTIN WILBERT

In 1912, when the Hague Convention spurred federal agitation for a national antinarcotic law, the United States Public Health Service looked into state laws regarding poisons and habit-forming drugs. The PHS had little influence within the federal government, but it was occasionally called upon to assist in a modest way centers of power such as the State Department; it was watched by the health professions lest it depart from its traditional role of combating communicable disease, treating merchant seamen, and gathering and disseminating information.[10]

With impetus gained from the national movement to establish a department of health with cabinet rank, the Public Health Service gradually expanded. From the Marine Hospital Service founded in 1798 it became in 1902 the Marine Hospital and Public Health Service, and in 1912 the Public Health Service. The Hygienic Laboratory, established in the late nineteenth century in New York City to perform some rudimentary scientific procedures, also grew and by 1904 was housed in its own building in Washington. Eventually the Hygienic Laboratory became the National Institutes of Health. Martin I. Wilbert, a pharmacist from Philadelphia, was chosen to be a technical assistant in the new laboratory's Division of Pharmacology, at that time the highest professional role a pharmacist had achieved in the federal service.[11] Wilbert performed well in the intricate development of the federal antinarcotic laws. Like other outstanding investigators of the PHS, his valuable papers were too often confined to the technical *Public Health Reports*. What influence Wilbert enjoyed was not due to his rank in the Public Health Service; in Philadelphia his scientific work had established the pharmacy of the German (now Lankenau) Hospital as a model for the health profession. His devotion to raising the standards of pharmacy led to enormous work with the American Pharmaceutical Association, its local branch, and brought him in contact with the medical profession. An original member of the AMA's Council on Chemistry and Pharmacy (1905), he served on it until his early death in 1917. His obvious disinterest in amassing wealth would have been established by his accepting a post with the PHS, if by nothing else. Wilbert had the reputation of being thorough, fair, and a constructive critic. When the National Drug Trades Conference met in Washington, D.C., in 1913, he was asked to represent the AMA in planning the antinarcotic law. Wilbert was the PHS expert in the field.[12]

In a 1912 compilation of state laws on habit-forming drugs, Wilbert declared,

> There are few if any subjects regarding which legislation is in a more chaotic condition than the laws designed to minimize the drug-habit evil. . . . In many of the states anti-narcotic laws are so comprehensive that practically every retail druggist would be subject to fine or imprisonment were an attempt made to enforce the legislation ostensibly in force, while in other states the laws are so burdened with exceptions and provisos as practically to nullify every effort to control the traffic in narcotic drugs.

Wilbert's description of the state laws reflected a common belief that local legislation had failed to halt the progress of habit-forming drugs in the United States. His reports left no question that these drugs represented a social danger and required further action, but he shied away from dramatic exaggeration.[13]

Wilbert and Hamilton Wright present a striking contrast. Wright fought for narcotic control on a grand scale, fending off devious international conspiracies and offending almost everyone he dealt with. Wilbert, an unassuming man with a rather quavering voice, nicknamed "Weepy Wilbert" by his colleagues and devoted to finding the most rational solution to a difficult problem, refused melodrama and aggressive actions. His long hours with committees exhibited "unlimited patience."[14] Wilbert was trusted; Wright was resented. Almost exact contemporaries, they died within a few months of each other, both relatively young and still in the midst of the narcotic control controversy. This period of state and local statute revision and treatment experimentation (1910–20) can be clarified by some examples from various places and by a close examination of the approaches tried in New York State.

LOCAL CONTROL: JACKSONVILLE'S NARCOTIC CLINIC

In Jacksonville, Florida, Dr. Charles E. Terry established a style of addiction control which within ten years became the most controversial in America. Dr. Terry, a dedicated public health officer who took an increasingly prominent role in the debate over narcotic control, became a leading exponent of the medical approach. He worked chiefly within the framework of professional or philanthropic health organizations such as the American Public Health Association and the Bureau of Social Hygiene. Terry eventually compiled a thousand-page anthology of information on narcotics.[15]

In 1912, however, Dr. Terry was the City Health Officer of Jacksonville, the largest city in the state, where he practiced an approach to drug addiction that became a debated alternative to various kinds of embargo, national or personal. He established a city drug clinic so that habitués could receive free narcotic prescriptions. His work is a direct forerunner of the methadone maintenance clinics which now exist in many American cities.

Dr. Terry decided upon this innovation after the failure of existing state controls. The Florida law had proven inadequate as revealed by prosecution undertaken by the State Pharmaceutical Association which all resulted in *nol prosses*. Therefore he asked the Jacksonville City Council to enact an ordinance regulating in an unusual way the common drugs of habitués. In order to locate physicians who would "lend their services to the fostering of these habits," he asked that prescriptions containing more than a normal dose of habit-forming drugs be copied and sent to his office. Druggists would be required to keep their drug prescriptions in ledgers which could be inspected by the health officer. Possession of the drugs, except under conditions of the ordinance, was made a misdemeanor. Most importantly, the ordinance permitted the health officer to provide free prescriptions to habitués if he thought it advisable. The prescriptions were provided to eliminate the excuse by druggists that sale without a prescription was necessary because the user was too poor to go to a physician. The requirement would also "bring the health officer into personal contact with the unfortunate addicted to drug habits." After conferences with the local medical society and city pharmacists, the law was passed by the council in August 1912. After a few early violators were promptly prosecuted and convicted, Dr. Terry felt the law was generally obeyed.[16]

After a year of operation, Dr. Terry had registered 646 habitual users, a number equal to about 1 percent of Jacksonville's population. Some, he does not say how many, were transient, but he guessed that this number would roughly equal those receiving drugs directly from their physicians and therefore escape the recording of prescriptions required by the ordinance. Although half the inhabitants of Jacksonville were white and half black, the number of white habitués outnumbered the blacks by almost two to one (416 to 230). He surmised that "with us at least, the whites are far more prone to drug addictions than the blacks." Among the habituated blacks, cocaine was favored by about half; among whites, by about a fifth; opiates took up most of the remaining fraction. Of all users, about 4 percent favored heroin, 20 percent laudanum, 25 percent cocaine, and almost 40 percent morphine. Females outnumbered males by about three to two, and tended to prefer opiates to cocaine.

The relatively low rate of drug use among blacks, and the willingness of Dr. Terry and the city government to supply the dreaded cocaine to them, is further evidence of the exaggeration of "cocainomania" in the American press and by federal government officials.

Dr. Terry gained the confidence of about one-third of the users, and although "mendacity is a common attribute of the drug fiend and information so obtained is not reliable," his conversations with addicts led to the conclusion that 55 percent of the habits had been acquired through treatment by physicians, 20 percent from advice of acquaintances, and 20 percent through dissipation. Only 2 percent arose from chronic and incurable disease treated with narcotics. Dr. Terry stated before the American Public Health Association:

Here were 112 men and women become confirmed drug habitués through the judgment of as many physicians who elected to submit their patients to this risk, in order to relieve varying degrees of pain caused by conditions which, for the most part, were in no way permanently benefited by the administration of an opiate, no small number of which were amenable to surgical interference or other well-recognized treatment, and where, in some instances, opiates, by every rule of intelligent practice, were distinctly contraindicated! . . . In many instances these first doses were not given at the bedside to allay severe pain, but handed out to office patients with apparently as little concern as a dose of calomel.

If this kind of righteous indignation could be aroused by an informed colleague, one cannot be surprised that the public believed the physician deserved to have his prescriptions of habit-forming drugs severely restricted. It is reasonable to assume that most of the physicians themselves shared Dr. Terry's harsh view of the dope doctor.

Dr. Terry also chastised the druggists who reaped an extravagant profit from their narcotic sales, and praised the form of New York's cocaine law of 1913 except for its omission of opiates. Any legislation must "take full cognizance of the practicing physician as a factor of prime importance in the formation of drug users and not content itself with restrictions thrown around the druggist." Effective prohibitive legislation "must provide for the free treatment of existing users." The users should be considered public wards for "at least one rational course of treatment." Dr. Terry had confidence only in public institutions after his experience with home treatments, private sanitaria, and private physicians. As a result of experience in his narcotic clinic, and a belief that medical treatment could be efficacious if given in a public institution, he declared that addiction was best left to health departments and not police departments. The police were distracted by many concerns and had only spasmodic interest in addiction "whenever chance or some too flagrant act brings the matter to their attention."

Clients were not feared by the clinic personnel but seemed an alien and pitiful group; Dr. Terry's description of chronic indigent addicts prior to the Harrison Act is of some interest:

The social misery, the inefficiency and communal depletion resulting from this civic malady, may not be properly realized by one who has not seen for himself this pitiful array of wrecks waiting, as in a breadline, for the free dope prescription, wives fearful lest their husbands discover their condition; fathers and mothers hiding, by every artifice a stimulated cunning may devise, their habit from their own children; young men and women asking in a whisper for a fifty-cent prescription for "coke," a vicious circle of carelessness, ignorance and cupidity involving a responsibility that has been shifted from shoulder to shoulder until no one seems willing to admit it, yet intimately associated with the public welfare and health conservation and deserving of the most careful investigation and expert treatment.

In Terry's early work, themes appear which he developed further over the next two decades.

STATE CONTROL: THE TENNESSEE NARCOTIC ACT OF 1913

Tennessee's revised narcotic law came into effect more than a year before the Harrison Act. Its most distinctive feature was the registration of addicts to enable them to have opiate prescriptions refilled "to minimize suffering among this unfortunate class" and to keep "the traffic in the drug from getting into underground and hidden channels." [17]

Like Dr. Terry, Tennessee's State Food and Drug Commissioner Lucius P. Brown believed that physicians were the leading culprits in causing addiction.[18] He warned that "a very large proportion of the medical profession has either lost sight of the fact that the habitual use of an opiate produces a true disease, or never knew it." The withdrawal symptoms, he said, were a specific disease, possibly fatal if not forestalled by the readministration of opiates. In this conviction he was following information, readily obtained from journals and textbooks, that was the chief argument for the medical approach toward addiction—it was a true disease, not a mere habit conquerable by exertion of the will.

Brown outlined the state's options: either provide opiates to indigent addicts to prevent suffering and perhaps death, or provide "state curative treatment for all indigent addicts, with permanent commitment of those incorrigible to institutions for the feebleminded." After registering addicts and gathering statistics in Tennessee, the option of cure or commitment proved "to be out of the question . . . because of the enormous number of persons involved." The reasoning is simply stated: if addiction is a disease, the victim can hardly be made to suffer for what he cannot help and, if the state cannot build gigantic sanitaria, the necessary drug must be provided. Issues of degeneracy, criminal behavior possibly induced by drugs, and moral turpitude leading to addiction were ignored by the Commissioner. The physician or druggist was seen as the chief wrongdoer and the state as the inevitable and reluctant caretaker.

In meeting the problem of addiction the state must prevent abuse of prescriptions. Numerous regulations were intended to assure that certified addicts received drugs at only one store and that the amount was recorded. When the permit was renewed an attempt was supposed to be made to lessen the amount of the drug allowed.

In the first twelve months of operation 2,370 persons were registered, of whom 86 percent used morphine. Only 1.3 percent used heroin, although it was thought that more heroin addicts remained unregistered, "inasmuch as this drug is used almost altogether for dissipation." Females outnumbered males two to one; the average age of addicts was 49 for both sexes and they had been addicts an average of eleven years. Although a fourth of the Tennessee population was black only a tenth of the addicts registered was black. Commissioner Brown suggested that this might be due to the fact that "the average Negro avoids as far as possible any contact with an official and to the fact that the Negro appears to use relatively less morphine, and more cocaine, than the white man." Cocaine was not included in registration because it was felt that no disease or "toxemia" was produced by it; one could stop cocaine without any dire physiological consequences. Commissioner Brown confidently placed the blame for the addict population: "Other investigations by me, as well as the experience of all other writers on this subject, would appear to indicate that well over 50 percent of existing cases of narcotic addiction are due to the indiscreet administration of drugs by physicians."

The Tennessee experience gives excellent information on heroin addiction. The suspicion that fewer than the actual number of heroin addicts were registered, and that heroin was used simply for dissipation, reflects attitudes toward the age group which used heroin: "youngsters from 15 to 25 years of age." Heroin was described as having "a very pronounced stimulant effect, and for that reason is largely used by boys and young men as a means of dissipation." The association between young men and boys and heroin was to be a repeated phenomenon in the decade 1910–20. Heroin's appeal for the adolescent seems to set it off from opium-smoking, morphine, laudanum, gum opium, etc. The age of heroin users was much lower than the average age of Tennessee's other registered addicts. Brown thought the habit, "as might be expected from the character of its devotees," would be difficult to cure and advised: "The sale of this drug ought to be hedged about with just as rigid and drastic restrictions as are possible to enact into law."

Neither Terry nor Brown was optimistic about cures in private sanitaria or by private physicians. Brown saw institutionalization as an impracticable ideal. For both, in fact, medical treatment did not mean cure, but prevention of suffering. But addiction maintenance would be associated in the public's mind with moral turpitude, the spread of vice and crime, indulgence in sensual delights, and the destruction of the human soul. In New York State, from 1913 to 1920, the full expression of these conflicting attitudes, as well as the interplay of mercenary and political influences, provides an instructive record.

NEW YORK STATE ANTINARCOTIC LEGISLATION

Accredited as a world authority on narcotics, Charles B. Towns proposed his own antinarcotic law to the New York Legislature in early 1913 and had it introduced by Senator John J. Boylan. Towns's bill had been endorsed by the Kings County Medical Society.[19] From the well established, Towns had little trouble,[20] but from the rank and file medical man who was then beginning to organize to better his economic and social status, he evoked hostility and resentment. The general practitioner's distaste for Towns and his antinarcotic bill is apparent in some provisions of his proposal which were too extreme to be approved in 1913.

Some elements were legitimate attempts to require that a prescription include the address and legible name of the prescriber, prohibit fraudulent professional credentials, and monitor transactions between wholesalers and retailers. All prescriptions for habit-forming drugs would be filled in on special forms serially numbered and retained for inspection by the pharmacist. Towns claimed that these measures would overcome the problems of fraud in obtaining narcotics and ignorance of the amounts of narcotics sold to physicians and druggists, and keep the continued supply of narcotics to patients under the control of physicians. Such restrictions could not be faulted except on grounds of excessive paper work for the busy physician and druggist. Towns did not, however, recommend an exemption clause for proprietaries, and this alone would have killed the measure. But perhaps the major opposition among physicians was created by his proposed restrictions on narcotic prescribing. For example, he would limit to three weeks the time a physician could freely dispense narcotics to a patient. Continuation thereafter would require approval from the local health department. This constraint was introduced to prevent the practitioner from indefinitely "treating" an addicted patient who could not be cured on an ambulatory regimen. Towns suggested that if a patient was addicted he should be offered medical treatment in a sanitarium, say for a week, and, if judged incurable, be furnished drugs cheaply by the local health authority.[21]

Such an unprecedented legislative restriction on the private physician did not go unnoticed and could not have been more effectively designed to stimulate the fear and enmity of the general practitioner. Although the direct loss of income might not have been great for most, the transfer of service responsibilities to health departments continued what the GP considered a trend of government competition for the patient's dollar. The cure of addicts would be shunted to sanitaria, probably operated by "hospital doctors," the unpopular elite of the profession.

By this effort to control the medical care of addiction, Towns set himself up as an enemy of the average physician in New York City. He was called a fraud who sought legislation that would injure the unfortunate addict, to Towns's pecuniary advantage,[22] attacked as practicing medicine without a license, and accused of hiring physicians on contract, a high-ranking sin among doctors. Towns's comrade, Alexander Lambert, was a strong proponent of health insurance, annual licensing of physicians, and the establishment of a standard fee schedule. Towns's antinarcotic law was opposed more for its threat to traditional freedom of medical practice than for its goal of restricting narcotic use. Thus two forces were set against each other—a growing public demand that physicians be restrained from complete freedom in narcotic dispensing, and the medical profession's fear that the state would dominate the practice of medicine.

At the same session of the New York Legislature that rejected Towns's suggestions, a new cocaine law was enacted through the leadership of Assemblyman Alfred E. Smith.[23] So many elaborate restrictions were placed around cocaine that there was little opportunity thereafter for its legal distribution in any significant amount by physicians or patent medicine manufacturers. The passage of the cocaine law reflected the total condemnation of that drug in American society. Opiates remained controlled by older laws with many loopholes.[24] A modern law that would keep step with increasing fear of opiates was not enacted until 1914.

Enforcement of the cocaine law had an important effect on the movement to control the availability of narcotics. The courts swelled with offenders who would not fulfill the requirements of the new and intricate law.[25] This result might placate public opinion, but a side effect of these arrests was the discovery that cocaine was only one of the delights offered in the "drug orgies" raided by police. Along with cocaine habitués, heroin users were found who were regulated only by the sanitary code of New York City. Heroin and cocaine became linked as drugs of dissipation that were without medical justification.[26]

The Boylan Act, New York, 1914

Public disclosure of drug abuse stimulated reformers to urge a new antinarcotic law for New York. Financial support for a committee came from Mrs. William K. Vanderbilt, Sr., who had interested herself in the drug cause, and thus the legal, correctional, and city officials who composed it were termed the Vanderbilt Committee. Although occasionally credited with the subsequent passage of the antiopiate Boylan Act, Mrs. Vanderbilt seems merely to have chosen a popular cause with which to associate her name. Not only was Towns again the major proponent of the bill, which John J. Boylan introduced, but Senator Boylan also described himself as the mouthpiece of Mr. Towns, and he strongly rejected any insinuations that Mrs. Vanderbilt influenced the bill's passage. "At one time," Boylan declared, "I sincerely feared that this 'assistance' from the group which bore Mrs. Vanderbilt's name would kill all effective anti-drug legislation for the session." [27]

The Boylan Act incorporated essential compromises which diluted the purity of the previous year's unsuccessful but more comprehensive bill.[28] The first compromise was an exemption from the law for proprietaries containing less per ounce than 2 grains of opium, ¼ grain of morphine, ¼ grain of heroin, 1 grain of codeine, or 10 grains of chloral hydrate. Prescriptions were to be completely filled out and could not include any of the controlled drugs unless the physician had first given the patient a physical examination. Also, pharmacists must verify by telephone or other means the authority of any prescription containing more than 4 grains of morphine, 30 grains of opium, 2 grains of heroin, 6 grains of codeine, or 4 drams of chloral hydrate. Narcotic prescriptions could not be refilled. Possession of narcotics without an authorized certificate prepared by the retailer would constitute a misdemeanor. Order blanks furnished by the state health commissioner were required in transactions between retailers and wholesalers. Records had to be kept of the retail transactions of any of the drugs and the record preserved for five years. Hypodermic syringes could be obtained only on prescription. The license of a registered professional could be revoked if he was addicted to the use of any habit-forming drug or convicted of any violation of the Boylan Act.

The Act permitted commitment of individuals regularly using habit-forming drugs to "a state, county, or city hospital or institutions licensed under the State Lunacy Commission." In order to preserve order in such institutions, there was provision for the transfer of recalcitrant addicts to institutions for disorderly vagrants, although they would be separated from other inmates.[29]

The Boylan Act may appear to have been a victory for Towns, but from his point of view there was at least one large defect. An action for commitment could be brought only against regular drug users who were *not* "under the direction and consent of a duly licensed physician." [30] Therefore the Act permitted the maintenance of addicts but restricted it to physicians. Nothing prohibited the physician from prescribing as large an amount of a habit-forming drug as he wished, although the prescription could not be refilled. In this respect the Boylan Act had created a potentially sizable number of patients who were bound to physicians by their need to obtain nonrenewable prescriptions and by the fear that without a personal physician they were liable to institutional commitment.

Between the enactment of the Boylan law on 14 April and its effective date on 1 July 1914, warnings were given by Towns to the "innocent" drug addicts—those who were not criminals and who might not even know they were addicted but were only aware that they had to keep taking certain medicines or proprietaries. He was quoted in the New York *Times*[31] as declaring that these new strictures would make it impossible for the involuntary fiends to secure more drugs from their physicians; but he was optimistic of results, if enough preparation were made for the influx of addicts to hospitals, since "it takes only five or six days to cure a drug fiend in a hospital." Such statements, in the face of the law which did in fact permit ambulatory maintenance, understandably confirmed the suspicions of doctors who had long been wary of Towns's sincerity and supposed lack of self-interest. But at least in this instance he did not blame the licensed professional for the drug habit, for he averred the principal cause of addiction was prior cigarette smoking, found in every case of the six thousand he had studied, long before the victim began to take drugs.

The *Times* asserted editorially on 1 July 1914 that drugs for habitual use were now outlawed. Education of the public about the provisions of the Boylan Act was apparently inadequate as reformers' dreams became reality. Hospitals were pressed to provide beds for users who volunteered for cure or were committed. Seventy-five beds were made available at Bellevue, fifty on Blackwell's Island, and some facilities were provided at the City Farm on Staten Island.[32] The City Inebriate Farm near Warwick in Orange County seemed a good place to set up a more permanent facility, but appropriations were difficult to obtain.

Urgency for treatment grew partly from the increasing number of drug-related arrests in New York. In 1914 there were 1,950 arrests for violation of drug laws in the city; 947 were convicted. In 1913 there had been only 511 arrests.[33] The increased arrests heightened concern; agitation for even stricter drug laws led in 1915 to amendments to the Boylan Act. Sales of drugs to minors so angered the legislature that such sales were upgraded to felonies. Record-keeping regulations for pharmacists were also tightened.[34] With the somewhat strengthened Boylan law and the federal Harrison Act coming into effect in March 1915, even more illicit drug transactions were uncovered. Although physicians could prescribe for addicts, it was said by such informed persons as Justice Cornelius Collins of the Court of Special Sessions that many physicians had stopped prescribing because they were uncertain about the law's provisions. The disinclination of doctors to maintain addicts, Justice Collins stated, was crowding court calendars to capacity with drug cases, and was causing more commitments for treatment and a widespread belief that the underworld was moving into the drug market to fill the vacuum left by the physicians.[35]

Once again the effect of police enforcement, particularly after the Harrison Act, was marked. Lieutenant Scherb, head of New York City's sixteen-man "dope squad," described the results:

> The poor victims who have been getting their dope from peddlers on the street are having a pretty rough time. From every report I get there is panic among them. Many of them are doubled up in pain at this very minute and others are running to the police and hospitals to get relief. Those who have been getting their drugs from dope doctors and fake-cure places are not so hard hit, because these traffickers have not been touched by the laws, but the poorer people, the men and women we call the "bums," who have always bought from street peddlers, are really up against it. The suffering among them is terrible.[36]

The cost of heroin on the streets rose from $6.50 an ounce to about $100 an ounce, according to the police. Hospitals took in those needing drugs and attempted cures by reduction.[37] But physicians at The Tombs prison reported in December 1914 that they doubted any quick cure, saying that it might take two months to get some users off drugs and that if they were then not isolated from drugs for at least a year, the outlook for cure was dim.[38] The problem of addiction became in 1914 and 1915 increasingly prominent and menacing to the public. Paradoxically, alarm was created by the enforcement of antinarcotic laws, which brought many users into court and caused the drug problem to appear greater than before enforcement. From Scherb's comment it is clear that the dope doctors and the fake-cure places were seen as islands of evil resistance in an otherwise fairly successful antidrug campaign. Public fear of dope peddlers grew with the increase in arrests. The medical profession, by obtaining a legal monopoly of the treatment and maintenance of addiction, also found itself a target for public animosity as other legal sources of supply were restrained.

The medical profession's response to their exposed position, like that of the pharmacists, was divided. Most doctors were not interested in having anything to do with addicts. They shared the prevailing view that addiction led to moral degeneracy and crime. The doctor who used minute amounts of morphine in his practice yearly was not concerned about the severity of narcotic restrictions. Charles Towns repeatedly got medical society support for his measures, which, if adopted as first drafted in 1913, would largely have excused private medical practitioners from the care of chronic addicts.[39]

But there were some physicians who rejected the attitude that addicts should be shunned. Without doubt some disagreed because there was a good income to be made from them. Others saw no harm in maintenance if it would enable a fairly normal life for a doubtfully curable individual. The *New York Medical Journal* denied in May 1915 that addiction was a vice, describing it as a "compromise or an adjustment to the conditions of life." [40] For some citizens, drugs were necessary to keep up with the American pace. Narcotic addictions would be the negative but perhaps unavoidable aspect of "the American way of life."

One source of organized resistance to the prohibition of addiction maintenance came from a physicians' group in New York City. These physicians opposed such a step as an element in a wider and more serious threat to the medical profession, which included health clinics, school nurses, fixed fee schedules, salaried and contract doctors, exclusiveness in granting hospital privileges, and an influx of other "foreign" ideas of social planning which would enslave and pauperize them. Recognition of this attitude places the narcotic debate in the context of larger professional and social issues.

In 1911, two groups of physicians in New York, the Yorkville Medical Society and the Medical Alliance, "began a systematic agitation for the protection and promotion of the economic interest of the medical profession." In the next two years more groups formed, and the need to coordinate their activities led to the formation in June 1913 of the Associated Physicians' Economic League, a federation of the Medical Alliance with the Brooklyn Physicians' Economic League, the Bronx Physicians' League, the Downtown Physicians' Protective League, and the Physicians' Protective League of New York. That same year the federation began publication of a periodical, the *Medical Economist,* which was either a propaganda sheet or a fearless defender of the GP, depending on one's viewpoint.[41] The periodical never gave Charles B. Towns or Alexander Lambert respite from criticism. It often declared the incompetence of the medical societies and urged its readers to fight for their views at Albany and City Hall. One of its proudest accomplishments, frequently cited as proof of the federation's effectiveness, was the exemption from ticketing and towing of physicians' cars while they were double-parked. Such practical accomplishments were its metier; it left science to the more effete medical societies.

The Associated Physicians' Economic League of New York spent much of its energy in the battle for antinarcotic laws favoring the general practitioner, but the fight to keep him as the primary agent of society responsible for the care and treatment of addicts was only part of a larger movement. The issues were economic betterment and the control of medical practice in ways acceptable to the GP. The specific faults denounced by the federation were contract practices (with social lodges, etc.), under which physicians were employed to treat a specific number of patients, each of whom paid the same modest premium. This contract physician violated the principle of payment for the amount or skill of work done: whether he worked two or twenty-four hours a day, he got the same salary. He also took patients away from fee-for-service physicians. The hospital dispensary which treated the poor at no cost was also a danger because of the ease with which the undeserving were believed to obtain enrollment. The league wanted only those demonstrably indigent to be treated; abusers of the system should be prosecuted. Unauthorized practice of medicine, by a prescribing pharmacist or by mail-order physicians, was similarly anathema, for which redress was sought in the legislature.

But even some regular private-practice physicians evoked the average practitioner's ire. Specialists maintained a stranglehold on the hospitals and on appointments to the hospital staff. The league complained that appointments were reserved for the influential. Even appointment as an intern seemed to be based on the applicant's race, religion, ancestry, and station, which had to be acceptable to the hospital directors. The system worked to the advantage of the few. The paying patients were bled by the consultant surgeon or specialist and hospital alike. In any event, the general practitioner was left out in the cold.[42] Through concentration on such evils, in a few years the league claimed a membership of several thousand, a sizable proportion of the practicing physicians in greater New York.[43]

Dr. Lester D. Volk rose in this movement to lead numerous forays against the federal government's efforts (successful after 1919) to separate the addict from the private physician. Earlier he had worked with greater success to mold the state antinarcotic laws in favor of the average practitioner. His remarkable career spanned the economic movement. In 1906, at the age of twenty-two, he had received his M.D. degree from the Long Island Medical School, but he soon became interested in law and politics. He was admitted to the bar and helped inaugurate the *Medical Economist,* of which he later became editor. His early interest in Theodore Roosevelt's Progressive Party and its radical social notions evolved into vigorous representation of the downtrodden GP. After a term as a Bull Moose assemblyman he declined renomination, switched from medicine to law, and established his second professional practice. After service as a medical officer in World War I, he enthusiastically and successfully championed veterans' bonuses and was soon elected as a Republican from Kings County to the House of Representatives. He served in Congress from 1920 to 1923, bitterly attacking Prohibition and the Harrison Act, particularly the regulations promulgated by the Treasury Department which prohibited maintenance or reduction supplies of narcotics to addicts. His public career ended after he had served as an assistant state attorney general from 1943 to 1958.[44]

Volk's appeal to the medical profession was modeled on the labor union movement:

> Membership in our leagues will mean to the physician what membership in his organization means to the working man and when we have once realized that we are not far removed from the level of the working man in our daily acts and duties, then we will lose the false sense of high position we so dearly love to assume towards the laity, but which we fail to maintain among ourselves. . . . Think organization, speak organization, and shout organization till by repetition it becomes a by-word.[45]

With regard to the narcotic problem, the league's first substantial success was to defeat, in cooperation with other medical societies, the proposal in the 1916 legislature known as the Boylan bill, which was more commonly referred to by the league as the Towns-Hearst bill because of its strong support from Towns and the Hearst papers (the New York *American* and *Journal*). This bill would have reclaimed some of the ideas advocated by Towns in 1913: three weeks was set as the usual limit for outpatient provision of an addict with narcotics, and an elaborate registration system for addicts was required; incurables would be furnished drugs by departments of health.[46]

The bill passed the Senate, but was not called up in the closing hours of the session by the Speaker of the Assembly. In order to settle the narcotics muddle which was becoming an annual donnybrook, the legislature authorized a joint committee of investigation composed of three assemblymen and two senators.[47] In time, the league's view of the narcotics problem would exert great influence over this committee. The investigation would mark the beginning of a decline in the influence of Towns and a temporary defeat in New York for those who wished to forbid maintenance of chronic addicts.

The Whitney committee began taking testimony in December 1916 in New York. As the various treatments for addiction were presented it became obvious that the medical profession had no consensus on how treatment should proceed or which treatment was most efficacious.[48] But maintenance was also deplored by such distinguished witnesses as the Commissioner of Health of the City of New York, Dr. Haven Emerson, who questioned the social and medical "propriety" of narcotics furnished to addicts by the Health Department.[49] Even under the amended Boylan Act, which permitted the maintenance of addiction under a physician's supervision, the Health Department did not encourage such treatment.[50] Justice Cornelius Collins testified to an increase in drug use in spite of recent laws, while other witnesses estimated the number of addicts in New York City alone to be about 200,000.[51]

The committee welcomed Dr. Ernest Bishop, who had worked with addicts at Bellevue and was especially interested in their medical treatment. Unlike Dr. Emerson, Dr. Bishop found nothing wrong with furnishing drugs to addicts of long standing. He had for several years strongly advocated the medical as opposed to the enforcement approach to addiction. His publications gave the impression that the practitioner could usually treat the opiate slave, not by a routine specific regimen of drugs but by the kind of individualized traditional treatment which the private doctor accorded his other patients. As the influence of Towns and his claims for a specific treatment seemed to imperil maintenance of addiction by the private physician, Dr. Bishop became more outspoken in his denial that a specific cure existed. He pointed out the inadequacy of institutions if all addicts presumed to exist were made to undergo isolated treatment. He asserted that addicts most probably were upright citizens who wished to be cured but had been discouraged by worthless treatments. He saw only one course: "the rational handling and care of existing conditions at the hands of reputable general practitioners of medicine." [52]

Opposition to maintenance came from equally concerned and sympathetic individuals who believed that the outpatient treatment failed because patients were not isolated from drugs or because of the ineffective ministration of charlatans. All sides agreed that institutions existed which were of value only to the proprietors. Justice Collins, a middle-of-the-road critic of Bishop's view, speaking in early 1919, tried to fend off suggestions that there was no effective treatment.

Although it may be said that while conditions make absolutely necessary a reliance, in the main, upon treatment by the general practitioner, that conclusion does not militate against institutional treatment, when and where available. There is, undoubtedly, an appealing necessity at this time for the establishment of hospitals or parts of hospitals devoted to the cure of drug addiction with facilities for after care, and a step in this direction will be a veritable godsend. [53]

The investigators' Preliminary Report to the Legislature in February 1917 used the approach, and in several instances almost the wording, of the report on addiction which had been adopted by the physicians' league. [54] Some of the chief positions taken by the Preliminary Report included:

1. "The problem of narcotic drug addiction has passed all bounds of reasonable comprehension in the state of New York and in the United States [and has become] the greatest evil with which the Commonwealth has to contend at the present time."

2. "Lack of understanding and appreciation of the disease of narcotic addiction and its treatment by a large majority of the medical profession has fostered conditions which make it impossible to determine a rational procedure for treating and curing the addicted by the state at this time."

3. "The constant use of narcotics produces a condition in the human body that physicians of medical authority now recognize as a definite disease, which diseased condition absolutely requires a continued administration of narcotics to keep the body in normal function unless proper treatment and cure is provided."

4. "Those afflicted with this disease express every desire to secure humane and competent treatment and cure and . . . drug addiction is not confined to the criminal or defective class of humanity."

5. "State investigation of . . . cures and institutions is recommended."

6. "Your committee believes it to be one of the first duties of the state, in dealing with this grave situation, to establish a supply of narcotic drugs, to which the confirmed addict shall have access, under proper state regulation, pending the establishment of rational and recognized scientific treatment for his disease."

7. "Proper and humane treatment and cure should be provided for the addict by the state and necessary legislation enacted to prevent the spread of narcotic addiction."

8. Evidence presented to the committee indicated that legal distribution had declined while public consumption had greatly increased; the committee concluded that the addict must be getting his drugs illegally and that this had occurred because pharmacists and physicians "either through misunderstanding of the law or the true nature of the addict's disease, have refused to prescribe or dispense narcotic drugs to the sufferer."

9. A more thorough system of recording transactions in narcotics should be developed and a register of addicts compiled, under proper safeguard for confidentiality.

10. Provisions for commitment should be broadened to include "commitment of said addicts to the care of a reputable physician . . . provided that the person so committed shall have on hand sufficient funds to defray the expense of such treatment."

Widespread rejection of the medical approach was ascribed to predominant attitudes: the majority of physicians and of the public were joined in their distaste for addicts. But the Whitney Committee was able to demonstrate to the legislature that, regardless of the emotional attitude, some compromise had to be struck between addicts' cravings and the availability of the drugs.

On the whole, the medical societies and the league approved of the law which grew out of the investigation.[55] The first Whitney law was signed by the governor on 9 May 1917. It superseded the Boylan law and specifically stated that physicians could treat addicts for their comfort, a circumstance permitted under the Boylan law but apparently considered insufficiently practiced. The relevant section reads in part:

It shall be lawful . . . for any duly licensed physician after a physical examination, personally conducted, to administer to, or prescribe for any person, whom such examination discloses is addicted to the use of any habit-forming drugs . . . in reasonable quantities dependent on the condition of such person and his progress toward recovery, provided that such physician acts in good faith, solely for the purpose of relieving physical stress or of effecting a cure of such habituates.[56]

The medical societies opposed registration of addicts and the requirement that a list of such patients be furnished each month to the State Board of Health.[57] But another provision may have assuaged some of their pain. Section 249 provided that an addict might be paroled by a magistrate to a physician rather than an institution if it "satisfactorily appears to such magistrate that such addict is able to defray the expense of competent medical treatment." [58]

One further major change (Section 249) relaxed the legal restraints on providing drugs to the addicted: local boards of health were permitted to furnish without charge prescriptions for drugs "to provide for necessities of such person, pending treatment."

Justice Collins believed this first Whitney law caused 50 percent reduction in the number of court cases for illegal possession and it checked underworld exploitation. Explicit provision for medical treatment by the local physician aided the situation, he believed, and he credited the "honorable practitioner of medicine [with] splendid service to the community." Yet a new problem developed, demonstrating a sort of hydraulic model of drug traffic. Once the underworld was partially blocked, the physician—at least unprincipled physicians—began to dispense narcotics with no regard for minimal doses or no attempt to cure but "to reap dishonorable profit, which in some instances is quite large." [59] Also, there was no scheme to prevent an addict from being treated by several physicians at the same time and thereby garnering a large supply of drugs for sale or personal use. Although preferable to an underworld supply, the promiscuous distribution by physicians called for some control.[60] This seemed to be immediately necessary because additional hearings of the Whitney Committee, in the winter of 1917–18, indicated growth of the habit. Estimates of addiction rates up to 5 percent of New York City's population were offered to the committee.[61]

A new fear arrived with American entry into World War I in April 1917. Concern grew that servicemen would become addicted by pushers, at the instigation of disloyal elements or spies at home or through use of morphine and heroin on the battlefield. Therefore, as severe as the problem might seem on the home front, when the soldiers returned conditions would be even worse.[62] What could be done? A disreputable minority of physicians took advantage of the legal encouragement for maintenance, but shutting off the prescriptions of the medical profession would lead again to underworld traffic. The new menace, heroin, increasingly afflicted youth in eastern cities so that the average age of the heroin addict in court was 22, with a very large number between ages 17 and 22.[63] The result of this deteriorating situation was another major legal revision, the Second Whitney Act, in May 1918. The new law established the independent State Commission of Narcotic Drug Control, with authority to issue and modify regulations as it seemed desirable.[64] An elaborate system of prescription forms was planned to get a firm hold on the number of addicts in the state and some gauge of their addiction.

The Final Report of the Whitney Committee, submitted to the legislature on 1 March 1918, reiterated the major contentions of the Preliminary Report. The report also concluded that the drugs of addiction, including heroin and cocaine, were useful and should not be totally banned. A central state authority should establish policy for the control of addiction in cooperation with federal authorities; and, "as soon as the financial condition of the state will permit," the state should provide an institution for treatment of addiction and its scientific study.[65]

Somewhat surprisingly the medical economic leagues favored a powerful commissioner of narcotics who would oversee and direct the treatment of addiction.[66] Perhaps its early support rested on the hope that Republican Senator Whitney, a man whose views the league accepted, would be appointed commissioner. But Frank Richardson was named by Governor Whitman, although Senator Whitney did become First Deputy Commissioner with responsibility for the New York City area. Then, upon the election of Democrat Alfred E. Smith as governor, Walter C. Herrick, a former state senator, became commissioner and Senator Whitney was replaced by Sarah Graham-Mulhall, an energetic reformer. To the resentment of some physicians, neither Richardson nor Herrick seemed to favor the private practitioner as an addiction therapist but sought to establish clinics throughout the state which would draw the addicted away from the GP into the purview of the state.[67] In these clinics addicts would receive their drugs, in some even be encouraged to take treatment in an institution. The clinics, scattered across the state, were in many cases patronage awarded to a physician of the right party—a franchise on addict prescriptions in his town. Some doctors made the venture quite profitable, others were uninterested in the job. But Herrick, by this kind of administration, opened the commission to charges of political spoilage and removed the addict from those vocal private practitioners who wished to treat addicts themselves. His increasingly elaborate restrictions and paper work further increased the anger of the professionals as well as the drug-takers.

The Department of Narcotic Drug Control became operative on 1 February 1919, taking over the work of the Bureau of Habit-Forming Drugs from the State Department of Health. The department was composed of a commissioner, three deputy commisssioners, a chief clerk, and five clericals. With this staff the department faced the 20,000 physicians, druggists, dentists, veterinarians, manufacturers, and wholesalers who would communicate via piles of order blanks, registrations, etc. Soon plans were made to establish narcotic clinics in cities and communities in the state where those suffering from the disease of drug addiction could receive treatment.

The plan of the first commissioner, Frank Richardson, was clear, and one which his successor Herrick also followed: physicians and druggists who took unfair advantage of these unfortunates were to be identified from the records, and when the narcotic clinics were established, but not before, the department would "feel justified in revoking the authority of the physicians and druggists to treat and dispense narcotic drugs to those addicted."

After the department had been functioning for a year, Herrick estimated that there were about 39,000 addicts in the state, of whom 13,000 were registered through the physicians by whom they were treated.[68] This total is substantially less than such figures as 200,000 which the Whitney Committee had accepted as reasonable. Herrick emphasized the involuntary cravings of an addict, contrasting him to the drunkard who "can, if he will, make a sudden determination and quit the habit forever." [69]

When the reports began to pour in, it became apparent that some physicians and druggists were buying gigantic amounts of narcotics or prescribing large amounts which appeared to be commercial transactions rather than the careful and regulated dosage the law implied by treatment "in good faith." The effect of such practice was detrimental to the program as a whole. Individuals opposed to the idea of maintenance held up these professionals as criminals and an example of what happens if thousands of variously trained physicians were allowed to do whatever their judgment indicated. The person who favored maintenance was troubled by the knowledge that these leaks in the system made restriction of narcotics to the chronically addicted very unlikely, and it was suspected that the leaks were also being used to create new addicts.

Among druggists, only a minority would deal with such prescriptions since "most of the reputable drugstores find the trade with addicts very disagreeable and fill only a few such prescriptions or none at all." Among those who did deal with prescriptions, many violations were discovered. Part of the basement of one New York drugstore was knee-deep in copies of used official prescription forms; 6,000 were filled in the month of November 1919 alone. In some drugstores only narcotics were available. It was said, the commissioner reported, that one of these druggists had made $75,000 in one year from this trade. Three stores in New York reported that during the month of November 1919 they had filled 6,148, 3,111, and 1,975 prescriptions, respectively; "ordinary drugstores" filled perhaps 50 each during the same month.

But it was among the physicians that the commission found its biggest headaches. Understaffed (there was only one inspector for New York City, at an annual salary of $1,320) the commissioner was constantly hampered in his investigation and regulation of the more than 10,000 physicians registered with the department. Those who were unscrupulous seemed as inventive as the addicts in their evasion of the law's intent. Physicians generally did not want to send in the names of patients who were addicts, for a variety of understandable reasons. Therefore they took advantage of exceptions in the 1918 Second Whitney Act, which permitted prescription on "unofficial" and unreported prescription blanks, to prescribe for large amounts of narcotics as if treating a "surgical case or a disease other than drug addiction." Herrick reported with irony:

> The peculiar thing about these unofficial prescription blanks is the fact that some doctors prescribe narcotic drugs as if they were really remedies or cures for diseases instead of being the means by which extreme suffering and pain can be deadened. An innumerable number of patients so treated were receiving no medicines other than these drugs. [*Second Annual Report*, p. 25.]

Of course, discovery of this state of affairs was dependent on investigation of the drugstores' and doctors' files by what inspectors were available—"a very difficult problem of administration." The reaction to this misuse of "unofficial prescription blanks" was the inevitable tightening and rephrasing of regulations so that the loophole was eliminated. Therefore the commissioner ordered in late 1920 the end of unofficial prescriptions and required all narcotics to be prescribed on official forms, copies of which had to be sent to the department within 24 hours of dispensing.[70] It had been estimated that 5,000 addicts were receiving their drugs under the unofficial system, some from more than one doctor and filling their prescriptions at more than one drugstore. But closing this gap only brought more anger from the private physicians who, one can assume, knew well what they were doing when they kept an addict's name from registration.

Although physicians such as Dr. Bishop and Dr. Volk advocated outpatient treatment of addicts on a maintenance or gradual reduction regimen, the Commissioner of Narcotic Control did not interpret the physician's task in so indefinite a manner. He constantly sought reports of cures from private physicians. These were so rare that the reduction method seemed only a feeble excuse for providing a permanent supply. Even the honest doctor could not prevent the addict from also being treated by another doctor, and when the reduced dose became uncomfortable, the addict would either insist and receive a higher one or go elsewhere permanently. One physician achieved some kind of record by giving out in one day 835 official prescriptions.

The number of such doctors and druggists the department had under careful observation was fairly small (e.g. thirteen physicians and twenty-two drugstores in New York City in 1919) but the number of their "patients" was large.

Having adopted the view that the ambulatory method did not cure and legalization of maintenance made effective control of drugs difficult for the state, Commissioner Herrick in April 1920 declared that institutional treatment should be preferred and whenever possible addicts should be sent to one for withdrawal of the drug. After about two weeks, the addict should then be sent somewhere else for rehabilitation, learning a trade or whatever, but not back to the conditions that encouraged drug addiction in the first place. In this regard, the existence of legal ambulatory treatment was particularly discouraging, because whenever the craving for drugs returned to the recently institutionalized addict he merely had to go to a physician or peddler and get back on the habit. Herrick recognized the need for aftercare and general rehabilitation, not just withdrawal of the drug. But his proposal was remarkably optimistic considering the discouraging results by 1920 from institutional care. Also, the provision for such care in New York State was meager, "embarrassing . . . the Department when it found reason to disapprove of a doctor's method of treatment and especially so in its attempts to get the addicts to turn over a new leaf." Herrick was caught in a now familiar dilemma—if maintenance was provided, abuse of distribution occurred and accurate control of the drugs was extremely difficult, cure a rarity; on the other hand, refusing maintenance and mandating institutional treatment was predicated on the false belief that institutions cure addiction, as well as patently increasing the number of illegal channels. It is interesting that as late as 1920 Herrick could make such a strong plea for institutional care; he explained away the failure of drug withdrawal by lack of good follow-up.

The department's staff was small and unpopular. In addition to the one inspector for New York City there was a stenographer and a file clerk. Deputy Commissioner for New York City, Sarah Graham-Mulhall, was forced to move from one address to another because of the feeling against addicts. She finally set up an office in her own home from which she was protected from dislodgment.[71]

The commission asked for more financial aid from the state in order to build a larger staff and to be more effective, but Commissioner Herrick was soon to discover that an opposite course would be taken and the commission along with all the state narcotic laws would simply be abolished. This resulted from a head-on collision between state and federal approaches toward narcotic control. Federal control had been strengthened by an amendment to the Harrison Act in February 1919, and in the following month a very strict ruling by the Supreme Court essentially outlawed the maintenance of addiction and even the reduction method and ambulatory treatment.

The Federal Assault on Addiction Maintenance

6

The Harrison Act became effective on 1 March 1915. Enforcement was assigned to the Bureau of Internal Revenue within the Treasury Department.[1] The revenue agents had had long experience with smuggling, evasion of tax stamps, and so on, by manufacturers and retailers and were thus prepared to regulate physicians and the drug trades. By 30 June 1916, 124,000 physicians, 47,000 retail druggists, 37,000 dentists, 11,000 veterinarians, and 1,600 manufacturers, importers, and wholesalers had been registered.[2] The accumulation of information from records was large, and any systematic attempt to scrutinize the records was impossible. When violations came to the attention of the revenue agents, they moved in. After evidence had been gathered, a federal district attorney took charge of the cases and sought indictments.

The first questions to arise were: Could any actions other than nonregistration and faulty record keeping violate the Harrison Act? If records were carefully kept and the dealer was registered and displayed his tax stamp, what other wrong could he do? Influential members of the pharmaceutical profession, like lawyer-pharmacist James Beal, replied with assurance that if the simple record requirements were obeyed, the federal government should be fully satisfied. Doctors and medical journals which had supported the Harrison bill believed that the otherwise annoying record keeping would strengthen the medical profession's control of these potent medicaments. Similarly, pharmacists saw HR 6282 as an aid in securing trade that might go elsewhere and a step toward the long-desired allocation to pharmacists of the sole right to dispense medicines.[3] But when federal agents tried to prevent addicts from being supplied for their comfort and not for diseases, some former advocates in the profession howled in anguish. Protests to the Treasury and Justice Departments quickly revealed the variety of their motives in supporting the Harrison Act, which ranged from financial advantage to the hope of reducing by 90 percent the use of narcotics in the United States.

ENFORCEMENT OF THE HARRISON ACT

In mid-January of 1915 the Treasury Department promulgated the regulations under which the Harrison Act would be enforced.[4] Although a regulation could not legitimately make a new law or add to what Congress had intended in the original act, details of the regulations would affect sensitive professional and trade issues. The first surprise to some physicians was the discovery that "in personal attendance" did not simply mean in the presence of a patient but required the doctor to be away from his usual place of business.[5] This regulation therefore required much more record keeping than some physicians had expected, but it had already been accepted by congressional lobbyists of medical and pharmaceutical interests in the summer of 1914.[6]

The regulations also declared that "a consumer, as such, will not be permitted to register under this law and can only obtain a supply of such drugs through a duly registered physician, dentist or veterinarian." [7] Therefore an addict could not register, as he did in Tennessee for example, and receive a regulated supply of habit-forming drugs. The new interpretation left registered professionals as the only legal source of supply. In turn, registrants were hedged in by record-keeping provisions (with heavy penalties for error) so that their prescribing philosophies could be monitored. The possession of narcotics through unregistered channels would be, the Treasury averred, prima facie evidence of violation of the Act; under Section 8 the possessor had the burden of proving that he had legally obtained the drug. As for addicts' possessing drugs to satisfy their cravings, the department would argue that even if the addict had a prescription for a maintenance supply, it only appeared to be a prescription: a valid prescription aimed at cure would be a "normal" dose. These administrative interpretations met with some difficulty in the courts.

One of the first public indications that the goal of federal enforcement was prohibition of narcotics for nonmedical addiction maintenance may have been a rather vague phrase in additional regulations published 9 March 1915. Druggists were warned to examine each narcotic prescription submitted to determine whether the physician's signature was forced "or that the quantity of drug prescribed was unusually large." [8] A likely explanation of this language would be that the bearer might raise the originally prescribed amount. But the department may have also sought to place on druggists some review responsibility over physicians, a burden the retail pharmacists almost invariably declined.

From the first days of the Harrison Act, revenue agents began to arrest physicians and druggists who provided drug supplies to addicts via "prescriptions," but the most common method of enforcing compliance was through stern warnings. In this regard, a druggist in Helena, Montana, wrote the Attorney General on 18 May 1915 asking for advice. He had technically correct cocaine prescriptions for six users, but "the revenue agents who are neither lawyers nor physicians tell me that these prescriptions are in excessive amounts." Since the physician insisted that the doses were not excessive for the users, the druggist was placed "in an anomalous position." He wanted "a straight-out, clear-cut answer and not a vague one that will still leave us to our own opinions and the resulting friction with different inspectors."

The Attorney General replied that this aspect of the Harrison Act was "a proper matter for the determination of the judiciary," and he could not comply with the druggist's request. His formal and brief reply covered a difference in opinion between the Internal Revenue Bureau and the Justice Department. Many U.S. attorneys actually agreed with the druggists that the law was vague in this matter, although this opinion was not publicly available.[9] The Treasury Department, however, believed it could decide the issue posed by the druggist by framing a new regulation, TD 2200, on 11 May. Part of this decision relates directly to narcotic maintenance.

> Where a physician, dentist, or veterinarian prescribes any of the aforesaid drugs in a quantity more than is apparently necessary to meet the needs of a patient in the ordinary case, or where it is for the treatment of an addict or habitué to effect a cure, or for a patient suffering from an incurable or chronic disease, such physician, dentist, or veterinarian surgeon should indicate on the prescription the purpose for which the unusual quantity of the drug so prescribed is to be used. In cases of treatment of addicts these prescriptions should show the good faith of the physician in the legitimate practice of his profession by a decreasing dosage or reduction of the quantity prescribed from time to time.[10]

The Philadelphia *Medical World*, a practical and economically oriented journal for the general practitioner, was outraged at the Treasury regulations which forbade maintenance. The editors had advocated the Harrison Act, but were apparently unaware of the goals or compromises involved in its passage. The *Medical World* distinguished between the professional treatment of a habitué, even if indefinite, and the "mere pandering to the desires of dope fiends." [11] Like the *Medical Economist* in New York, the Philadelphia journal did not condone the mere selling or catering to dope fiends, but on the other hand it felt that physicians were well within their rights in maintaining addicts until a cure came along.[12] The distinction between maintaining and pandering seemed to be in the way in which the narcotic was transmitted to the patient. If the addict merely picked up a prescription and gave over his quarter or half dollar, and if, say, more than twenty addicts did this a day in a physician's office, then he was pandering. But if the number of addicts was small, and if the prescription was given in a less hurried and more professional manner, particularly should there be any attempt to discourage use of narcotics to produce euphoria, the patient was "treated." This distinction appeared to be the primary dividing line between respectability and infamy; the physiological state of the patient and the effect of the drug were irrelevant. Thus the strength of the journal's argument for distinguishing the "dope doctor" from the physician who "treated indefinitely" was not apparent outside the profession.

Later the *Medical World* shifted its attack on the new regulation by conceding that "doctors of the right kind do not dispense narcotics to habitués. Few, if any, of the panderers to the dope fiends are within the medical profession, and those that are should be expelled." Dispensing, however, was the point at which the Commissioner's rulings were now declared "unjust and not warranted by law." [13] Such federal restrictions were unusual in 1915 and seemed threatening to the profession's independence. The country practitioner was especially hard hit by the inconvenience to his own dispensing; the city specialist who approved of the Harrison Act was not in a position to see the plight of his less fortunate colleagues.

The Treasury Department's opposition to maintenance was not much of an aid to the Justice Department, which even by the date of TD 2200 (ten weeks after the Harrison Act became law) was having considerable trouble convincing federal district judges that registered physicians did not have the right to prescribe as they wished to anyone they wished. To be valid, the Treasury decision had to arise from the statute, and was subordinate to it. Therefore cases had to be argued on the words of the statute. The Harrison Act made no mention of addicts and, although the wording seemed clear to the reformers, it did not define for indifferent or hostile interpreters "legitimate practice of medicine" and "good faith" in prescribing. The manifest lack of federal power to regulate medical practice as well as the need to unify professional support of the Harrison Act may have required these vague phrases.

The chief problem the Justice Department encountered in the attempt to prohibit maintenance of addiction was that federal courts thought any federal regulation of medical practice unconstitutional. The negative attitude of district judges to the government's interpretation of the Harrison Act was found in numerous jurisdictions (Montana, Pennsylvania, and Tennessee) within the first few months of aggressive enforcement against addict-maintaining physicians.[14]

The Justice Department usually followed a set procedure whenever a professional was arrested. The federal attorney did not charge the physician with malpractice but sought an indictment that would include the physician, the druggist, and the addict. Section 8 of the Harrison Act made possession of narcotics by any unregistered person unlawful unless they were obtained from a physician who prescribed in good faith. The Act also placed the burden of proof upon the defendant. Therefore the physician and the druggist could be charged with conspiracy to place the drugs unlawfully in the possession of the addict by prescribing and dispensing, the prescription not having been made in good faith but only to maintain the addict's habit. Or, an indictment would charge the physician with aiding and abetting the addict to secure drugs which he could not legally possess.[15]

A conspiracy indictment had the advantage of potentially punishing the sequence of wrongdoers at the retail and consumer level. It rested on the assumption that the maintenance of addiction was illegitimate medical practice and could not be conducted in good faith. Of the many questions that district attorneys directed at the Attorney General and the Treasury Department, none questioned this moral assumption. Rather, the question raised was whether the Harrison Act could sustain violations of this morality as an illegal act. Public complaints against dope doctors also assumed that the maintenance of addiction was a convenient and profitable activity by physicians and druggists without any pretense of cure. Examples of such transactions were numerous and blatant in many communities. The legal attack on maintenance was begun on the first day of March 1915, without any hesitation or doubt among Treasury officials that this was a chief goal of the Harrison Act, an interpretation that proved ill founded when tested in the courts.

The first setback occurred in Pittsburgh, in May, where the district judge declared that since the Harrison Act did not permit an addict to register, he could hardly be held to possess narcotics illegally. The department quickly obtained a writ of error from the Supreme Court and sought to have the decision reversed. In June a similar decision was rendered by Judge John E. McCall in Memphis, much to the dismay of the United States attorney who was desperately trying to stop flagrant sales of narcotics through "drug stores" which existed primarily to fill narcotic prescriptions.[16] In one instance the physician moved his office into the front of the shop and wrote out prescriptions for customers who had them filled on the spot. In ten weeks the store filled over a thousand prescriptions for powdered opium, heroin, and cocaine. United States Attorney Hubert F. Fisher complained to the Justice Department:

> Prescriptions which are and have been so promiscuously written by physicians can hardly be called "prescriptions" meant by Congress in passing this Act, still the words are in the Act and a registered physician signs the paper which is relied upon by the druggist.[17]

The first warrants for arrest in Memphis closed down dealers in drugs which could not be registered under the Harrison Act, but this move, Fisher continued, "had the effect of narrowing the fight down to the sale by the drug stores, upon prescriptions by physicians. . . . Prior to March 1, Memphis had been a bad place for the sale of cocaine, opium and heroin, the lax enforcement of the State antinarcotic law having brought about the promiscuous bootlegging of prohibited drugs." The Harrison Act improved the situation somewhat but seemed to afford no avenue of attack against drug-supplying doctors and druggists.

A similar problem arose in Florida when one pound of granulated opium was prescribed for a person not registered under the Harrison Act. The district judge upheld the constitutionality of the Act but directed a verdict of not guilty to the jury. The judge believed that "there was nothing in the law to limit the quantity that a physician might prescribe," that by the law this was left to the discretion of the physician. The court also held that a doctor was not required to prescribe only such quantity of the drug as might be sufficient for immediate needs of the patient; in other words, if the patient was a habitué, the "physician could prescribe such quantity of the drug as in his opinion was necessary for the use of the patient for several days." [18]

By September 1915, Assistant Attorney General William Wallace, Jr., chief strategist for the Harrison Act indictments, conceded to a questioning Denver attorney that "the present condition of the enforcement of the law is not entirely satisfactory." The U.S. attorney for Colorado had grave doubts that a registered physician could be successfully prosecuted for prescribing "narcotic drugs to a patient who is a habitual user thereof without any intent to cure." After analysis of the Act's wording the attorney concluded that "it would seem to us to be a fair construction of the Act that a written prescription by a registered physician absolutely protects the physician from a charge of violating the Act, regardless of the fact that he was prescribing the same to drug fiends without any intention of effecting a cure." Nevertheless, the attorney was under pressure by internal revenue agents to present a number of such cases to the next grand jury.[19]

A month later the government received bad news from Montana where Judge G. M. Bourquin dismissed cases against consumers who he felt were not permitted to register under the Act and therefore could not be punished for not registering.[20] In Kansas City, Kansas, the district judge had taken the presentation of indictments of alleged violators of the Harrison Act as an opportunity to deliver a strong statement in favor of civil freedom and against the encroaching powers of government bureaucracies. Although taking the arguments under advisement, the government attorneys realized that the public statements of the judge, prominently reported in the local press, were not good omens. The Attorney General sent detailed arguments to the local district attorney with the plea to "urge these arguments with all your power upon Judge Pollock, as it is important that the government should not suffer a defeat on the question of the constitutionality of the Act." The District Attorney in Baltimore received similar encouragement, although Assistant Attorney General Wallace admitted that the situation "is a difficult one because the United States Judges feel doubt as to the constitutionality of the law, and in most instances seem to be opposed to it." [21]

The fight to preserve the Act's constitutionality represents a retreat from aggressive prosecution of addict-maintaining physicians to a defense of the very existence of the Act itself. The instructions sent to district attorneys in late 1915 increasingly emphasized arguments for constitutionality and expressed displeasure with the progress of enforcement against physicians and druggists who were registered and prescribing for addicts. The internal revenue agents' enthusiasm for blocking addict maintenance was suffered patiently by the attorneys, who saw it as a very difficult legal issue.

One of the most instructive discussions of the physician's right to prescribe for addicts occurred between the U.S. attorney for Nevada and the collector of internal revenue in San Francisco. The collector gave the attorney voluminous evidence of two Reno physicians who had prescribed for addiction maintenance, and commented that the physicians seemed to be in direct conflict with TD 2200. In a detailed analysis of the Harrison Act, section by section, the attorney stated that although "the conduct of these physicians is most reprehensible, and not in the course of their professional practice" nevertheless,

> It is not clear to me that the writing of a prescription, even though there may be lacking good faith on the part of the physician, and it is not issued in the course of his legitimate professional practice, is embraced in any of the prohibitory sections of the Act, a violation of which constitutes a criminal offence.

In response, the collector, having received the same advice from the San Francisco district attorney, reluctantly agreed that such cases could not be prosecuted without a change in the statute. The Attorney General's office, reviewing this correspondence, advised as usual to proceed for conspiracy to violate Section 8 or to charge the physician with aiding and abetting the unregistered addict to have the drug in his possession. But the Justice Department recognized that if the Supreme Court ruled against the government's interpretation of Section 8 and affirmed the decision of the district judge in the Pittsburgh *Jin Fuey Moy* case, these recommended approaches would be invalidated.[22]

U.S. v. Jin Fuey Moy, 1916

With opposition from district judges throughout the nation to the Treasury's interpretation of Section 8, and with the Justice Department believing no other approach would be successful against maintenance physicians, the hearing before the Supreme Court on 7 December 1915 assumed considerable importance. The *Jin Fuey Moy* case, which so affected the early enforcement of the Harrison Act, was an attempt by the government simply to stop a physician from supplying an addict with drugs. Dr. Jin Fuey Moy, of Pittsburgh, had prescribed a dram (about 1.8 grams or 1/16 ounce) of morphine sulfate to Willie Martin, an addict. The physician, according to the government, conspired with the addict to place in the addict's possession morphine, not for medical purposes, "but for the purpose of supplying one addicted to the use of opium." Since it was illegal for anyone not registered under the Harrison Act to obtain morphine except by prescription written in good faith, Martin's possession was a violation of Section 8. The government's argument was the one favored by the Justice Department and contained the assumption that maintenance of addiction was not compatible with medical practice in good faith.

The district judge had quashed the indictment on grounds that Martin was not required to register under the Harrison Act since he did not "import, produce, manufacture, deal in, dispense, sell or distribute" the morphine, but merely consumed it. Therefore he could not violate the Harrison Act by merely having morphine in his possession.

The Act was understood by the lower court as strictly a revenue act and, if it went beyond revenue or interstate commerce powers, it might violate the provisions of the Constitution of the United States. Unconstitutionality, presumably, would arise by government's attempting to regulate directly the practice of medicine, a power reserved to the states.

In June 1916 the Supreme Court's decision in the *Jin Fuey Moy* case confirmed the Justice Department's doubts of the legality of directly attacking the maintenance physician. By seven to two the Court rejected the government's arguments for broad police powers under the Harrison Act.[23]

The Court's majority opinion, written by Justice Oliver Wendell Holmes, Jr., maintained that there was no indication in the wording of the Harrison Act that it was passed in fulfillment of treaty obligations and, even if it were, the details of Section 8 were not required by treaty. When one considers the years of agitation by the executive branch to get a domestic narcotic law to fulfill America's international pledges, the drafting of the law in the State Department and its intimate relation with the American-inspired Hague Convention, one can sympathize with the government's and Dr. Wright's anguish at this decision.

If the law was not in aid of a treaty and did not deal with a totally foreign substance, Congress had much less power to legislate in this area than the government claimed. The Court held, "Only words from which there is no escape could warrant the conclusion that Congress meant to strain its powers almost if not quite to the breaking point in order to make the probably very large proportion of citizens who have some preparation of opium in their possession criminal or at least *prima facie* criminal and subject to serious punishment." Like the lower court, the Supreme Court was critical of the provision in Section 8 which placed on the citizen burden of proof that the narcotic in his possession was obtained within the provisions of the Harrison Act. The Court would not even consider "prescribed in good faith" open to a broader interpretation, since the phrase was "so vague that it may have had in mind other persons carrying out a doctor's orders rather than the patient." [24] Justices Mahlon Pitney and Charles Evans Hughes dissented.

In the Treasury's annual reports of 1916, 1917, and 1918 vigorous requests were made to Congress to counteract this emasculating decision, by amending the Harrison Act. [25] The commissioner warned in reference to the *Jin Fuey Moy* case:

> This decision makes it practically impossible to control the illicit traffic in narcotic drugs by unregistered persons, as the mere possession of any quantity of the drugs is not evidence of violation, and therefore the government is forced to prove in every case, even where the circumstances indicate sale and dispensing, actual sales by this class of offenders, which it has been found difficult to do. [26]

According to the Internal Revenue Bureau, a large number of unregistered persons had been convicted under Section 8, now found inapplicable, and although they were quickly released from prison, there was evidently no statutory authority to return their fines. The law must be amended, the Treasury warned, if the nation was to be protected from the drug evil. In addition to making general statutes applicable to the Harrison Act, with regard to seizures, forfeitures, etc., other strengthening seemed necessary—specifically, the imposition of a tax on narcotics by weight and provision for stamped packages. Lack of a stamp would be evidence of illegal possession unless the drug was obtained through legitimate prescription. This would at least make cases against possessors of large amounts of unmarked narcotics easier to prosecute. Substantial revenue would also make the Act more believable as a tax measure since the courts had interpreted the antinarcotic law as a revenue act. Next, registration should be explicitly restricted to those lawfully engaged in dealing under the Act: alteration of records, forging of prescriptions, and lack of record keeping should be punished by suitable penalties.

Finally, Congress should provide some medical agency for treatment, a plea that would be repeated in subsequent annual reports and by many writers on the drug problem, but which would, for a variety of reasons, not be provided by the federal government until 1935, twenty years after the Harrison Act. In the belief that treatment was essential, the Internal Revenue Bureau would in 1919 support the establishment of clinics for temporary maintenance and seek the cooperation of the Public Health Service to take over federal responsibility for institutional treatment of indigent addicts deprived of drugs.

Although the Revenue Bureau appeared anxious to go after narcotic violators, attention directed at Harrison Act enforcement was modest until a separate Narcotic Division was established in the Prohibition Unit on 1 January 1920. This separation was reasonable, since the federal staff was not large and the primary responsibility of the Alcohol Division was to oversee the largest single source of internal revenue for the United States government. In the fiscal year 1916 the aggregate receipts from internal revenue were $513 million, of which the largest item was from distilled spirits ($153 million) and the second, fermented liquor ($88 million). Individual income tax accounted for only $68 million. Thus the Alcohol Division was too occupied to police the almost infinite details of the Harrison Act.[27]

The original and strict interpretation of the Harrison Act, which had been softened by the *Jin Fuey Moy* case of 1916, was reasserted in March 1919 by the Supreme Court in two crucial decisions. By a five to four decision the Court reversed a District Court dismissal of an indictment against Dr. Charles T. Doremus of San Antonio, who on 11 March 1915 had provided five hundred one-sixth grain tablets of morphine to a known addict. The lower court held that the restrictions on Dr. Doremus's practice were irrelevant to the collection of revenue and therefore exceeded the Constitutional powers of the federal government (*U.S.* v. *Doremus,* 246 Fed. Rep. 958, decided 2 January 1918). On appeal, Chief Justice White and Justices McKenna, Van Devanter, and McReynolds agreed with the district judge; Justices Day, Holmes, Brandeis, Pitney, and Clarke constituted the majority. This triumph of the reformers confirmed the constitutionality of the Harrison Act's tax on physicians and concomitant control over the manner in which the drugs could be dispensed, that is, "in the course of . . . professional practice only" and through "prescriptions" (*U.S.* v. *Doremus,* 249 U.S. 86, decided 3 March 1919).

Having affirmed the Act's constitutionality, the Court on the same day decided the other important issue: Could the legitimate practice of medicine include the maintenance of addicts? In this case a retail druggist, Goldbaum, and a practicing physician, Webb, had been indicted for conspiracy to violate the Harrison Narcotic Act by providing maintenance supplies of morphine to an addict with no intention to cure but "for the sake of continuing his accustomed use." A similarly divided Court concluded that to call "such an order for the use of morphine a physician's prescription would be so plain a perversion of meaning that no discussion of the subject is required" (*Webb et al.* v. *U.S.,* 249 U.S. 96).

THE RED SCARE OF 1919

The change in judicial outlook between 1915 and 1919 with regard to addiction maintenance was not the triumph of a minority but the majority's success in making a minority view intolerable. What had been a respectable viewpoint by 1915, although not the dominant attitude of the public—the value of addict maintenance by physicians or others—by 1919 and 1920 had come to seem a great danger and folly. Advocacy of maintenance was repressed as sternly as socialism. Vigorous protests from a few physicians, congressmen, politicians, and laymen were completely ineffective in modifying legal opposition to supplying drugs for the pleasure or comfort of addicts.

Between the *Jin Fuey Moy* decision in 1916 and the vigorous attack on addiction in 1919, profound social changes had occurred in the United States. World War I had been fought, the 18th Amendment had been adopted, and the liberalizing movements of La-Follette, Theodore Roosevelt, and Wilson had declined into a fervent and intolerant nationalism. As a corollary perhaps to the last change came an enormous fear of Bolsheviks and anarchists, which has been termed the Red Scare of 1919–20.

The Harrison Act appeared to both Republican and Democratic administrations a sound measure to protect the nation from the ravages of addiction. Its form as a tax measure was a familiar ruse to attain a moral end by constitutional means.

Having already been defined by most Americans as immoral or at least the cause of wasted lives, addiction by 1918 was perceived as a threat to the national war effort. Anything so perceived was likely to be in trouble. Any action interpretable as support for the enemies of the United States was punished severely, and the nation adjusted itself to a high level of intolerance and suspicion.[28]

The socialist Eugene V. Debs, who opposed the war and draft because he believed the whole matter a capitalist enterprise, was imprisoned for his actions under the Espionage Act of 1918, and his ten-year sentence was confirmed unanimously by the Supreme Court in a decision written by Justice Holmes and rendered a week after the basic antimaintenance decisions of Webb and Doremus.[29] Debs's arrest in 1918 came as the popular fear for national survival began to reach a sustained height. The growth of aggressive nationalism could be exemplified by Theodore Roosevelt's change from a strong liberalism in the campaign of 1912 to an anti-German spirit after 1915.[30] A. Mitchell Palmer, a leading Wilsonian, a champion of progressive child labor laws and the League of Nations, led the infamous raids against anarchists and Bolsheviks in 1919 which ignored rights of free speech, assembly, and due process and resulted, to his chagrin, in no evidence to justify his hysterical roundup.[31] Such astounding shifts in attitude were partly created by a fear based on explicit revolutionary and anarchic statements from domestic agitators. The Bolshevik success in Russia with a small number of dedicated Communists, and the happy anticipation by American Communists that a similar revolt would occur here, strengthened the fears of Americans already on guard against the dangers of the Kaiser, immigration, and a growing radical labor movement.

This intensely fearful period in American history must be borne in mind in evaluating the suppression at that time of dissent on the issue of narcotic control. Since narcotic use was officially described as leading to antisocial acts and individual degeneracy, the current fear of such conditions helps explain the public's angry opposition to anyone advocating the maintenance of such an evil.[32] As a consequence, the federal government could easily shut down the New York State maintenance clinics which were the product of several years of planning by its legislature. Furthermore, it helps explain the remarkable change of opinion in the Supreme Court to the point that the maintenance of addiction—the pandering to the sensual desires of habitués—was considered so obviously an immoral notion that the majority of the Court thought it not worthy of discussion or justification.[33] Indulgence in narcotics tended to weaken the nation and was associated with other un-American influences which would dissolve the bonds of society.

In this spirit the mayor of New York established a Committee on Public Safety in May 1919, to look into two specific problems which he saw as related: the heroin epidemic among youth and the bombings by revolutionaries.[34] Since narcotics use even in more peaceful times had evoked the image of a Negro cocainomaniac or a seductive Chinese, it was not that the popular image of the drug user changed but that the minority opinion in favor of maintenance became intolerable. As in so many issues in the period 1918–20, free expression of minority opinion was extinguished and maintainers of "dope fiends" went the way of the IWW.

Three weeks into the rabid year of 1919, the thirty-sixth state ratified the National Prohibition Amendment; one year would elapse before it became effective. Therefore the year 1919, which marked the crystallization of a national antinarcotic policy against maintenance, was also the year of preparation for liquor prohibition. Maintenance of addiction could no more be defended than maintenance of alcoholism. Both classes of indulgence were to be treated not by maintenance but by a remedy appropriate for social cancers: surgical extirpation.

THE SPECIAL NARCOTIC COMMITTEE
OF THE TREASURY DEPARTMENT, 1918–1919

Shortly after submission to the states of the 18th Amendment in December 1917, the federal government began planning revision of the Harrison Act to overcome the Supreme Court's adverse decision in the *Jin Fuey Moy* case. In March 1918, Commissioner of Internal Revenue Daniel C. Roper proposed to Treasury Secretary William McAdoo a special narcotic committee to study the problem of control and to recommend changes in the law and its administration. Roper alluded to the war, now a year old for the United States, as an especially appropriate background for restraint of drug use. Regulation of national habits for the purpose of creating wartime efficiency was a familiar expedient.[35]

The Treasury Committee, appointed 25 March 1918 by Secretary McAdoo, was a respectable and fairly representative group which combined bureaucratic expertise, congressional influence, and medical knowledge. Its purpose was to rectify adverse Court decisions so that the government could proceed with greater effectiveness against addiction maintenance. This goal was achieved, although not solely through the committee's influence.

The committee represented the federal government's position on drug control in 1918 and 1919 and provided antimaintainers with a very impressive voice. The chairman, Representative Henry T. Rainey of Illinois, was a powerful Democratic leader who would later become Speaker of the House.[36] The three other members were Dr. Reid Hunt, professor of pharmacology in Harvard Medical School and former Chief of the Division of Pharmacology in the U.S. Public Health Service (1904–13); B. C. Keith, Deputy Commissioner of the Internal Revenue Bureau, a coordinator of legislative efforts with regard to narcotics; and A. G. DuMez of the Public Health Service, who had become, after Wilbert's death the previous year, the service's chief expert on narcotics. Clerk to the committee was a physician, Dr. B. R. Rhees. A drug industry representative was contemplated but not appointed. Admiral Charles Stokes of New York City, former Naval Surgeon General, who had developed a "cure" for addiction, was kept off the committee although he energetically sought an appointment.[37]

In August, Representative Rainey introduced a bill prepared by Deputy Commissioner Keith which, although only partially adopted, succeeded in strengthening the Harrison Act through provisions added to the Tax Act of 1918, the second general tax revision to raise funds for the war. Rainey failed in his hope to revoke Section 6 of the Harrison Act, which provided for exemption of a limited amount of narcotic in proprietaries, but he did make recording of sales and manufacture of proprietaries mandatory. Also a tax of one cent per ounce or fraction thereof of narcotics was inserted into the Act in compliance with the Internal Revenue Commissioner's repeated recommendations to make the Harrison Act an unquestioned revenue measure. Thereafter, possession of a package without a tax stamp, unless obtained on a physician's prescription, was prima facie evidence of illegal possession. This would help close one loophole created by the *Jin Fuey Moy* decision which made any amount of narcotics legally possessible by an unregistered person. The revision would still permit maintenance, but it would open an avenue of attack against possessors with large amounts of narcotics who made no pretense of having obtained the drugs through prescriptions. Lobbyists pleaded with the House Ways and Means Committee to preserve Section 6. At the time, Rainey complained that the committee members were "being flooded with telegrams by interested druggists throughout the country, anxious to retain the privilege of selling the dope which they now sell under Section 6." Section 6 survived, but Rainey's other amendments passed and came into effect on 24 February 1919.[38]

Rainey held no hearing on the Harrison amendments, for which he was criticized by the drug industry, but he pleaded that there was too much urgent business for such activity in wartime. He also feared hearings that would enable the pharmaceutical industry to whittle away again at the law's effectiveness.[39] Some indication of the distance Rainey kept from the day-to-day business of narcotic sales was his discovery several years later that his amendments did not prevent grocery stores and other nonmedical commercial establishments from selling proprietaries with narcotics in them.[40] But his lack of firsthand knowledge was no hindrance to his being an effective ally of the Treasury Department.

A preliminary report was issued by the Treasury Committee shortly before Rainey's amendments were introduced in the Congress.[41] This official statement had the effect of helping persuade Congress that amendments were quite necessary. In June 1919 the final report, *Traffic in Narcotic Drugs*, was published, although its contents had been known for months and had been discussed in the newspapers. The report, dated 15 April 1919, was preceded by a partial disclaimer from the Treasury Department to the effect that it could not vouch for the accuracy of the statistics nor could the conclusions be taken as final. But the report was considered as "comprehensive a survey as is possible under the circumstances of the problem from the humanitarian as well as from the administrative viewpoint." Heroin, with its appeal to "boys and girls under 20," and the other fiend-maker cocaine, were singled out for special concern.[42]

Analysis of a questionnaire survey directed at the 125,000 physicians and 48,000 pharmacists registered under the Harrison Act formed a major element in the report. About 30 percent of the doctors and 40 percent of the druggists replied. The physicians reported 73,000 addicts under treatment and the committee extrapolated this to estimate 238,000 addicts if all physicians had replied. In a similar fashion the druggists were estimated to have filled 18.3 million narcotic prescriptions during the previous twelve months, although the amounts and purposes of the prescriptions were not ascertained.[43]

The extrapolation method and the questionable reliability of replies on such a controversial subject make the results suspect. Cooperation from other information sources was even less satisfactory.[44] Of some interest, however, was the reply from 79 nonprofit institutions providing treatment for drug addiction. The respondents estimated the average length of treatment to be two years and ten and a half months. About a quarter of the state, district, county, and municipal health officers responded. Most had no information nor any means of gathering any, but those who had, reported a *decline* in addiction over the previous three years.

The responding doctors were almost evenly divided on the question whether addiction was a disease or a vice. The majority of physicians used "gradual reduction" treatment and a quarter employed "special procedures." At least 192 cities and counties were discovered to have provision for treatment of addicts in almshouses and penal institutions. From private hospitals and sanitaria the replies dropped to almost 5 percent—of the 4,568 superintendents asked for information only 227 could provide any for the committee. From these few the average length of treatment for addiction was recorded as only six to seven weeks at about five dollars per day. Encouragingly, 61 percent of patients in private institutions were described as "permanently cured," and up to 74 percent "benefited to some degree." As a cross section of observers' opinions, the report conveys conflicting notions, simplistic explanations, and general

confusion on the nature and treatment of addiction at the time the
federal government moved dramatically to end addiction maintenance.

From the extrapolation that physicians had under treatment about
a quarter million addicts, and assuming that "only a small portion of
the total number of addicts present themselves for treatment," and
considering the other estimates given for the addict population, the
committee concluded that "the total number of addicts in this country probably exceeds 1,000,000 at the present time"—the most commonly quoted statistic from the report.[45] This estimate of addicts
became questionable the year of publication. New York City's
Health Commissioner had informed the committee that the number
of addicts in the city was 103,000. Yet when he established heroin-
dispensing clinics in April, liberally providing heroin to children
as young as age 15, no more than 8,000 habitués could be located in
a year. The committee's estimate of more than a million addicts in
the United States thus appeared exaggerated when compared to the
data from New York, the accepted center of the nation's addict population. It is difficult to escape the conclusion that the committee's
report grossly exaggerated the number of addicts in the United
States.

In addition to an extravagant estimate of addicts in 1919, the committee pictured a bleak future. Prohibition of liquor was singled out
as a factor that would tend to increase drug use. Although the
committee was unsure whether Prohibition enforcement would result in a general turn to narcotics, the "consensus of opinion of
those interested in the subject appears to be to the effect that the
number of addicts will increase."[46]

In summary, the report declared that opium addiction has a
disease aspect. Addiction results from continued use of opiates for
ten to thirty days, and the addict thereafter takes his drug to remain
as normal as possible. But addicts are weak creatures, lacking in
moral sense, and when deprived of their drug may commit crime
in order to obtain it. The report offered one comfort; the opium
addict was not always lost to all sense of decency and honor and
could even be an upstanding person except in the area of addiction,
to which he was enslaved, and he could not discontinue without
outside assistance. With the new amendments to the Harrison Act
and the Supreme Court's ruling in March against maintenance, it

was expected that many addicts would become desperate for their drugs. Therefore the committee insisted that provision for medical care be made and that federal and local governments enact legislation to provide it.

But the form of medical care remained uncertain after decades of inquiry. Research was needed, the committee concluded: "at the present time there are numerous forms of treatment for drug addiction, none of which appears to have been given a thorough trial by the medical profession as a whole, or to have received the unqualified support of those members of the profession who have had no financial interest in the matter." In this understated manner the committee admitted a quandary: although addiction would probably rise, for all the usual reasons as well as liquor prohibition (which was only half a year away), there was not even one accepted medical treatment for it. In fact, deprived of their drug the addicts might become violent. This warning was received by a nation in the throes of a panic reaction to Bolshevik bombings directed at institutions and national leaders, violent and widespread labor strikes, IWW agitation, and anarchist plots. Rarely in recent American history could such a declaration by the federal government about an alleged million-member subgroup carry as much threat of danger to the nation.

The legal battle for the control of "nonmedical" narcotic use had already been won by the reformers when the report came out in June, so it became something of an apologia for activities well under way. Once again Treasury agents went into action against maintainers, but without the legal resistance of 1915. Although arrests were made, suspension of drugs to habitués, particularly opiate addicts, was not intended to be abrupt. Treasury officers feared that if there were a million addicts, abrupt drug restriction would lead to crime or to the death of many addicts. Therefore, when dope doctors or druggists were arrested, some attempt was made to provide the addict-clients with a temporary supply of drugs. The carefully planned establishment of clinics for this purpose indicates that the federal government and particularly the Bureau of Internal Revenue did believe there were many addicts and that treatment should be offered. A federal responsibility for the addicts' plight was accepted by the Revenue Bureau, but this was not sufficient to persuade Congress to enact any of the Treasury's proposed remedial legislation.

The Treasury Department moved quickly to use its new powers in New York. In April 1919 several New York City physicians and druggists, who had been supplying hundreds of addicts, were arrested. These professionals had been under watch for several months but it was not until the *Webb* and *Doremus* decisions that the government thought it could successfully prosecute addiction maintenance. The raids were led on the federal side by Major Daniel Porter, who was slated to head Prohibition enforcement in New York City when the 18th Amendment became effective the coming January.[47]

The city was prepared for such arrests, if any preparation was necessary, by early 1919. Respected and presumably well-informed authorities had issued increasingly severe warnings of the narcotic situation. In February, Admiral Stokes, former Naval Surgeon General, simply and directly equated alcoholic and narcotic addicts. He confidently expected an increase of drug addiction with the beginning of Prohibition. Moreover, he could not offer much hope of easily curbing addiction. Cure by outpatient methods would not work, Stokes admonished, because cure could be effected only by a change in the habitué's environment.[48]

A month later, Health Commissioner Royal S. Copeland issued information on drugstore narcotic sales which revealed that a small percentage of the retail outlets (33 of about 2,500 stores) had sold in the single month of December 1918 72 ounces of cocaine, 876 ounces of morphine, and 1,690 ounces of heroin (an ounce of either opiate can supply the daily needs of three addicts for a month if the average daily dose is assumed to be 5 grains). Along with these statistics he dramatically warned of the effects of addiction on the daily life of the city. Dr. Copeland echoed Admiral Stokes's prediction that Prohibition would increase the number of addicts. Already, he asserted, one of every thirty New Yorkers was addicted (i.e. about 150,000). With the city threatened by such evil, Dr. Copeland confessed he had little sympathy with those who obstructed drug control by talking about the addict's legal privileges—one should pay at least as much attention to the constitutional rights of the victims of the addicts' crimes as to those of the addict. His most outspoken criticism was reserved for his own profession: physicians who sell prescriptions to addicts "should be boiled in oil." [49]

The federal agents who had arrested the physicians and pharmacists coordinated their activities with the city's Health Department so that clinic as well as hospital facilities would be available as soon as the regular ration of drugs was cut off from several hundred patient-addicts. Major Porter led the raid in the evening of Wednesday April 9. Next morning a narcotic supply clinic opened at 145 Worth Street. Addicts who had been patients or customers of the arrested suppliers were told they could get their drugs at the Health Department and for much less than they had been accustomed to pay.[50] Of course, plans to set up maintenance clinics had been contemplated under the second Whitney law and the Commissioner of Narcotic Drug Control had signaled his intention of establishing supply stations wherever needed in the state.[51] But unlike the state clinics, the city clinic did not permit maintenance for any lengthy periods but sought cure as rapidly as possible, just as the Treasury Department planned for the nation.

On the first morning, 12 addicts arrived at Worth Street for drugs, by the second day 135 had volunteered for hospital treatment. Federal and city officials had minimized the agonies of withdrawal among the addicts and they had ready not only an outpatient clinic generously providing narcotics but also institutional facilities. The hospital beds soon proved inadequate and only after enduring repeated disappointments and rebuffs by communities around possible hospital sites would the Health Department be able to provide sufficient beds. While waiting for a bed the addict was maintained.[52]

Complete hospital care and rehabilitation would be a public and crucial large-scale test of the assumptions which underlay institutional treatment and outpatient narcotic dispensing stations. If institutional treatment did release addicts from their craving, and if addicts did in fact want freedom from their bondage, then a model addiction treatment program would have been established for the nation. If the assumptions of the Health Department were erroneous, there would be a major setback for the proponents of medical treatment for the elimination of addiction.

THE FRANCE BILL AND THE PUBLIC HEALTH SERVICE

A clinic proposal from the Treasury Department was part of a more elaborate program contemplated by the Bureau of Internal Revenue. It included potentially more extensive and curative aspects in the use of Public Health Service hospitals for treatment of addiction, PHS officers for liaison and consultation with the various states, and matching funds to the states for the care of addicts through institutions, leading to definitive cure.[53] The clinics inspired by the Treasury Department were the doorway to institutional cure. In some respects this antinarcotic proposal resembles a recently approved (1918) venereal disease program of the Public Health Service which provided matching funds and coordination of a national attack on VD.[54]

The chief proponent of the comprehensive federal plan was Daniel C. Roper, a Democrat from South Carolina, who had ably served as chairman of the party's organization bureau in the second presidential campaign of Woodrow Wilson. He had been Commissioner of the Internal Revenue Bureau for over two years when the drug crisis loomed. Roper's determination to strike at narcotics was tempered by sympathy. In his autobiography he writes that the rejection of 8,000 draft-age addicts in New York City prompted a campaign to rid the nation of the dope menace, and he helped institute a campaign against dope. He concluded that "if the public, always incensed at the doping of race horses, could be aroused into one half the same state of indignation over the destruction of human beings by improper drugs, the problem would be easier of solution." The Special Narcotic Committee may have been part of this drive to inform the public, a motivation which would help explain the committee's exaggeration of the menace in its report. He described his own early experience with the narcotics question during his term as clerk of the House Ways and Means Committee (1911–12) when antinarcotic laws were under discussion, and the more personal impact of the death of the manager of his South Carolina farm from an overdose of narcotics given to him by a local druggist for "nerves." [55]

Roper did not believe the tax agency of the government was an appropriate instrument to direct the control of addiction, nor did he believe the Revenue Bureau should have to assume Prohibition enforcement, which Congress had settled on it over his strenuous objections.[56] He had sought to strengthen the laws by establishing the Special Committee the previous year, but he did not hesitate to declare that the treatment crisis was federally created. As the reality of rigorous antimaintenance enforcement came closer, he sought aid for the medical emergency from the federal health organization. He warned the Surgeon General in June 1919 that when supplies were shut off, there would be a great outcry.[57] Commissioner Roper began to prepare legislation later introduced by Senator France of the Senate Public Health and Quarantine Committee.[58] New regulations for the Harrison Act containing recommendations for the temporary supply of addicts were promulgated on 15 July.[59] On 31 July Roper wrote the collectors of internal revenue across the nation advising them to work with local authorities to take care of the addicts who would be abruptly taken off their drugs.[60] He feared deaths from sudden withdrawal or perhaps violence. In accord with this directive, clinics or other arrangements for drug supply were established in various parts of the nation. Some areas probably handled the problem quietly by permitting certain physicians to prescribe, or registered addicts to receive, maintenance doses. In some localities a formal clinic was established by the municipal government, sometimes in a police station, as in New Haven, or in the Health Department, as in Cleveland. These clinics were intended to remove addicts from the hands of private physicians who might have been continuing the addiction for their own profit.

The France bill was a substantial proposal which would require both congressional appropriations and the active cooperation of the Public Health Service. The PHS reacted with some reluctance to the commissioner's notion that their hospitals and men should assume responsibility for addicts. The PHS saw addiction as a traditional public health problem, one in which it had a limited role —certainly no responsibility for direct services except to merchant seamen. In its view all health issues must be shared by the states. The PHS even hesitated to give advice to the medical profession with regard to treatment or its possible legal complications; it simply disseminated information. The PHS countered Roper's plea by suggesting the pattern already set up to combat venereal disease.[61] Like addiction, VD was a hidden social vice with less than ideal treatment, whose spread alarmed responsible citizens everywhere. Under law, federal matching funds were awarded to localities for the establishment of public clinics. The PHS therefore suggested that funds for addiction treatment be awarded on a matching basis by the federal government, but that clinics and treatment be the responsibility of the states. By following the precedent of the VD program the PHS would not be committed to supply treatment, about which it had serious questions, but would still perform a vital coordinating function.[62]

The Surgeon General's alternative was accepted by Roper, but legislation authorizing increased federal activity in the health field was opposed by the medical profession as a portent of state medicine. In the AMA the France bill received the support of the liberal element, but this faction's power was rapidly waning, particularly in legislative matters.[63] The Sheppard-Towner Act of the same Congress, providing matching funds for maternal and child health passed, but it was never fully successful because of the opposition of national and state medical societies. The France bill faced similar opposition. And in addition to opposition on the grounds of political principle, the number of addicts seemed fewer than predicted, and their possible panic less than anticipated. But other reasons existed for congressional disinterest in new appropriations for any purpose. The Republican-dominated Congress wished to establish a record for budget trimming in preparation for the congressional and presidential elections. Then in 1920 the nation slipped into an economic recession. The France bill, a well-intentioned national program to combat addiction, could hardly have bid for appropriations at a less propitious time, and it never became law. Submitted to committee on 15 August 1919, the bill was slightly amended and recommended for passage on 10 October, but it failed of passage in the Senate.[64]

The clinics envisioned by the federal government were not to be indefinite maintenance stations but an emergency measure; addicts were to be offered hospital treatment. The PHS, however, did not share the conviction that medical treatment was a necessary step in addiction control. Its narcotic experts were doubtful of specific treatments and cures at least by late 1918, well before Dr. Hubbard questioned medical treatment after his experience with the New York City clinic. A. G. DuMez, a member of the Treasury's Special Committee, in an internal memorandum for the PHS, outlined a program leading to its more active involvement in the narcotic problem. It was proposed, in the ancient tradition of the PHS, that it compile statistics on the numbers of addicts, conduct educational campaigns, and investigate the mechanism of addiction, methods of treatment, etc. For this purpose he recommended a staff composed of a writer and lecturer, a lawyer, a pharmacologist, and two stenographers; he did not recommend direct services to patients.

Summarizing the narcotic problem, DuMez saw the recent years offering more hope than in the past when addiction was considered a mere vice by the public and the vast majority of the medical profession. Now (1918), he believed that almost all recent knowledge pointed to the conclusion that the habitual use of opiate drugs leads to a diseased condition which "requires a continued use of the drug or special medical treatment leading to complete withdrawal." [65] But no specific treatment had been established; in fact, considerable doubt had been thrown on the Towns-Lambert method because "these men operate a private sanitorium for the treatment of addicts and have been charged with being influenced by the monetary remuneration received therefrom." In this confidential report to the Surgeon General, DuMez was suggesting a way for the PHS to assume leadership and giving a broad overview of the addiction problem. DuMez also reported that the physician was generally considered the number one cause of addiction in the United States even by the majority of medical writers. The lack of any clear-cut and satisfactory treatment was evident from his statement.[66]

A few months later DuMez undertook to review the "treatment of narcotic drug addiction" for the Surgeon General. In this instance his criticism of the various treatments is more direct. Again he points out that "it is only [since the Harrison Act] that the medical profession has awakened to the fact that addiction to the use of narcotics produces changes in the organism which cannot be controlled by the will power of the individual." After reviewing the standard cures advocated by sanitaria and medical men, he concluded with a pessimistic statement that the claims of some institutions of 80 percent cures have been investigated and found greatly exaggerated. When such treatments have been carried out in state institutions, "only about 10 percent of cures have been reported. . . . Our present methods of treating drug addiction must be considered failures." [67]

Therefore, before the New York City clinic opened and the Supreme Court decision outlawed simple maintenance, a responsible and informed physician was convinced that no satisfactory medical treatment existed for drug addiction. DuMez's report would influence the PHS in conducting national treatment programs in its own or other hospitals. His dismal and well-documented review of addiction treatment would not encourage the Surgeon General to enter an intensive campaign for a medical approach. The PHS concluded that any method that got the addict off drugs, including abrupt withdrawal, would work as well as the celebrated cures, thus moving the antinarcotic program toward reality.

If no cure was more effective than just keeping the addict away from drugs, then the problem really was: How do you keep addicts away from drugs? And this question was not medical, it was an enforcement problem. In the early years of strict enforcement, after 1919, the PHS, with the exercise of commendable objectivity, had excused itself from claiming knowledge of how to cure addicts and drew the conclusion that the nation should rely on legal enforcement to control narcotic supply.[68] The Internal Revenue Bureau, on the other hand, frustrated in its attempts to curb addiction through enforcement, looked to medical treatment as the answer.

THE NARCOTIC DIVISION OF THE PROHIBITION UNIT

The center of antinarcotic activity in 1919 remained in the Bureau of Internal Revenue in spite of its efforts to share responsibility with the Public Health Service. Evidently the PHS did not actively seek any of the responsibility the tax collection agency had acquired in 1915, partly because of its role which excluded direct patient services to civilians and partly because the government's health agency had no faith in medical antinarcotic treatments. The failure of the France bill relieved the PHS from statutory responsibility to treat any addicts other than those among its legal wards. The responsibility of the Treasury Department, however, was increased by the strengthened legal assault on addiction, although Roper continued to protest that addiction was not a police problem.[69]

In October the Volstead Act, passed over President Wilson's veto, provided the detailed legislation under which the 18th Amendment would be enforced. As a compromise with the wet opposition, enforcement was given over to the Internal Revenue Bureau over Roper's well-publicized protests. Another part of the compromise excused Prohibition agents from civil service requirements. Agents were appointed through political patronage and were generally such poor choices that even in the first flush of enforcement fervor they were described as inadequate and incompetent by federal judges and grand juries. The Prohibition Unit, headed by National Prohibition Administrator John F. Kramer, included the Narcotic Division, headed by a former official of the Alcohol Tax Division, Levi G.

Nutt.[70] The Narcotic Division headquarters and the field force were under civil service.*

In 1920, the Narcotic Division's chief problem was what to do with the various maintenance clinics operating in the nation. Whatever strategy Nutt established would be more effectively carried into action than in any previous year, for in fiscal year 1920 expenditures for enforcement rose to $515,000 (almost double that for fiscal year 1919) and provided for 170 narcotic agents to work out of district offices.[71]

As a preliminary to fundamental decisions on national narcotic enforcement, the Revenue Bureau in late 1919 sent questionnaires to leading physicians and scientists in America asking their opinion on the present state of narcotic treatment, the wisdom of ambulatory treatment, and the existence of specific antibodies in the blood of chronic addicts (a physiological hypothesis for addictive phenomena). Collectors of internal revenue were also canvassed for their opinions on the best way to enforce the Harrison Act.[72] For a period of several months the narcotic unit, with the help of expert opinion, considered its basic enforcement policy.

Most medical opinion opposed the antibody theory because it had not been substantiated by evidence; this strengthened the unit's doubts that addiction was a special disease with unique bodily changes requiring long-term or indefinite maintenance. The negative response also increased suspicion against clinicians such as Dr. Bishop, who were vigorous opponents of the government's anti-maintenance stand. The government's opponents were perceived as a serious hindrance to law enforcement; this was regrettable, for physicians who argued that addiction was a special disease held to a view which until at least World War I had been respectable.

The medical authorities by a large majority pronounced themselves opposed to ambulatory treatment and in favor of institutional confinement; the former was basically faulty and unworkable, the latter was favored because the addict would be held in a state of abstinence and treated medically for his withdrawal symptoms.

Collectors of internal revenue were also critical of ambulatory clinics, but there was division of opinion among them on the wisdom of maintenance clinics. Some thought them quite reasonable and

---

* In 1930 the Narcotic Division became an independent agency and remained under the Treasury Department when the Prohibition Bureau was transferred to the Justice Department.

successful, others considered them dens of iniquity. There was in fact less consensus among the agents than among the medical experts against ambulatory clinics.[73]

The collected evidence pointed to a more strict nonmaintenance policy but, before taking further steps, the Narcotic Division received formal support from the AMA in opposition to the ambulatory regimen. At the annual meeting of the AMA in New Orleans in April 1920, the Committee on Habit-Forming Drugs introduced a resolution opposing ambulatory clinics.[74] The resolution was approved by the Council on Health and Public Instruction, and then by the House of Delegates of the AMA.[75] The AMA's action, like the response from medical experts to the questionnaire, did represent current medical thought, and we have no evidence that coercion or deception was exercised to get this support.

The Narcotic Division's next step was to investigate the clinics and determine in each case the prevailing conditions and the results obtained. In sum, there was evidence that no significant number of cures had been obtained and that the clinic approach was subject to a variety of abuses. There were some clinics without discernible abuses and with strong community support, but these also did not cure. Of course, this investigation was conducted with the government's attitude toward maintenance clinics already determined and backed by expert medical opinion.

The Narcotic Division, under the leadership of Levi Nutt, decided in late 1919 or early 1920 to close maintenance clinics and oppose maintenance in every case except among the aged and medically incurable. This was accomplished with ease in some cases, after several years of effort in others, and was grounded on a variety of considerations. (1) There was no medically proven specific treatment for narcotic addiction, while there was the assurance by the PHS and other medical authorities that any withdrawal method would result in getting the addict off drugs. (2) The danger of death in withdrawal cases was exaggerated, and authenticated cases of such deaths were difficult to locate. (3) After any method of withdrawal, addicts would usually return to drugs if they were available. (4) The chief source of drugs was still thought to be a small percentage of physicians who would write out a prescription for anyone. (5) The clinics were merely another supply source for those who wished drugs for comfort or pleasure.

Legal restraints on physicians had to be inflexible in order to prevent easy prescribing of drugs by a determined minority; outlawing maintenance was a weapon commensurate with this need. But legal maintenance clinics, if permitted by the federal government, would make indictment of the erring physician very difficult to obtain. How could the federal government arrest the dope doctor when he was doing nothing legally distinguishable from the clinic operated by a local health or police department? And, if maintenance was a good public health or police practice, it would be difficult to prevent regular physicians from following an accepted therapy. The federal government did not have authority to restrict maintenance to certain physicians or to well-operated clinics—maintenance would have to be allowed nationally or not allowed at all. Discrimination on the basis of "responsible" prescribing placed the federal government in even more constitutional uncertainty than strict anti-maintenance, a policy which rested on a five-to-four Supreme Court decision, since discrimination was in effect the licensing of physicians.

There was little evidence that the maintenance clinics effected cures. Even the clinics that were operated without abuses and by competent medical direction did not claim a large number of cures, but rather "social adjustment" for the addicts. From the inception of the State Department's campaign the government had not sought to stabilize the addict population at one of the large figures commonly quoted, say a million citizens, for the effects of addiction were thought to be moral degeneracy and paralysis of productivity among the addicted. To maintain a million or so addicts was not tolerable to a nation fearful of numerous unassimilable minorities. And there was also the deep fear that to maintain so many addicts —in such widespread and loosely controlled supply sources—would lead to a great increase of addiction among the rest of the nation, particularly the youth. Therefore the government sought to reduce or to eliminate addiction. To do so, the legal and enforcement agencies had fought a long battle since 1915 to outlaw maintenance. This was eventually accomplished in March 1919.

It was reassuring in 1920 to note that addicts were apparently fewer than had been estimated in earlier antinarcotic campaigns. The number seemed much more controllable by police methods than had been previously thought. For these reasons, then, there was little fear that disaster would befall addicts or the nation if legal and illegal drug supplies were suppressed.

Nevertheless, legal provision was still made for rapid withdrawal under a physician's supervision, and hospitals and institutions in many areas were made available for indigents; private sanitaria remained open for paying customers. Since the federal government believed there was no valid medical treatment other than withdrawal, no need existed for distribution of specific remedies or the specialized training of physicians. Enforcement agents had to keep in mind that the supreme goal was to get addicts off their drugs within some reasonable limit. In 1921, thirty days was taken to be reasonable, an adoption by the federal government of a California statute.[76] If the addict could not come off in thirty days, he was indeed in trouble. He could no longer get legal supplies of drugs; possession would now be evidence of guilt. The best way to aid the addicts who had tapered off, or did not have the will power to do so, was to eliminate drug supplies. Naturally a first step would be the end of legal sources of indefinite maintenance—that is, the narcotic clinic and the physician's right to prescribe narcotics as his judgment dictated.[77]

Abuses of clinics had occurred, sometimes flagrantly, and these served the Narcotic Division as ammunition for public denunciation or quiet intimidation. But the clinics were closed if they maintained addicts and even if no abuses were discoverable.

The Narcotic Clinic Era

7

Dr. Terry's narcotic clinic in Jacksonville, Florida, may have been the first one established in the United States by a government agency, but it is likely that some arrangements for collective care of a locality's addicts had been made before that time. Poor addicts were the chief clients for clinics; those who preferred not to publicize their addiction could get their drugs more expensively elsewhere—legally and without much difficulty until about 1919.[1] The clinic for addicts was an extension of the program of clinics set up by health departments to treat tuberculosis, mental illness, or syphilis.[2] Some narcotic clinics were part of a general health clinic; others were separate and specialized.

When Internal Revenue agents made the rounds of police and health departments in the summer of 1919 urging the establishment of narcotic clinics, about a dozen cities complied. The Connecticut clinics set up in 1918–19 in Hartford, Meriden, Norwalk, Waterbury, New Haven, and Bridgeport, and the clinic in Providence, were started on the recommendation of the district collector of the Internal Revenue Bureau. The New York State clinics, in contrast to the city clinic, were established by the Department of Narcotic Drug Control about September 1919 and generally were operated under political patronage except in a few of the largest upstate cities. In some instances "clinics" were established in cities with little need except a deserving physician with the proper political connections: Port Jervis, Saratoga, Watertown, Binghamton, Corning, Elmira, Hornell, Middletown, Oneonta, and Utica, as well as Albany, Buffalo, Rochester, and Syracuse. The New England and New York State clinics accounted for almost half of the nation's total. The rest of the clinics (forty-odd) usually had a history and character unique to each. They were unevenly scattered about the nation: in Louisiana (New Orleans, Shreveport, and Alexandria), Georgia (Augusta, Atlanta, and Macon), California (Los Angeles and San Diego), Ohio (Cleveland and Youngstown), Tennessee (Knoxville and Memphis), and one each in Clarksburg, West Virginia, Paducah, Kentucky, and Houston, Texas.[3] Clinics were contemplated in St. Louis and San Francisco and some were probably established in other cities, but, if closed before mid-1920, they never reached the attention of the Narcotic Division.[4] Major cities which do not seem to have had a clinic system include Boston, Philadelphia, and Chicago.

The known clinics, except in New York, never had very large clienteles. The other clinics in operation in 1920 probably did not have as many as 3,000 clients at one time and perhaps as few as 2,500.[5] New York had registered 7,500 addicts before it was closed in early 1920. The average age of clients in all clinics other than New York was about 40 for both sexes and men outnumbered women by two to one. Individual clinics had substantial variations in clients' age and sex ratios.[6] But these few clients compared to the earlier estimates of 200,000 to 4,000,000 addicts nationally meant either that the clinics were not a major factor in the maintenance of addiction, or that there were many fewer addicts than estimated. Although the clinics were not a major source of drug supply for the addict, they were nevertheless obstacles to the agents' efforts to indict the major purveyors: physicians, druggists, and peddlers.

THE NEW YORK STATE CONTROVERSY OVER ADDICTION CONTROL

Clinics that had been established through the authority of the State of New York were the result of extensive legislative hearings and public debate. An independently established agency, the Department of Narcotic Drug Control, supervised clinic establishment. Even the New York City clinic became ex officio a part of the New York State system, and the commissioner of health in the city was an agent of the State Commission. But the State Commission aroused opposition from several powerful groups. As the rein of the commission tightened to catch the small number of errant doctors and druggists, irritation rose in both professions at harassment and paper work.[7]

The commission also found itself immersed in a bitter controversy over the fear of state meddling in the practice of medicine. This affected their activities and reacted against the progressive ideology that infused the AMA leadership until about 1918.[8] An issue that mobilized a massive campaign of opposition was health insurance. The fear of government control did not come from private practitioners and private health insurance companies alone, but also from Samuel Gompers and other labor leaders who saw health insurance, paid out of wages, as the federal government's opening wedge to gain control of the union movement.[9]

The Harrison Act and the crackdown on doctors in 1919 seemed proof to many physicians of their suspicions that the federal government viewed them as culprits whose practice needed to be over-seen. They also saw the specter of state medicine gaining total control of their profession.[10] Although the medical profession had succeeded in putting out of business about half the medical schools of the country on valid grounds of incompetence (and thereby lessening the competition), they believed that the government wanted to reduce physicians practically to employees.

Dr. Lambert, of course, supported a strict interpretation of the Harrison Act as sturdily as he approved insurance: he saw these two reforms of American medical practice as improving its quality and distribution. Both were designed to curb simple profiteering and to force the profession into responsible service to the nation. He failed in his lifetime to achieve government-sponsored medical insurance, but his interpretation of the Harrison Act prevailed.

How did opposition to the Harrison Act fail, and attacks on health insurance succeed? Partly because the Harrison Act was directed at a social subgroup viewed as a menace to society and a small fraction of the medical profession which was, in the crucial period of 1919–20, a source of fear and revulsion.[11] The medical profession's attack on the Harrison Act was up against a general fear of dope fiends; its opposition to health insurance was in harmony with a more widespread fear of state control.

When the Narcotic Control Commission drew its net tighter and tighter around the wrongdoers by methods which also affected the practice of almost all physicians, fears were expressed by these professionals that the government was harassing citizens and exercising an extravagant and unjust power. In New York State the evolution of the clinics and maintenance policy was in opposition to the reform movement of Brent, Wright, and Lambert, which did not favor "coddling" the addict, and it went particularly against the mood of the time. The dominant public attitude by 1920 was strong and fearful: to maintain an addict was to maintain or create a menacing personality.

The repression of maintenance put state and federal bureaucracies in a difficult spot. The orders for vigorous enforcement and elimination of addiction came from above, but they were faced with the reality of a complex social problem which so far had not responded to medical or legal measures. As pressure increased during 1919, responsible state and federal officials in New York State met to talk following conclusions and recommendations to the Commissioner of Internal Revenue. The New York City meeting was one of many across the nation which were prompted in the summer of 1919 by the new Treasury Department regulations. The Internal Revenue officials for Connecticut, Rhode Island, and New York, along with the district attorney for the Southern District of New York, Walter R. Herrick of the New York State Department of Narcotic Drug Control, and two deputy commissioners, met twice in September 1919.[12]

Maintenance clinics were in full operation, while legal agencies sought indictments against peddlers and addict-maintaining physicians. While national enforcement policy was still flexible, the middle management of narcotic legislation discussed their dilemma.

Peddlers and health professionals posed different but difficult problems. The impact of peddlers on drug control was not to be underestimated. The battle could not be won without modification of enforcement procedures. When "peddlers were practically driven off the streets, the physicians and druggists were doing a thriving trade." But when the law closed in on the physician and druggists, there was usually an immediate revival of the street trade.

They seemed legion; as soon as one was arrested another took his place, attracted by the opportunity to make "large profits by selling adulterated drugs at high prices." At any one time the number of street sellers was large, and the ease of moving from more dangerous and less profitable enterprises to peddling drugs was inviting to the criminally bent. It was easy to convict peddlers, but the sentences imposed were usually light and were not effective deterrents, nor did they frighten peddlers into revealing their sources. Large operators were difficult to detect and were willing to take chances because of their "enormous and easy profits."

Erring health professionals, on the other hand, were easy to detect but difficult to indict or convict. They would claim that prescribing narcotics was professional treatment and could evoke a jury's sympathy by describing the sufferings of the addict deprived of his drug. It was particularly irritating to the enforcement group in New York that doctors and druggists often asserted that addictive drugs must be supplied until "provision of adequate means for cure." This argument, Commissioner Roper was informed, "is apt to have weight with the average juryman, who feels that the government should not undertake to shut off the addict's supply without making provision for his relief."

In response to these problems attorneys, revenue collectors, and state administrators pleaded for an expansion of institutional facilities to care for and treat addicted individuals. Suppliers could not be put out of business because the gains were greater than the legal deterrents. Even some physicians and druggists specialized in addict treatment because it brought in "so much more than their legitimate practice." Therefore, the side of the equation that had to be attacked was the addict's need for narcotics. Yet any steps taken to provide treatment "should be accompanied and followed for some period of time by a vigorous and continuous campaign of law enforcement."

Again and again the state and federal officials called for institutional restraint and effective treatment. The group warned that laws "will fail unless they include sufficient provision for the cure of addicts." And cure could come about only by "supplying and maintaining hospitals or custodial institutions adequate for the accommodation of all persons addicted to the use of drugs." But the experts required for their program something that would not be given: "appropriations of considerable size" for hospital establishment and maintenance. The conference in New York City had succinctly posed the policy issues faced by the newly formed Prohibition Unit and its Narcotic Division. If massive appropriations were not forthcoming from federal, state, and municipal governments for institutional restraint, what inexpensive steps could be taken that would reduce narcotic addiction?

The Supreme Court ruling of March 1919 which forbade nonmedical maintenance had been urged by the federal government in a period when the possibility of curative treatment was widely accepted. But now that nonmaintenance was law, cure was thought to be very unlikely by any method, or possible only through expensive institutions. The France bill, which proposed a nationwide program of addiction treatment facilities through federal assistance, would never receive congressional approval. The states and cities themselves were in a deepening postwar depression causing diminishing tax revenues.

Therefore a traditional enforcement attack against suppliers was launched, which naturally included municipal and state agencies, narcotic clinics, and private health professionals. If all other parts of the national and international program worked as hoped, the restrictions on clinics and health professionals would plug a legal loophole in drug supply. If the grand plan of the federal government failed, enforcement at least would have eliminated "legal" addiction, one part of the fundamental goal of federal narcotic reform.

When the Narcotic Division adopted the view that no addiction maintenance was justified or tolerable except for medical reasons, the New York State Narcotic Drug Commission was an obvious target for attack. The commission had established many maintenance clinics; some functioned efficiently and honorably and some were glaring examples of mercenary political patronage. Defects in the New York clinics would make their closure that much more simple, but all clinics were to be closed regardless of the quality of operation. Closure of the clinics would place the maintenance decision with the private practitioner, an easier target for intimidation or indictment than a state or city health department.

THE NEW YORK CITY HEROIN CLINIC, 1919–1920

In July 1919, while the New York City clinic was rapidly expanding, the Bureau of Internal Revenue urged its agents to cooperate with other local authorities in supplying the emergency needs of addicts whose supplies had been cut off by enforcement of the amended and strictly interpreted Harrison Act. Dr. Royal S. Copeland, Health Commissioner, and Major Porter, head of the federal narcotic agents in New York City, agreed on the danger of addicts to the city. The Commissioner estimated 150,000 to 200,000 addicts there, of whom many were "recently discharged soldiers." Heroin was the favored drug and 70 percent of the heroin users were under age 25.[13] Major Porter warned the city that enforcement of the Harrison Act would be strict and without compromise. His determination matched his belief that the drug habit had grown to become the "biggest problem of the nation." [14]

As addicts arrived by the hundreds at the Health Department's Worth Street clinic, a counterattack to this usurpation of their prerogatives was launched by the Physicians' Protective Association. The association condemned the decision that physicians must give decreasing doses of narcotics. Dr. Copeland was two years late in handling this problem, spokesmen for the association maintained, and a reputable physician, not a clinic, was the proper source of treatment. Opponents of the clinic argued that only about 10 percent of addicts were criminal and did not want treatment. The rest, estimated by the association to be 212,500, should be treated by private physicians—not the city, county, or state.[15] A group in the New York County Medical Society also tried to raise opposition to the Health Department's program but failed to rouse substantial numbers of their associates.[16] The association's hostile response to the legal attack on narcotic maintenance had very little effect on the city's Health Department. But the ineffectiveness of the addict-maintaining physicians to reverse enforcement policy was only partially due to their small numbers. One of the strongest arguments against any toleration of addiction was the fear that Prohibition would create even more addicts than the enormous number suspected in early 1919. The Association Opposed to National Prohibition, in one of its last efforts before defeat, published an interview with the New York City Commissioner of Public Charities in which he expressed fear that Prohibition would result in a great increase in drug addiction.[17] Others, like the late Dr. Wright, had also used this reasoning to show that liquor prohibition was ill conceived. But when the 18th Amendment had been adopted and upheld by the Supreme Court, the argument served only to make the crackdown on addicts seem more necessary, lest the known millions of tipplers (far more of them than addicts) would sink even lower to become morphine or heroin or cocaine habitués. In this sense Prohibition, which divided the nation, unified the public in a condemnation of narcotic abuse and maintenance.

In early and mid-1919 the care of addicts was welcomed, if carefully monitored, by the city's Health Department because it feared it could not cope with more addicts than it already had.[18] At the same time, federal officials did not yet want to impose restrictions on state and municipal agencies or threaten their employees with arrest.

The state's Narcotic Control Commission moved to assist the city's health commissioner by announcing that a triplicate system of prescriptions for addicts would be inaugurated—the physician would keep one copy, and the addict would give two to the pharmacist who would retain one and send the other to the State Narcotic Commission.[19] The addicts would be registered and by this means each would receive only the amount his physician deemed appropriate.

This system would still permit maintenance, and did exist until September 1920 when the new antimaintenance policy of the Internal Revenue Bureau enforced a regimen of decreasing dosages.

Registration was a problem for the Worth Street clinic. How could one be sure that an addict, out of the hundreds who came every day, did not cheat? Many ingenious solutions were proposed. Staining the hands with silver nitrate was favored for a while, but it was dropped because it imposed a criminal-like stigma on the addict. Finally a registration card was adopted with the addict's photograph, signature, identifying marks, statistics, and dosage chart, which would be signed by only one designated physician or clinic for each addict. But such registration also led well-to-do addicts or more resourceful ones to get their drugs from physicians or peddlers.[20]

In the first days, the Worth Street clinic was quite accommodating. The limit of morphine or heroin to one person was 15 grains; cocaine could also be obtained on request. There was no way to tell what the usual dose of an addict might be and therefore, within the stated upper limit, his word was accepted. After the first day cocaine was not offered, on the grounds that it was not addictive and no special concern needed to be shown for its users. Most of the addicts were young and favored heroin. By the first of July, after two and a half months of operation, 2,723 addicts had applied to the clinic: 80 percent were under age 30, 57 percent under 25, and 27 percent 19 or younger; 507 females and 385 non-white had received drugs, making both categories small minorities. Leading nationalities were American, Hebrew, German, Polish, Irish, and Russian. About 60 percent had a trade or profession; the rest were unskilled. Seventy-nine percent used heroin; about half had been addicted less than six years; 70 percent attributed their use of the drugs to "bad associates" and only a few to illness or pain.[21]

By January 1920, 7,464 addicts had been registered, of whom almost 1,600 were females and slightly over 1,000 black. The age profile had gradually shifted to older addicts, so that now only 10 percent were under 19 and 38 percent 24 or under. Two-thirds were under 30 years of age. Over 5,000 had been born in the United States and 60 percent had been addicted for over five years. Fewer than one out of four voluntarily entered the hospital for treatment. Addicts' occupations varied, the most frequent, in order, were drivers, laborers, housewives, household help, and clerks; but there were also actors and actresses, journalists, printers, plumbers, and even one grave digger, shoe cutter, song writer, syrup maker, embalmer, detective, and picture framer. The early rush to register slacked off as the year wore on. Young addicts predominated in the early months when the average daily attendance rose to 800 clients.[22]

Near the close of the clinic in March 1920, the count had declined to 150 daily and the average age had climbed.[23] These changes can be partly explained by the treatment regimen. From the beginning the average heroin or morphine dose was about 10 grains with a maximum of 15. Every other day half a grain was dropped until the addict became uncomfortable (at a dose range of 2 to 8 grains). He was then offered a bed in the Riverside Hospital on North Brother Island, a municipal institution which had been used for tubercular patients. If hospital treatment was refused, the clinic continued the dose reduction until it reached zero and the addict was discharged. If no bed was available when the minimum comfortable dose was reached, that dosage was continued until the client could be hospitalized. The clinic treatment program did not appeal to those who did not wish to be cured, and most youngsters were in that category.

By 1920, official attempts to locate addicts failed to reveal a prevalence anywhere near the previous estimate. State registration of addicts in New York City reached 7,000 in 1920, one-third, the state believed, of all addicts in the five boroughs.[24] Still, 21,000 would be only a tenth of the Health Commissioner's dire estimate of April 1919. Dr. Alexander Lambert, commenting on the experience of the city clinic in January 1920, remarked:

> It is evident that the number of narcotic addicts has been enormously exaggerated and instead . . . of comprising 1 percent or 2 percent of the population, it is evidently not more than one-quarter of 1 percent. The Harrison Law strictly applied in New York has produced but about 6,000 addicts, instead of the 100,000 or 200,000 as was claimed and expected.[25]

In the same vein one of the chief clinic physicians, Dr. S. Dana Hubbard, criticized predictions of panic and mass unrest. The numbers of addicts estimated in New York City "are mythical and untrue and . . . therefore the fear of a panic of these miserable unfortunates was negative." [26]

That many fewer addicts existed than had been feared was good news for health and enforcement agencies, but a second question, to which the New York experience would provide an answer, was the success rate of treatment. For the cure of addicts at Riverside Hospital, gradual reduction was employed with physiological support provided by hyoscine after a thorough "elimination" by purgatives. After coming off the opiates in three to five days, the addict was given four to five weeks of rest, exercise, and good food in fairly pleasant surroundings.[27] Although the city's program included rehabilitation and medical treatment in the hospital setting, results were very discouraging; within a few days of discharge, most addicts were back on drugs. The addict craving to get off his drug was rarely seen, the doctors reported: "Over 95 percent of all drug addicts treated at Riverside Hospital, from the beginning of the service until now [1920] have shown by their acts a non-appreciation of the service, and have repeatedly attempted to be discharged before the end of treatment, or have in some way interfered with its prosecution while there." The department's annual report for 1920 recommended that: "such cases as are of a truly pestilential character [be] detained in institutions that can provide custodial care, for that is the most important therapeutic agent necessary in taking them off the drug," and that the treatment service close.[28]

The Health Department's negative response came after a year of providing extensive treatment to addicts along the lines of the best medical opinion—and failing. Just to provide hospital beds required the utmost political effort of the Health Commissioner. The problem of addiction probably lay deeper, and the disillusioned doctors in the Health Department apparently believed that addiction was the result of a depraved personality not amenable to medical therapy.

One of the reasons for the failure of Riverside Hospital was the availability of drugs when the patient was discharged. Legal supplies being offered, the addict could simply visit a physician or register at one of the state clinics to resume his habit. Legal maintenance was therefore not viewed with any kindness by the Health Department. As one member complained, "Treatment of the narcotic drug addict by private physicians prescribing and druggists dispensing, when the individual is going about, is wrong. The giving of a narcotic drug . . . for self-administration should be forbidden. Few doctors use this form of treating addicts and it is believed that those doing so must be either ignorant of proper methods, or do so in bad faith."²⁹ The solution suggested by the department was to make drugs as difficult as possible for the treated addict to obtain, not to entice him with legal maintenance.

Conclusions drawn from the New York experience influenced the Treasury Department's attitude toward all clinics.³⁰ Perhaps the most important lesson was that not many addicts existed or, if more existed than attended a clinic, they could not be lured there even by heroin at two cents a grain. Therefore the clinic was not needed as an emergency station when supplies were cut off by enforcement. Furthermore, the clinic did uncover the fact that at least 75 percent of addicts did not crave institutional treatment. Those who were taken off the drug and given a month's rest, exercise, and good diet returned to addiction at the rate of nineteen out of every twenty.

The Health Department now realized that the underlying flaw in its treatment of addicts was that drugs could easily be obtained in the streets. Shortly after the clinic closed Dr. Hubbard declared an urgent "necessity for the general and uniform enforcement of the statutes. There will be no panic or falling in the streets, or robbing of stores or crowding physicians' offices by the addicts affected. If they cannot obtain a supply, they will reform, and it is certain that not a fatality will be recorded." Abrupt withdrawal or "cold turkey" was declared "not only possible but practical" as demonstrated by its routine employment in Kings County Hospital. Dr. Hubbard was optimistic about the solution of the addiction problem since the addicts he saw were mostly young, few had any physical reasons for using the drug, and many needed only a "fair chance" to change their ways since they may never have had a square deal. Dr. Hubbard avowed that he was more than pleased with the clinic's efforts.³¹

Dr. Arthur R. Braunlich, Visiting Physician to the Riverside Hospital, believed that "All addicts will relapse with little or no excuse, or one so flimsy that it sounds absurd." He put the matter in scientific language: Addicts' pathological craving seemed to be "due to the impression made by the former use on the memory cells of the brain [which] becomes more pronounced if the former patient knows he can get the drug or has hopes of getting it. To take away all possibility of getting the drugs is, in my opinion, the only way of getting a cure." Dr. Braunlich concluded "In other words, under certain conditions, a man who has once been a habitué is in danger of relapse, even though he has not had morphine for years." ³²

In a report in the *JAMA*, Dr. Hubbard was more optimistic about cure in institutions and used words that are reminiscent of those used by physicians who had advocated outpatient treatment by the general practitioner. "The process of removing the drug and all physical craving is simple, safe, and can be quickly done—a matter of days only, not weeks, months or years, as some would have us believe." This, of course, ran counter to Dr. Braunlich's more pessimistic view of prolonged episodes of craving, lasting perhaps a lifetime. But Hubbard believed his optimism was justified and that success in treatment depended merely on the elimination of drug availability. This could be accomplished through enforcement of laws and prohibiting any practitioner from maintaining treatment on his independent judgment, or worse, for financial gain.[33]

This was a curiously cheerful conclusion after the fact that most of those treated in Riverside Hospital had reverted to addiction, even after the best that current medical therapy could offer. Although it was undoubtedly true that without narcotics there would be no addiction, the belief that cure would result from an active enforcement of the laws was so far unproven in the United States. Indeed, an institution which one would think most likely to support the "medical approach" until the bitter end—a municipal agency with a national reputation for advanced and effective programs for public health—abandoned it with finality in 1920.

In its well-publicized denunciation of the medical approach, the Health Department did not deny the disease concept of narcotism, but the syndrome appeared as an unmysterious disease about which one would like to know more, but merely from a purely scientific point of view. Therapeutically, however, the condition was said to be understood sufficiently so that success in detoxification could be obtained from present methods of treatment: "In the vast majority of instances—99 percent—excellent results may be obtained by simple abrupt withdrawal." No esoteric knowledge, no complicated specific cures were necessary, just stop the drug—and, if one wanted to be more gentle, use hyoscine support. Addicts difficult to cure, perhaps one-fourth of all those addicted for nonmedical reasons, should simply be hospitalized or institutionalized "and held there, until a medical officer considers it safe for [them] to return to society." Although the role of the medical officer approximates that of a warden, it is only fair to recall that this severity toward addicts came from a health department which had made a vigorous and optimistic effort to treat addiction and had been confounded. The doctors then turned to quarantine as the magical tool to correct the deficiencies with which they were intimate. Control of narcotics was a practical police matter. Either drugs should be available for maintenance and therefore to anyone who wanted them, or they should be eliminated to stop addiction "by sufficiently stringent laws strictly and efficiently enforced [since] as long as addicts can obtain cheap supplies of drugs without personal risk, very few will apply for hospital curative treatment."

Hubbard denied that criminal addicts were criminals because of their addiction; the habit was not the cause of immoral character but just another reflection of unsavory environment. Causation of addiction certainly was more complex than a direct relationship with criminality.[34] Hubbard's analysis foreshadows a reevaluation of the addict that became more common among psychologically minded physicians in the 1920s, replacing physiological explanations.

Even Dr. Lambert, who had so elaborately confirmed the Towns treatment, now found the primary cause of addiction in the user's personality.[35] Such reasoning followed further study of deviance and social disorder. Increasingly, the cause of social or individual disorder was located in psychological dynamics—deep-rooted and long-standing character formation which antedated the appearance of the manifest antisocial behavior. Since by this interpretation basic character would have been formed long before drug abuse, addiction could only be one manifestation of personality and certainly not the cause of deficient character. The influence of psychoanalytic thought, and the rise of social work and psychology, would offer support in the 1920s to the belief that the causes of addiction lay deeper than its manifestations. While investigators evolved their psychological explanations, the Supreme Court, the Treasury Department, and Congress had put into effect methods to eliminate drug availability through traditional methods of law enforcement.

THE NEW ORLEANS CLINIC, 1919–1921

Although the New York State clinics were easily closed by the Narcotic Division, those in Louisiana, where the legislature had similarly authorized addiction maintenance, more effectively held off closure. In the favor of clinics in New Orleans, Shreveport, and Alexandria was their more efficient operation and the lack of blatant political manipulation. Under authority of the Board of Health, the three clinics came into being in the spring of 1919, just after the decisive Supreme Court ruling which led to arrests and fear among addicts and some physicians.

Shreveport maintained the most important of the Louisiana clinics. In the early 1920s the clinic presented the Narcotic Division with one of its most worrisome holdouts to closure, and it was closed only after three full investigations. Its performance is still heatedly debated by opponents and advocates of a national maintenance system. Its dispensary, under the direction of Dr. Willis P. Butler, has been totally damned by the Federal Bureau of Narcotics and warmly praised by, among others, sociologist Alfred Lindesmith.[36]

Louisiana has another reason for importance—Dr. Butler's nemesis, Dr. Oscar Dowling. Dr. Dowling was the president of the State Board of Health under which the clinics operated. From favoring the clinic plan in 1919 he became one of its most implacable enemies by 1922 and assisted the Narcotic Division in closing not only the three clinics in Louisiana but any others that caught his attention. His influence was not confined to the state since he was a member of the AMA's most powerful governing body, the Board of Trustees, from 1913 to 1925, and its chairman in 1923 and 1924. He served on AMA and American Public Health Association committees which studied drug abuse, and in 1921 he chaired the Committee on Drug Addiction of the State and Provincial Health Authorities of North America.

Initially Dr. Dowling favored clinics as a humane service to the community and thought that any defects were not in their goal but in faulty operation.[37] Before becoming a staunch opponent of clinics, he discovered that in spite of an apparent friendship with Levi Nutt, the best-run clinic would not satisfy the Narcotic Division. Prohibition Commissioner Kramer also warned him that as president of the Board of Health he might be indictable for authorizing clinics.[38] This threat helped transform him into an eager lieutenant who would use his office to help close the resisting New Orleans and Shreveport clinics. About the Alexandria clinic little has been learned, but evidently its closure never presented a problem.

Louisiana clinics had their origin in state legislation of 11 July 1918.[39] The State Board of Health employed a consultant, Dr. Charles Rosewater of New Jersey, to survey the narcotic situation. He estimated 18,000 addicts in Louisiana and saw the situation as very serious.[40] Thereupon the legislature acted. Similar to the First Whitney Act in New York State, the law provided for official narcotic prescription blanks for addicts, commitment to institutions either by complaint or voluntarily, and investment of the State Board of Health with power to set up regulations for the prosecution of the law.

In March 1919 there was an appeal by addicts to the State Board of Health for drugs, apparently prompted by the early effects of the Supreme Court decision. In the temporary absence of Dr. Dowling, Dr. M. W. Swords, secretary of the board, began dispensing drugs in New Orleans to a few addicts each day. The number grew in a few weeks to several hundred. Dr. Swords saw this service as a response to the needs of addicts and as a precaution against their purchasing drugs at greater cost from peddlers.[41] The State Board of Health asked the attorney general of the state for advice on the legality of selling drugs to addicts, since there was no appropriation to cover the expenses, and was told that it was permissible—in fact, that it was the board's clear duty to do so in order to reduce the likelihood of property and personal damage by addicts.[42]

Within a few months an old building was fitted out with examining rooms, segregated into three areas for white men, white women, and the non-white; application cards; history forms; etc. Dr. Swords said he tried to reduce the addicts to a minimal maintenance dose and keep them comfortable until institutional care became available. But the State Legislature declined to establish an institution, and New Orleans had available only the house of detention and the jail. Dr. Swords became an ardent advocate of the clinic as the only alternative if no institutional care was possible.

Dr. Dowling began to recommend closing the clinics, especially after the mid-November 1920 visit of Nutt to the city to urge the district attorney to that same goal.[43] Yet the rest of the board, Dr. Swords and the new governor, John Parker, were hesitant: first provide an institution, and then we can phase out the clinic, they argued.[44] Local narcotic agents responded that the police superintendent had promised a vigorous crackdown on peddlers, as soon as the clinic (now operating in violation of the Harrison Act) was closed, but not before. The U.S. attorney complained that the clinic greatly hindered prosecution under the Harrison Act since the clinic did openly what private physicians were told they could not do. Therefore the federal agency demanded the clinic cease operation and it conducted in late 1920 a quick "investigation" to implement this order.[45]

The board took up the consideration of closing the clinic on 15 February 1921. An intensive investigation by a narcotic agent was planned for the interval until the board meeting. Swords had believed that the previous brief investigation was biased and designed not to ascertain facts but to build a case against the clinic.

W. T. Truxtun, the revenue agent in New Orleans, angered by Swords's attack on the first report, did his best to present a thorough case to the governor: 223 addicts were registered on 2 December 1921. Eighty-one of these had criminal records, including offenses against state and federal drug laws. Some were prostitutes, three had given false names, five were treated by Swords under pseudonyms, and the rest were suspect, although Dr. Swords had stated that the clinic supplied only respectable working residents of New Orleans. Dr. Swords also claimed to have dispensed only morphine, but it was discovered that he had provided one addict with a daily ounce of laudanum. Also he had received from wholesale drug houses 2 ounces of cocaine and 2 drams of heroin. Three drams of cocaine had been consumed and the rest (29 drams) was "stored by Swords outside the walls of his institution, in the possession of the state chemist, who it is to be assumed had no knowledge of medicine whatsoever." [46] One dram of heroin had been distributed without record and the other dram was also in possession of the state chemist. A few other faults were found: at one time, although not recently, Dr. Swords had dispensed drugs to six persons with addresses in other states, and in several instances registrants were alleged to have sold their morphine to other addicts not enrolled. It was not denied that 80 percent were employed, as Dr. Swords claimed, but the clinic's hours—9 to 3 on weekdays and 9 to 12 on Saturdays—were said to be inappropriate for workers.

Examination of Truxtun's report reveals that he found only a small percentage of faulty dispensing and his most substantial statistics, the number of registrants with criminal records, was actually irrelevant to whether, if addicted, people with criminal records should receive narcotics until treatment in an institution was available.[47] Truxtun's statement to the governor suggests that he was determined to put the clinic and its director in an unfavorable light.

Dr. Swords complained that he had not received from the inspecting government officials "the courtesy and consideration that you would naturally expect of a representative of a government of a free people, particularly when I represent not an individual, but a sovereign state." But Dr. Dowling believed that the agents, particularly Truxtun, were working hard to discover the truth, and his firm views on clinics were also the official position of the American Medical Association, adopted during its convention in New Orleans in April 1920.[48]

With Governor Parker in the chair, the State Board reconvened in mid-February 1921 to consider the narcotic agents' investigation of the clinic. The board had used the interval to conduct its own investigation. Four of the seven board members united in recommending the establishment of a hospital where addicts could be confined and treated, but continuation of the clinic until then. With a hospital the clinic would operate "as an outpatient service for the purpose of dispensing morphine to incurables, aged and infirm and those cases in waiting, preparatory to being admitted into the hospital for treatment." The committee specifically commended Dr. Swords and Dr. Butler "for their splendid services rendered." The police and federal agents as well as Dr. Dowling did not budge, and the board retreated from its support of the clinics.[49] By the end of March the board ordered closed the New Orleans, Alexandria, and Shreveport clinics which provided maintenance narcotics.[50] Shreveport's clinic, however, continued to operate for two more years under authority of a city ordinance.

THE SHREVEPORT CLINIC, 1919–1923

Like the New Orleans Clinic, the Shreveport Clinic was high on the list of sites to be investigated by the Narcotic Division in early 1920. The first full-scale investigation of Dr. Butler's clinic was completed on 27 March 1920.[51]

The investigation viewed the clinic as a means leading to institutional treatment believed to be curative. It was not presented to nor perceived by the agents as a maintenance clinic. The strong support of enforcement and other public officials was impressive, and the agents "were very favorably impressed with the clinic, and also with Dr. Butler, who seems very efficient, and seems to have one idea of curing the addicts by treatment in the hospital."

A second investigation was made on Nutt's verbal orders in October 1921. By this time the clinic was becoming conspicuous—

almost all municipal and state clinics in the nation were now closed.

Two agents, one of whom was Dr. B. R. Rhees, secretary of the recent Special Narcotic Committee of the Treasury, went to Shreveport. First they visited the drugstores. No prescriptions were found for narcotic addicts, a significant fact to the investigators; the reputable druggists of Shreveport unanimously praised Dr. Butler as "honest and sincere in his efforts to help the City of Shreveport." Then they visited three prominent doctors and again approval was unanimous—they were no longer bothered by drug addicts except an occasional visitor to the city. The physicians warned that "there would be serious objection to the clinic's discontinuance." The agents saw little if any opportunity for morphine to be improperly disposed of. Every grain was accounted for. One hundred twenty-nine patients had been declared incurable and were receiving maintenance supplies. Each incurable was so certified by three or more physicians.

Various officials were also interviewed. Federal District Judge Jack again affirmed his high opinion of the clinic, which now had been operating for over two years. He warned that he would vigorously oppose any steps taken toward a discontinuance of the clinic, because from his own knowledge it had lessened crime in the city. The city judge was even more outspoken than the federal judge in his praise of Dr. Butler. He particularly favored care of the incurable addict which enabled him to work and not be a charge on the city. Both the chief of police and sheriff said that crime, such as petty thievery which might be resorted to to pay for illicit drugs, had lessened since the inauguration of the clinic. The U.S. marshal was of the same opinion.

The agents discovered a political environment which they found unique among communities with clinics: "There is absolute cooperation between Dr. Butler, the Police Department, the City officials, and the Federal officials." They recommended that the clinic not be discontinued since it was "operating under the full sanction of officials charged with the preservation of peace and order in the City of Shreveport and the Parish of Caddo." [52]

Shreveport's survival attracted national attention. Dr. Charles Terry, now Executive Director of the Bureau of Hygiene, sought a large number of statistics from Dr. Butler and grew to admire the operation and success of Butler's clinic.[53] For *American Med-*

icine Butler wrote a detailed description of the clinic, which was published in March 1922.[54] Now other cities began to ask if they also could set up such clinics. Shreveport became an obvious irritant and threatened to cause a revival of clinics throughout the nation—yet no fault in the clinic operation could be located. Two full investigations had found only praise for Dr. Butler among all the officials of the area, local and federal, and even the agents had been won over.

Dr. Butler began to infuriate some of the narcotic officials. The narcotic agent in charge of the Kansas City Division claimed he "made probably five or six visits to Shreveport, Louisiana, and stayed something like a day or two each time with no other business except to see if any point of approach could be gotten from which to ferret out and disclose the true working conditions and sentiments connected and controlling in the operation of the Shreveport Clinic." Finally the chief narcotic agent in the division decided that there was an explanation for the existence of this terrible situation: Dr. Butler was not only the head of the clinic but also "of an organization of propaganda in support of the clinic, and covertly in opposition to the Harrison Narcotic Law." [55]

The clinic's demise began in late August 1922, when an agent, H. H. Wouters, happened to be in Shreveport allegedly on business having no connection with the clinic whatsoever. He reported that a group of four citizens approached him and asked his aid in shutting off illicit supplies of narcotics sold by a peddler. They told Wouters that none of the local authorities could be trusted and that the illicit dealer was believed paying "full tribute to one of Dr. Butler's so-called inspectors." The next morning, when Wouters consulted with the district attorney, he was instructed to conduct any narcotic investigation with the aid of the sheriff, Dr. Butler, and his inspectors. As a dutiful agent, Wouters saw only one course: "I did as requested, with the result that no case was made against the apparent illicit dealer." A "reputable businessman" from whom the agent stated he got a lot of his information, told Wouters that he was being "double-crossed by the gang" and that Wouters's undercover buyer would be kicked off the peddler's veranda that night when he tried to make a purchase. And so he was. That was enough to arouse Wouters' suspicion of Dr. Butler and his distrust of the "authorities." Even more strange events occurred. The night of his first day in Shreveport, "as my custom when going into a strange city, I circulated around in the rough section during the evening." The next morning, when visiting Dr. Butler's clinic, he saw "a half dozen prostitutes that had solicited me the previous night, in line, getting their daily allowance." He told the doctor he did not think much of that nor of his clinic.[56] On his part, Dr. Butler found the agent "as vile and vulgar a man as I ever had to converse with." [57]

The immediate cause of the formal investigation, although prompted by Wouters's August visit, was made on the verbal order of Nutt, who had received an anonymous letter from someone purporting to be a clinic registrant. Under the date of 10 September 1922, the letter, signed "Use your own judgment," informed Nutt that Dr. Butler coached the registrants whenever an agent came to town because "he knows we get more than we need and we sell what we have to spare." Nutt was concerned about this letter and asked Wouters to make an investigation at his earliest opportunity.[58] The agents in September interviewed about 50 of the 129 registrants and convinced themselves that the clinic was just a fraud,[59] while being careful not to reveal their animosity toward the clinic to such supporters as Judge Jack or the U.S. attorney.

The true reason for the clinic's existence, they decided, was to maintain a large payroll of clinic employees. If the addicts were really cured, or given morphine for only genuine illnesses, Butler would be out of business and his payroll ended because the addicts maintained the clinic. The agents based this conclusion not only on their acute suspicion of Dr. Butler but also on their interviews with about 40 percent of the registrants. How these registrants were chosen is not indicated, but the agents found in them easy proof of the need for closing the clinic, if only the local officials would lose their confidence in Dr. Butler. The interviews reveal the issues deemed pertinent by the agents, their reasoning, and their characterization of long-term addicts. A few of them, excerpted from the agents' report, follow.

E. W.—39 years old, occupation sign worker, not working. Came to Shreveport 3 years ago from Joplin, Missouri. On clinic ever since he came to Shreveport. . . . Had been receiving 11 grains daily from Dr. Butler ever since coming to Shreveport. Said he would take much less if it cost more. "To our minds, Wilson is a drug addict, pure and simple."

Mrs. M.—had lived at another address for 6 months than the one listed by Dr. Butler. Came from Indiana 3 years ago, got 10 grains daily after starting at 8. Weighed 186 pounds when she came to Shreveport and lost 50 lbs. "Looks good and healthy but claims she feels bad if she doesn't get her daily allowance of morphine . . . a typical drug addict [with] no visible means of support."

Mrs. S.—37 years old, 8 years an addict, received 10 grains daily, had no visible means of support. Appeared to the agents as "a good healthy plain everyday drug addict."

J. R.—54 years old, morphinist for 20 years, " a physical wreck" receiving 10 grains daily. Although "appearing in very poor condition" the agents were "naturally unable to tell if he was affected with any ailment" but warned against his use as a witness in any prosecution due to his "physical appearance." He told the agents that two inspectors from Washington a couple of years ago said "there were very few people receiving narcotics on the clinic that were entitled to same, but that he was one of them."

B. J.—Prostitute, 32 years old, addict for 12 years and on clinic rolls for two. "Admits that on several occasions she has been off the drug, but not since she has been going to Dr. Butler; receives 12 grains daily." Although claiming a little of many diseases, she did not strike the agents as ill, but in reality "the picture of health; strongly built, and to our minds is a simple vicious addict." The agents were "solicited by her when we entered the premises."

W. M.—"a well-known bootlegger in liquor and narcotics" who had been driven out of Oil City by "a Public Committee" (the Ku Klux Klan). He had his daily dose of morphine picked up by his son against the time he should return. But the wife and son could not locate the drug for the agents when asked for it.

M. P.—52 years old, storekeeper, "a respectable man" who had been receiving 6 grains daily from the clinic for the past year. He would like to stop taking the drug and could do so "providing it is hard to get same." Claims a lot of healthy people got morphine from Dr. Butler who did not need it.

F. V.—30-year-old woman, "old opium smoker" who had switched to morphine. Came to Shreveport in 1920 (the year the Houston

Clinic closed) "to satisfy her addiction for the drug." Claimed
to have given money for hospital treatment to Dr. Butler which
he would not furnish, although she would like such treatment.
She had purchased drugs from outside sources, particularly from
"Jew R," who, it was claimed, paid $50 a week protection money
to one of Dr. Butler's "narcotic inspectors."

S. W. H.—39 years old, claimed to have been off morphine several
times for as long as 2 weeks at a time "when he was unable to
obtain it."

Investigations continued, and the case built against Dr. Butler
depended on information given by persons whose veracity or motives were not closely examined. The collection of accusations could
have come from a small group that profited from peddling and saw
the clinic as competition, or from a group which simply disliked
the clinic or Dr. Butler for political reasons. The grounds on which
antagonistic information was credited seem to have no internal consistency.

In conveying Wouters's report to the Prohibition Commissioner,
the narcotic agent in charge of the Kansas City Division warned of
the danger of the Commissioner should he ever meet Dr. Butler in
person. Dr. Butler, he said, was a deliberate violator of the law
and the most subtle medical opponent of the Harrison Narcotic Act
in that part of the country. If Dr. Butler should visit Washington he
should "be given to understand that the law must be adhered to
by the high as well as the low in the social strata." Wouters had
written earlier (29 September) to Assistant Prohibition Commissioner Blanchard in fear that Butler might come to the Capitol,
that he was "One of the greatest soft soapers that I have met for
many years and I am afraid, to use another slang expression, that
you may be carried away by his smooth ways. . . . He must not
be given the slightest encouragement at Washington." Wouters
asked that his letter be circulated to Nutt so he could be prepared
if Butler should come to see him.

Study of Wouters's report in Washington led to agreement that
"the District Judge and the U.S. Attorney evidently feel kindly
disposed toward this clinic, on account of propaganda." [60] The
Narcotic Field Force decided to send a "diplomatic" representative
to the federal officials before contemplating prosecution. For this
task the narcotic agent in charge of the Richmond, Virginia,

Division, G. W. Cunningham, was dispatched to confer with the judge and attorney. But even before Cunningham could get to Louisiana to meet with federal officials, Nutt had visited New Orleans and had spoken with Dr. Dowling on 4 December. Apparently Nutt had asked Dr. Dowling to write and put pressure on Butler for various reports on the supply of narcotics for the clinic, to remind him that the State Board had ordered the clinic closed, and to ask for the specific authority under which the clinic operated.[61] Dr. Butler replied on the 18th, explaining that he was not representing the State Board in any narcotic matter and that the hospital operated on the basis of a city ordinance which he enclosed. He stated that the district judge and U.S. attorney had given him verbal support and had expressed the belief that he was not violating any federal law.

On 30 January 1923, a conference was held, attended by Dr. Butler, the U.S. attorney, and three revenue agents, at which time it was mutually agreed to close the clinic on 10 February, leaving time for the "legitimate" clients to get their drugs elsewhere. The conference was not what Dr. Butler had expected. Two days later he wrote to Edward Wilson of the Atlanta *Georgian*:

> No records were gone over, no patients, officials, or doctors were called and nothing was gone into except the closing of the dispensary. I have felt all along, and still do, that I am right, but rather than enter an endless controversy without reasonable hope of what I consider right to prevail I agreed to discontinue the so-called clinic.
>
> All was very harmonious, and I must say the Inspectors appeared to be very nice gentlemen, far different from Mr. Wouters. I was told that I am not in any way accused of wrong-doing or bad faith, but that the work that I am doing here caused trouble because other places contended that if Shreveport be allowed to have a "clinic," they should also be allowed such a privilege.
>
> Mr. Cunningham read a part of Wouters's report in the conference. The addict's word was accepted by Wouters as truthful without corroboration, and without an investigation of facts that records, histories, and examination findings would reveal. For instance, several cases who have resided here for years were classed as not belonging here. Cases almost dead were called curable, so they report.[62]

Butler tried to transfer clinic addicts to private doctors or to give them institutional treatment, which was still permitted under state and federal law. For some he believed incurable he continued to write prescriptions on his own authority.[63] In June 1923 the Shreveport *Journal* investigated the city's drug traffic and claimed that morphine and cocaine were being freely sold, whereas before the closing of the clinic the traffic was practically unknown.[64] No clinic has had more controversial history or has provoked such irreconcilable attitudes as Shreveport's. Fortunately, much of the record has been preserved in the government's and Dr. Butler's files, so that a balanced reconstruction is now possible.

Willis P. Butler, a graduate of Vanderbilt Medical School in 1911, was thirty-five when the clinic opened in mid-1919.[65] Three years of clinic operation proved to be an early and anomalous incident in his long career in forensic and clinical pathology. Like Dr. Copeland, he interested himself in politics, but on a smaller scale, and was elected Parish Coroner and Physician for twelve four-year terms. He served as president of the Caddo Parish Medical Society, on the governing council of the American Public Health Association, and he is a founder of the American Society of Clinical Pathologists and the American College of Pathology. He survived the Narcotic Division's personal attacks and continued to receive professional and popular support in his various activities. The end of the clinic experience must have been unpleasant for him, but strong local support and his political and organizational ability as well as his high level of medical training make the clinic's closure one of the nation's most interesting power struggles over narcotic control.

As late as 1955, thirty-two years after its closure, the federal narcotics agency was still condemning Dr. Butler's clinic for permitting "75 percent of the drug addicts in Texas [to make] their headquarters there," and detailing many serious allegations against the Louisiana operation. Dr. Charles E. Terry, however, who had spent seven years as the executive of the Committee on Drug Addiction of the Bureau of Hygiene collecting information on the problem of addiction, wrote Dr. Butler in 1928:

In looking back over the work that has been done here and there throughout the country, I know of no single piece that can compare with yours as a constructive experiment in the practical handling of cases. The only criticism that I would make is that you did this work probably about twenty years ahead of the time when it could be appreciated, and I have little doubt but that in the next ten or fifteen years your plan will be in widespread operation in this country. If it is not, it will simply mean that rational education of both official and lay groups has been slower than I hope it will be.[66]

Alfred Lindesmith, in comparing the Federal Bureau of Narcotics' account with that in Terry and Pellen's *The Opium Problem* (1928) concludes in 1965, "There is hardly a single general statement about the clinic in the Bureau's account which can be accepted as accurate and which does not require serious qualification." [67] The Shreveport clinic remains the rallying point for those who believe a clinic system should have been established across the nation after 1919.

Three other clinics are representative of the several types that existed in 1920. The Atlanta clinic had a long history dating with interruptions back to the first days of the Harrison Act in 1915. In New Haven, a clinic created by the Police Department with the approval of the Internal Revenue Bureau functioned with local satisfaction but was closed by the Narcotic Field Force, although it had no discernible defect. Albany typifies some New York State clinics, operating with profit and significant political patronage, giving out cocaine as well as opiates, and therefore easy to condemn and to close.

THE ATLANTA CLINIC, 1915–1923

Establishment of the Atlanta clinic in 1915 is evidence that the Harrison Act had an effect on the customary sources of addictive drugs. The Treasury Agents' aggressive attack on addiction maintenance by physicians probably led Atlanta, as well as Jacksonville, Florida, and other cities to make some special provision for the indigent and "incurable" addict. At least since 1919 the "City Physician's Office Service to Drug Addicts" had operated out of the Department of Health, housed in the Atlanta City Hall.

The Narcotic Division's head, Levi Nutt, visited Atlanta on 23 March 1921 and informed the local revenue agents that the maintenance clinic there was illegal.[68] Special Agent Erwin C. Ruth then arrived to investigate the clinic.[69] This investigation, in the pattern of many others, described the origin, conduct, and reputation of the clinic, provided a list of addicts, some medical information on each, narcotic dosage, age, etc. The Atlanta clinic provided narcotic prescriptions for about 200 addicts. These would usually be filled at one of the two drugstores which did a fairly substantial business in the drugs, the first selling in the twelve months prior to the inspection 1,004 ounces of morphine and 17 pounds of opium. The average addict's daily dose varied between 5 and 10 grains of morphine. The two physicians who were employed full time for the medical needs of Atlanta's indigent divided between them the addict clients and wrote free prescriptions. Nonresidents of Atlanta were not regularly served but transients might be given an emergency supply to help them on their way. There were few instances when any substantial reduction in dosage occurred.

Ruth's report in mid-April recommended that morphine be dispensed in strict conformance with the Harrison Act, that is, for those medically incurable but not for the maintenance of simple addiction. As a result of Ruth's investigation, the Atlanta clinic dropped half its registrants and retained ninety-five who were described, at least by the city physicians, as incurable for medical reasons or of such long-standing addiction that they must be continued on the rolls. In January 1922 Nutt met in Washington with the chief Atlanta narcotic agent and reemphasized the need to halt the Atlanta maintenance program. Within a few days, T. E. Middlebrook had launched the second investigation of the clinic, with particular attention to the "incurables."

The recommendations of the second investigation were more severe. Middlebrook requested that city physicians be informed that any privileges previously given by narcotic officers were withdrawn and that the physicians be put on notice that prescriptions from then on would be scrutinized with great care. In cases of narcotic law violation, prosecution would be recommended. "I believe," the Atlanta narcotic agent wrote, "that if we stop the city physicians from prescribing that other physicians will be afraid to take [addicts as patients] and in that manner will stop the traffic in dope that is now going on in Atlanta." [70]

In late 1923 Dr. Lawrence Kolb, Sr., in the early years of a lifetime spent in the study of addiction, visited Atlanta at the request of Nutt to examine those few habitués still receiving drugs at the clinic. His task was to determine who might be cured and who should be left on the rolls. In November he interviewed and examined several dozen patients and prepared reports on them.[71] His trip to Atlanta is significant for the fact that it occurred at the request of the Narcotic Division. The report enabled local narcotic officers to take more clients out of the clinic, but little confidence was placed in his judgment that some addicts merited clinic treatment who were not already on the clinic rolls.

By 1925 the Atlanta clinic had faded away. It had succumbed to repeated investigations and threats to the physicians, although no indictments are known to have been sought or obtained. Whether its demise affected the level of drug use in the area is not known.

THE NEW HAVEN CLINIC, 1918–1920

By 1916 a private physician in New Haven had been designated by an internal revenue agent to write prescriptions for addicts at fifty cents each. This practice gradually accumulated complaints. The cost for a prescription seemed rather high, and purchase of the drugs at pharmacies designated by the physician was additional.[72] Police Chief Philip T. Smith alleged that drug peddling thrived in spite of the system and that addicts turned to thievery and prostitution to obtain money for drugs. Chief Smith did not oppose the idea of maintenance, but he favored less mercenary methods by the prescribers and dispensers. On 17 August 1918 a new system was inaugurated: addicts were directed to City Hall where they were registered and given drugs at modest prices under the care of police surgeons and pharmacists who were paid by the Police Department.[73]

The prescription fee was dropped to twenty-five cents and the morphine dispensed to the addicts at four cents a grain. Even at these lower charges a daily profit was made of $15 to $20. The profit went into a fund used to send addicts to respectable institutions for treatment. To register, an addict must reside and work in New Haven and be approved by the Chief; 68 addicts attended daily in August 1918 and this grew gradually to 91 when the clinic was investigated by Revenue Agents H. S. Forrer and O. W. Lewis.[74]

The *New Haven Register* reported the addicts' plight before the clinic was established: they would come to the private physician's home for regular prescriptions and "It was getting so the children and residents of the neighborhood recognized them as they wended their way to the doctor's office and pointed them out and subjected the unfortunates to unnecessary embarrassment." [75] It would appear that addicts in New Haven were more menaced than menacing.

The Police Department clinic operated from August 1918 until September 1920. Police Chief Smith saw advantages to a clinic: he traced addicts who failed to report and could thus locate perpetrators of thefts and burglary. Several drug peddlers were apprehended by tips given by clinic registrants. No scandal seems to have been associated with the clinic, doctors, pharmacists, or mode of operation, and, in fact, it received high commendation from Agents Forrer and Lewis in 1920. Its only fault lay in that it violated the Harrison Act by providing addiction maintenance. [76]

The clinic was closed in September 1920 along with other Connecticut clinics after the operators were threatened with indictment in letters prepared by the Prohibition Commissioner, but not without some remonstrance from Chief Smith, which Agent Ruth, who checked to be sure the clinics were closed, believed was actually an admission of the clinic's failure.

> The clinic at New Haven was closed September 13th and the Chief of Police arranged to have the addicts attending the clinic sent to a private house with a physician in charge. Only two addicts applied for treatment at said house. The Chief of Police stated that most of the clinic addicts are yet in the city and are purchasing their drugs from peddlers. The Chief also stated that the "dope peddlers" doubled their prices on "dope" just as soon as the clinic was closed, admitting that there were peddlers in the city during the time the clinic was in operation. Drug stores are not filling narcotic prescriptions for drug addicts. [77]

THE ALBANY CLINIC, 1919–1920

The Albany clinic illustrates some of the less desirable features of clinics operated under the authority of the New York State Narcotic Control Commission. It was one of the first established by the commission (18 April 1919), a week after the New York City clinic had opened. It operated about a year and a half, until September 1920, and had, in June 1920, 120 addicts in attendance. [78]

The clinic had its origin in a meeting in early April 1919 of Deputy Commissioner Whitney, Albany's mayor, the city's health officer, and a local physician. They agreed that the physician would conduct the clinic and be compensated fifty cents for each narcotic prescription. According to investigators Forrer and Lewis, who spent about a week looking into the clinic in June 1920, when Commissioner Herrick replaced Commissioner Whitney, the first physician appointed, who had sought to reduce maintenance dosages, was replaced for political reasons by two other local physicians. After this change in July 1919 no further records or receipts from the sale of prescriptions were kept. The clinic met from noon until two o'clock six days a week for several months until it was instructed by the commissioner's office to meet only on Mondays, Wednesdays, Fridays, and Saturdays. The case histories and records were confusing to the inspectors and they finally concluded that a conspiracy existed among the clinic doctors, the Narcotic Drug Commission, and a local drugstore which filled all the prescriptions. The evidence for this was suggestive. Other drugstore owners claimed that an addict would be cut off the clinic list if he did not take his prescription to this one shop. Other facts indicating a conspiracy around the clinic's operation included the chief clinic doctor's private practice; he prescribed for well-to-do addicts although he denied at first that he treated any addict outside the clinic. One of his private patients was thought by the police to be a peddler who had once been arrested on this charge. The doctor is reported as defending the patient's maintenance on grounds that he "has the appearance of suffering from tuberculosis" although records showed that no sputum examination or other scientific test had been made to establish the diagnosis.

The drugstore made up addicts' drugs in advance and sold them at the clinic for eight cents a grain or fraction thereof, two or three cents per grain above the price of other drugstores. The estimated annual income to this shop after deductions for costs was slightly over $17,000. In 1920, Levi Nutt, the head of the Narcotic Division, had an annual salary of $5,000 and an average agent earned less than half that. A feature that was rare among American clinics was the sale in Albany of cocaine to the addicts. In May 1920, 113 of the 120 addicts received prescriptions for 2 grains of cocaine along with prescriptions for morphine which averaged 7½ grains. At the rate of fifty cents for each of the prescriptions, the addicts paid a dollar at each clinic visit. At four visits a week this income was about $450 each week or about $23,000 annually.

The police spoke against the clinic on grounds that it cured no one and attracted addicts "from all parts of the country" who turned to crime to pay for their drugs. Furthermore, a number of the addicts were prostitutes with criminal records. But the Police Department's complaints are not fully substantiated by clinic statistics. Data for 3 June 1920 furnished to the inspectors by the clinic physicians revealed no addresses for cities farther away than Troy or Schenectady, and about half the addicts had attended the clinic since its opening, making the claim that it attracted addicts from around the country to be, if true, less threatening than it might seem, even without consideration of the small numbers involved. Altogether 47 nonresidents of Albany attended the clinic and of these all but one were from addresses within 15 miles. Thirteen attending had chronic diseases which might justify maintenance morphine. Men and women were evenly divided; a quarter of the women and a tenth of the men were nonwhite. The average age of the women was 30, of the men 34, the range 21 to 58. The daily dosage of morphine for women varied from 5 to 9¾ grains and for the men from 5 to 10 grains, the average dose for the whole clinic 8 grains.

Almost all the New York State clinics were good profit makers. The suspicion that politics played a major role was borne out by the repeated discovery that one had to be a political partisan in order to get a clinic franchise. The large profits from conducting a clinic ostensibly for the cure or curbing of drug use made the whole system a farce to the revenue agents. A showdown took place on the morning of 1 September 1920, in Commissioner Herrick's office. Present were Deputy Commissioners Riordan and Graham-Mulhall, Supervising Federal Prohibition Agent Simonton, and District Collector of Internal Revenue Frank J. Fitzpatrick. Herrick was told that the clinics in New York and in several other states had been investigated, and the reports were then considered at a conference held in Washington. As a result, all the clinics were to be closed except possibly Buffalo's.

The commissioner was willing to correct defects in the operation of the clinics, but not to close them. He believed that such clinics should operate until institutional treatment was available. But to this argument the agents replied that the present clinics were making almost no use whatever of the institutional treatment that was available. Moreover, there was no reason to hope for more facilities, since "it was extremely doubtful whether the State or Federal legislatures would provide the necessary funds for narcotic institutions—certainly not for a year or more, and probably not for many years." This regrettable reality determined as much as any other factor the decision to close narcotic clinics. Evidently by late 1920, federal agents were willing to admit the probable failure of the national program proposed by the France bill and were frank about the impossibility of relying on institutional treatment to end addiction. Then Simonton sternly informed the Commissioner that the Prohibition Unit had "adopted a definite policy in the matter." If he would not cooperate, the Treasury was prepared to take legal action. "I then," Simonton wrote, "exhibited to him, for the first time, one of the letters signed by Commissioner [of Prohibition] Kramer (the contents of which you are, of course, aware), and informed him that I had been instructed to deliver these letters personally in the event he refused cooperation." [79] The letters, dated 25 August 1920, were addressed to the various clinic physicians and informed them that they were in violation of the Harrison Act and should desist from treating immediately or face prosecution. This final threat was effective, for it was supported by the recent Supreme Court decision which clearly prohibited maintenance. The clinics were closed, and early the following year the New York State Commission itself was abolished by the legislature.[80]

Thus ended the many efforts by the New York State Legislature to devise a satisfactory drug control law. For six years after 1921 the state had no narcotic legislation, the problem being left up to city ordinances and federal statutes. A separate and distinct approach to addiction met head-on the reformers' plans for nonmaintenance and lost. No effective opposition to the federal stand against maintenance had been mounted by New York State, nor had Washington officials shown any hesitation in closing the clinics, although the clinics had state legislative sanction and were operated by a state agency.

The attack on the drug supply now became the chief goal of the Treasury Department in 1920. Imports and exports would be controlled by federal legislation and international treaties. Strict law enforcement would curb availability in the United States except for legitimate medical uses. Addicts could be treated in institutions and withdrawn from drugs; they could then return to their communities where they would not relapse, because of the danger of arrest and the high price or absence of narcotics. In this view, the narcotic clinic was a disruptive institution: it sanctioned the indefinite maintenance of addiction when the goal of the Narcotic Field Force was its elimination. The clinic not only made indictment of other suppliers of narcotics more difficult or impossible, it openly sustained what the public desired to eliminate. It was not thought that closure of the clinics themselves would miraculously solve any problem, of course. It in fact was anticipated that many long-standing addicts would seek out other supplies when the public source was shut off. For clinic closure to have its full effect, the rest of the control program would have to be successful.

The decision to move against municipal and state narcotic clinics seems to have been taken after deliberation in the winter of 1919–20. Implementation was not to be hasty or crude.[81] The Prohibition Unit's legal counsel cautioned against any attempt to close clinics by means of criminal proceedings unless prior wholehearted support had been obtained from local district attorneys and public officials, since grand jury indictments against municipal and state authorities would be difficult.

Perhaps, the division hoped, a simple indictment without prosecution would effect closure among the recalcitrant.[82] But no clinic closure ever required indictment. Persuasion or threat was all that was necessary. In New York, not only clinics but the entire State Narcotic Control Commission was quickly put out of business since its primary task had been to monitor addiction maintenance by private physicians and clinics. In 1921 the act establishing the commission was repealed and no new narcotic laws were enacted by the state legislature until 1927.[83]

The clinics were closed, but other parts of the federal program—keeping drugs out of America and gaining international control of narcotic traffic—would not be an outstanding success. Yet in 1919–25, the time of the anticlinic campaign, there were obvious loopholes in the laws which could be plugged, permitting further time to pass before these amended laws proved to be illusory. As long as some legal manipulation remained possible, the solution to the narcotics problem could always be seen just a step away. The psychological value of these legislative tinkerings was similar to the many modifications of the Towns-Lambert and other "cures." Many years had passed before the specific cures were seen to be worthless. For the progress of the human spirit, or at least the maintenance of the reforming spirit, the value of unproved treatments and legislative improvisations can be considered a powerful tonic.

The Troubled Twenties

8

The successful campaign to close the clinics can be credited to the establishment of a semiautonomous federal agency, the Narcotic Division of the Prohibition Unit, which could mount a coordinated and enduring attack from its headquarters in Washington with its own field force of about 170 agents divided among thirteen districts.[1] The head of the Narcotic Division, Levi G. Nutt, remained in his post from 1920 until early 1930, outlasting several Prohibition commissioners who succeeded one another as the enforcement of dry laws failed under widespread dishonesty and public contempt. One reason for the poor quality of prohibition enforcement was that jobs were openly filled by political patronage. Even Warren Harding informed Congress in 1922: "there are conditions relating to [Volstead Act] enforcement which savor of nationwide scandal. It is the most demoralizing factor in public life." [2]

The Narcotic Division, however, was under civil service. Scandal in its operation occurred less often, although indiscretions discovered in 1929 led to Nutt's removal in 1930. For the first decade of the Narcotic Division's existence, enforcement of the Harrison Act was eclipsed by the drama of national liquor prohibition. Narcotic agents were eventually embarrassed by their association with dry agents, and there were several recommendations by the AMA as early as 1921 that Nutt's agency be separated from Prohibition affairs.[3] There were other loud dissidents, Internal Revenue Commissioner Roper among the earliest, who saw no reason for making the tax agency of the government responsible for Prohibition enforcement. Finally, in 1930, Prohibition was transferred to the Justice Department, and narcotic affairs were vested in a new unit, the Federal Bureau of Narcotics, which remained in the Treasury Department until 1968, when it too was turned over to the Justice Department and considerably revamped.

Levi Nutt, a registered pharmacist who joined the Treasury Department in 1901, had been an official of the Alcohol Tax Unit, which administered the Harrison Act. Enforcement of the Harrison Act had been, until 1920, a difficult task because the Bureau of Internal Revenue rapidly acquired immense new responsibilities for income taxes and other sources of revenue to prepare for and prosecute World War I, while congressional provision for increased personnel and reorganization lagged behind.

The Prohibition Unit was established on 22 December 1919, after passage of the Volstead Act had outlined enforcement of the 18th Amendment.[4] The first Prohibition commissioner, John F. Kramer, and his force of about 2,500 agents were deeply involved with the great experiment and left narcotic enforcement to the much smaller and distinct Narcotic Division. Expenditures for narcotic enforcement rose from about $270,000 in fiscal year 1919 to slightly more than $500,000 in fiscal year 1920, and for several years thereafter it ranged between one-half and three-quarters of a million dollars annually. The number of agents and inspectors rose from about 170 in 1920 to almost 270 in 1929, and hovered around the latter figure during the Depression.[5]

From 1915 on there were fewer convictions and arrests of registrants under the narcotic statute than of unregistered peddlers and smugglers. Because the problem was more circumscribed, and narcotic agents numbered a tenth of dry agents, narcotic violations were fewer than Volstead violations during the 1920s.[6] But because of the severity of judges and juries, the federal prisons were flooded with narcotic violators. By mid-1928 almost a third of 7,700 prisoners in the one female and four male penitentiaries were Harrison Act violators, more than the combined total for the next two categories— liquor prohibition and car theft.[7] This superabundance of narcotics prisoners led, at long last, to federal hospital care for addiction. The Public Health Service was given the thankless task of caring for addicts in narcotic "farms" at Fort Worth, Texas, and Lexington, Kentucky.

The Narcotic Division used threats and intimidation, when necessary, in dealing with uncooperative physicians, and the flow of convicted offenders to federal prisons made these tactics effective. Physicians had been repeatedly called prime offenders in the national narcotic menace, and agents were not disposed to condone "dope doctors." Before World War I the AMA minced no words: the evils of addiction were so great that they

> convince the most ardent advocate of states' rights that legislation regulating the sale of all dangerous habit-forming narcotics should be national in scope and absolutely uniform throughout the country. In matters which affect the health of the nation at large the laws should be made by Congress, and their execution should be in the hands of federal rather than state authorities.[8]

Yet after the 1919 *Webb* and *Doremus* decisions, and subsequent enforcement by zealous agents, reputable physicians became uncomfortable. The social and economic position of the registered physician was so sensitive, trials so time-consuming, and appeals so long and costly, that hostile agents could make cases against physicians with impunity and nearly ruin them whether charges were warranted or not.[9] Narcotic agents were so unpopular and feared that upon his appointment as Commissioner of Narcotics in 1930, H. J. Anslinger told his agents to "discontinue investigating the corner drug-store and the family doctor and get after the smugglers and racketeers." [10]

Both the Narcotic Division and the now wary AMA followed closely each court decision subsequent to the major pronouncements of 1919. The issues of intention and good faith were dealt with by the Supreme Court in March 1922. A New York physician was indicted for prescribing a large amount of heroin, morphine, and cocaine for a patient, an equivalent for nonaddicts of three thousand ordinary doses. The physician was arrested for providing several days' narcotics for the addict's self-administration. The defendant claimed that he was treating drug addiction, but the Court's majority of six concluded that such an enormous number of doses could only be used, as phrased in the earlier *Webb* decision, "to cater to the appetite or satisfy the craving of one addicted to the use of the drug," and thereby swept away any pretense that the physician's written order was a prescription. The Court held:

> Undoubtedly doses may be varied to suit different cases as determined by the judgment of a physician. But the quantities named in the indictment are charged to have been entrusted to a person known by the physician to be an addict without restraint upon him in its administration or disposition by anything more than his weakened or perverted will. Such so-called prescriptions could only result in the gratification of a diseased appetite for these pernicious drugs or result in an unlawful parting with them to others.

Justices Holmes, McReynolds, and Brandeis dissented, stating in the words of Justice Holmes that the good faith of the physician, which was not contested by the federal government, would protect the defendant regardless of his acts, "however foolish." [11] Yet the Court, by a somewhat larger majority than in the *Webb* and *Doremus* cases, had eliminated even the intent of the physician as a defense if he should prescribe large amounts of narcotics for an addict.

Uneasy physicians began to protest to their professional organizations and to their congressmen against the threat of indictment which hung over them. Congressman Lester Volk of New York, the physician-lawyer who had been a prominent leader of the medical-economic interests in his state, demanded in January 1922 that Congress investigate the narcotic laws and their administration. Volk condemned a small group of physicians who had formed a "conspiracy" to deprive the medical profession of its accustomed legal rights. He named Alexander Lambert, S. Dana Hubbard, A. C. Prentice, Royal S. Copeland, E. Eliot Harris, and an attorney, Arthur D. Greenfield. These men had dominated the national medical organizations and their committees on drug addiction and had given a false picture of medical opinion on the issue; they also supported the federal government's encroachment on states' rights.[12] But the investigation never took place; Volk lost his seat in Congress to Democrat Emmanuel Cellar in the November elections. In the medical profession, however, opposition to federal activity was also becoming more open. Dr. James F. Rooney, a vigorous spokesman for the private practitioner and an opponent of legislation that would restrain any of the prescribing rights of physicians, was elected president of the New York State Medical Society in March 1921, and the AMA was beginning to waver in its support of federal intervention in medical affairs. By May 1922 the House of Delegates of the AMA emphatically condemned state medicine and urged that such schemes for partial state medicine as the Sheppard-Towner Act for maternal and child care be vigorously opposed.[13]

Several victories were won by opponents of federal control of narcotics in medical practice. In 1922 the Treasury Department's refusal to register addicted physicians was declared beyond the department's authority, as was its practice requiring one year to pass after a felony conviction before re-registration was granted to a druggist or physician.[14] In 1925 a Missouri district court decided that a druggist could fill a physician's prescription although he might have reason to believe that the patient was an addict and was receiving enormous amounts of narcotics.[15]

Then in January 1926 the Court took the unusual step of inviting a new test of the constitutionality of the Harrison Act. The Court declared that several recent decisions, including the child labor tax case and *Linder* v. *U.S.*, "may necessitate the review of that question [the Act's constitutionality] if hereafter properly presented."[16]

The Treasury Department's revised enforcement program was submitted to Congress in March 1926 for adoption by amending the Harrison Act.[17] This time the federal government had to face alert and active opposition from both trade and medical interests. The opposition had been encouraged by two recent Supreme Court decisions which seemed to reverse the trend toward control of the practitioner's judgment in narcotic use. In April 1925 the Court had unanimously reversed the conviction of a Spokane physician who dispensed three tablets of cocaine and one tablet of morphine to an informer of the Narcotic Division. The doctor claimed the informer had described severe abdominal pains such as would come from an ulcer or cancer, while the government claimed the doctor knew the informer was an addict and gave medication merely for her comfort. The Court unanimously held:

> [The Behrman Decision of 1922] cannot be accepted as authority for holding that a physician who acts *bona fide* and according to fair medical standards may never give an addict moderate amounts of drugs for self-administration in order to relieve conditions incident to addiction. Enforcement of the tax demands no such drastic rule, and if the Act had such scope it would certainly encounter grave constitutional difficulties.[18]

Against this background of increasingly critical court decisions which might lead to a decision against the constitutionality of the Act itself, the Treasury Department sought to strengthen it by congressional amendments. If states' rights appeared to be violated, the constitutional basis for these amendments would lie in fulfillment of the international treaty obligations of the United States under the Hague Convention, and would be in accord with the 1920 Supreme Court decision *Missouri* v. *Holland*.[19] When hearings began in the House in May 1926 the administration asked for seven amendments to give the Narcotic Division authority:

1. To prevent addicted physicians from registering under the Harrison Act and to withhold registration for a year from any registrant who had been convicted of a Harrison Act violation.
2. To remove the necessity of proving venue in the absence of a tax stamp on a package of drugs.
3. To forbid "ambulatory treatment" and to require full recording of all drugs dispensed or distributed except in an emergency.

4. To place some responsibility on the druggist to determine that a prescription was written in good faith.

5. To provide that records of "purchases" of exempt narcotic preparations as well as other kinds of transactions be reported and recorded.

6. To confiscate automobiles used in narcotic violations.

7. To make forging or altering narcotic prescriptions an offense.[20]

The Treasury case, chiefly presented by Narcotic Division Counsel Alfred L. Tennyson and Nutt, had hard going. After two days of testimony the government withdrew the third and fifth recommendations; the ultimate result was that none of the amendments was enacted.[21]

The Supreme Court's request for a test case of the Harrison Act's constitutionality was later granted. In April 1928 the Supreme Court held, by a six to three decision (*Nigro* v. *U.S.*), that the Harrison Act was indeed constitutional.[22]

After hints of unconstitutionality in the *Daughertey* v. *U.S.* decision, the AMA *Journal* editorially wondered whether the demise of the Harrison Act would be an "unmitigated evil" and compared its invasion of states' rights with that of the Sheppard-Towner Act. The purpose of the Harrison Act, "the suppression of the narcotic habit," had never been proven by the Act's proponents to be closer of attainment than in 1914, according to the journal.[23] Oscar Dowling, who had so dutifully cooperated with Nutt in 1920–23, found by 1925 the relationship between the Narcotic Division and the physician in need of repair.[24]

Still, the controversy over the Harrison Act, contained as it was between the health professions and the government, did not reach the proportions of the national debate over prohibition of liquor. There were parallels, however, between enforcement problems in both liquor and narcotics. To improve the disgraceful state of liquor enforcement, two remedies suggested at the inception of Prohibition were finally enacted: civil service requirements for all employees except the Commissioner, and a separate Bureau of Prohibition in the Treasury Department (but still including narcotic enforcement). Representatives of the Treasury Department appeared in April 1926 before Congress with a list of proposed amendments, but its requests were about as successful as Nutt's of the following month.[25] Assistant Secretary of the Treasury General Lincoln C.

Andrews, who had taken effective control away from the Anti-Saloon League's sympathizer R. A. Haynes in April 1925 and reorganized the unit's operation, asked Congress for more authority to control medicinal liquor, to search homes for stills, to stop and search American ships beyond the twelve-mile limit, etc.[26] Congress, however, would only set up a separate bureau and authorize civil service standards. It then adjourned without providing funds to carry out civil service examinations. This was very frustrating to the head of the Anti-Saloon League, Wayne B. Wheeler, who had testified at the hearings in April that the fact that the law was difficult to enforce was the clearest proof of the need for it.

With bureau status acquired in April 1927, and an increase in appropriations of more than two million dollars, the Prohibition Bureau continued its difficult task. Eventually civil service standards were established and all previous appointees had to take the examination in late 1927 in order to keep their jobs; to the embarrassment of the bureau, three-quarters of them failed. Through various maneuvers like temporary appointments, and by taking other candidates outside the bureau who had qualified, the field staff was gradually filled out in most positions.[27]

Establishment of a separate bureau meant little change in procedures for the Narcotic Division. Nutt, now named Deputy Commissioner of Prohibition, continued to send prisoners to federal penitentiaries in large numbers and claimed that the situation was under control. He declared that there were probably fewer than a hundred thousand addicts in the United States and denied accusations that the problem was out of hand.[28] Annual appropriations for narcotic control gradually rose during the decade from about half a million dollars in fiscal year 1920 to $1.6 million for fiscal year 1930.[29] By 1930 the style of enforcement had settled down to fairly well-recognized procedures and legal boundaries. The clinics were out of business, doctors were aware of the danger of maintaining addicts and the likelihood of entrapment, and drug companies submitted their manufacturing and trade reports regularly. The narcotic agency led a fairly routine life, punctuated only occasionally by a scandal or a major arrest.

ANTI-NARCOTIC ORGANIZATIONS

The end of World War I reawakened some of the interest which had led to American activity abroad in earlier years. Once again

trade with the Orient drew attention to the economic role of opium
traffic and addiction. The end of the war also meant that nations
could again consider effective restraints on illegitimate opium traffic,
particularly that directed toward America. The United States was
at first very pleased to cooperate with Great Britain in adding Section 295 to the Versailles Treaty, making ratification of that treaty
equivalent to ratification of the Hague Convention. The League,
which President Wilson anticipated the United States would join,
was given the international responsibility which the Netherlands
government had previously discharged for the Hague Convention.[30]
If the United States had joined the League, undoubtedly American
leadership would have been preserved, but the failure of the Senate
to approve the League Covenant meant that America would be for
the first time outside the official body responsible for international
opium control. This situation would lead to many complications,
for American distrust of foreign sincerity with regard to opium
control would be reinforced by distrust of the League.

Within the United States several lay groups sought to eliminate
the narcotic menace.[31] The International Narcotic Education Association (1923), the World Conference on Narcotic Education
(1926), and the World Narcotic Defense Association (1927) were
all creations of the remarkable Richmond P. Hobson, Spanish-
American War hero and prohibition propagandist, who publicized
the danger of narcotics in every conceivable way. He was particularly anxious to get his message into school textbooks, on radio programs, and into the halls of Congress, where he had once served.
The officers of these groups were socially prominent and politically
active men and women who eagerly joined him to awaken America
to the dire menace of narcotics. Any suggestion that the number of
addicts in America was not immense (like the reassuring report of
Kolb and DuMez in 1924 that there were probably only 110,000
addicts in the nation) was met with strong rebuttal.[32] Hobson was
one of the most active popularizers of the belief that narcotics,
particularly heroin, prompted crime and drove users to commit the
most horrible acts. He possessed charm and an impressive manner,
knowledge of the Prohibition movement (he was the highest paid
of the Anti-Saloon League's "special speakers") and a desire to crusade. The *JAMA* complained of his distortions and exaggerations;
Nutt maintained as early as 1926 that he thought there were even
fewer addicts than the Kolb and DuMez estimate, but the Hobson

associations kept on fighting, spreading fear and producing statements that were faithfully repeated by other national organizations, fraternal orders, and radio networks; all felt that by relaying Hobson's message they were serving their nation.[33]

The last week of February 1927 (picked because it contained George Washington's birthday) was denominated by Hobson as Narcotic Education Week. In a national radio broadcast of 1928, the time donated by the National Broadcasting Company, he marked the close of the second annual observance of this call to national awareness by telling about heroin addicts, "the Living Dead":

> To get this heroin supply the addict will not only advocate public policies against the public welfare, but will lie, steal, rob, and if necessary, commit murder. Heroin addiction can be likened to a contagion. Suppose it were announced that there were more than a million lepers among our people. Think what a shock the announcement would produce! Yet drug addiction is far more incurable than leprosy, far more tragic to its victims, and is spreading like a moral and physical scourge.
>
> There are symptoms breaking out all over our country and now breaking out in many parts of Europe which show that individual nations and the whole world is menaced by this appalling foe . . . marching . . . to the capture and destruction of the whole world.
>
> Most of the daylight robberies, daring holdups, cruel murders and similar crimes of violence are now known to be committed chiefly by drug addicts, who constitute the primary cause of our alarming crime wave.
>
> Drug addiction is more communicable and less curable than leprosy. Drug addicts are the principal carriers of vice diseases, and with their lowered resistance are incubators and carriers of the streptococcus, pneumococcus, the germ of flu, of tuberculosis, and other diseases.
>
> Upon the issue hangs the perpetuation of civilization, the destiny of the world and the future of the human race.[34]

The next year Hobson broadcast: "Ten years ago the narcotic drug addiction problem in America was a minor, medical problem. Today it is a major, national problem, constituting the chief factor menacing the public health, the public morals, the public safety." [35]

While attempting to create maximum fear over narcotic addiction and its connection with crime, the International Narcotic Education Association claimed increasing success in their proposed changes in school textbooks to alert youth to the criminal and destructive influence of narcotics.[36] Hobson also sought a fund of ten million dollars from public contributions so that his campaign could be put on a permanent, sound footing. He remained active in the 1930s, alerting the nation to a need for stringent marihuana laws, and even devoted the 1937 Narcotic Education Week to that topic, just before hearings on the Marihuana Tax Act began in the House of Representatives.[37]

Another major narcotics association was modeled after the burgeoning national groups with local chapters which focused on a particular disease (e.g. the National Tuberculosis Association founded in 1904; the National Committee for Mental Hygiene, 1909): The White Cross, Inc., was founded in Seattle in 1921 as a direct outgrowth of narcotic interest within the China Club, composed of leading Seattle residents who were interested in improving trade with China. Members discovered in 1920 that foreign morphine was being shipped across the United States to Japan to be smuggled into China and also that some American narcotic drugs were going to Japan for eventual use in China. The China Club persuaded two Washington congressmen to prepare legislation to remedy a situation which was embarrassing to American businessmen.[38]

Once the China Club had tasted success in Congress, a cadre of local groups and members of the Seattle Chamber of Commerce metamorphosed itself into the White Cross International Anti-Narcotic Society. The White Cross was most active on the West Coast, but affiliates existed elsewhere in the nation. Like the Tuberculosis Association, the leadership became interested in treatment at the local level. By 1926 the White Cross was endorsing the work of Dr. Butler, and it eventually came to espouse narcotic clinics at which addicts could receive their daily supplies.[39] Clearly this group aimed in a direction opposite that of the International Narcotic Education Association, which did not believe that drugs causing "degeneration of the upper brain . . . in a few months" should be regularly supplied, thereby perpetuating "the Living Dead." [40] In the late 1930s, when a bill to permit narcotic clinics like Butler's was under consideration in the Washington State Legislature, the full efforts of Commissioner Anslinger and the Hearst *Seattle Post-*

Intelligencer were used to defeat the proposal.[41] When Hobson died in 1937 his coterie lacked leadership and the associations dissolved; the White Cross became defunct after World War II.

Hobson's associations did not disseminate accurate information on narcotic addiction, but they were a means by which addiction in the United States came to be regarded with fear and disgust. Hobson effectively associated heroin with crime and violence. It is worthwhile to note that Hobson, although not respected by someone like Anslinger, was used as an active propaganda force; he knew influential people and would persuade anyone who listened to him that the Federal Bureau of Narcotics' fight was vital and should be maximally supported. Organizations like the White Cross, which had members at least as sincere and seem to have had more direct contact with the addict than the Hobson organizations had, were fought because they tried to reestablish maintenance, a once-respectable mode of care but one which would have wrecked the prohibitive enforcement law on which federal narcotic controls were based.[42] Overall, the propaganda spread by zealots like Hobson was accepted as true, and addicts were perceived as an immense evil which should be blotted out of society.

The emergence of lodges and service clubs, the Moose, Kiwanis, Knights of Columbus, and some Masonic orders, as supporters of antinarcotic legislation and disseminators of narcotic information was another characteristic of domestic antinarcotic activity after World War I.[43] The China Club's interest is easily understandable, but other groups, with no specific association with narcotics except that addiction was a threat to their communities, joined the crusade in the coming years. Politicians who were lodge members, like Representative Stephen G. Porter of Pittsburgh, were able to garner national support for stringent measures through their fraternal contacts. Hobson sent millions of pamphlets and information sheets to service clubs, encouraging their interest in fighting the menace.[44] Other organizations, like the WCTU and the International Reform Bureau, continued their prewar support of antinarcotic laws. Fighting narcotics became a very respectable and time-consuming activity for clubs in search of a suitable menace. Picturing the opium addict as a beast who threatened homes and safety gave the crusade a little excitement, confirmed the public need for their efforts, encouraged appreciation, and harmed no one except perhaps the addict.

AMERICAN INTERNATIONAL INITIATIVE IN THE 1920S

The China Club's alarm at Japanese smuggling of drugs into China, combined with anxiety over domestic prosperity, led to a legislative proposal that would affect international trade in narcotics. "We are poisoning our best customer," warned the secretary of the China Club, "a customer that is potentially able to take more American goods than any other nation." Trade with China, which Seattle greatly coveted, had been increasing, but evidence of American complicity in the Japanese drug traffic threatened to worsen our relations with China. Unless we prohibit these drugs from leaving the United States, Underwood warned, "we will continue to be a party to one of the greatest crimes in history, and at the same time destroy one of our best markets for American goods." Just as American altruism at the Shanghai Commission had put British trade in an unfavorable light, this postwar action embarrassed Japan. In autumn 1920, as the postwar economic depression worsened, members of the China Club met with Representative John Miller and Senator Homer Jones to prepare a simple amendment to the narcotic laws which would ban all exportation of narcotics from the United States, whether of domestic origin or in transit. The Surgeon General would be given authority to permit crude opium and coca leaves to enter for manufacture into necessary domestic narcotics.[45]

Hearings were held on Miller's bill, HR 14,500, in December 1920 and January 1921, during the last session of the 66th Congress. The subcommittee of the Ways and Means Committee, which heard testimony, was chaired by Representative Lindley Hadley, also of the state of Washington. Representative Rainey, who had framed the most recent amendments to the Harrison Act, had been defeated in the recent Harding landslide along with many other Democrats, yet he participated until his last day in Congress as a member of the subcommittee.

Witnesses provided considerable information on the current problem of American narcotic control. Provision of morphine for Chinese addicts was only one danger that arose from our loose import-export laws. Closer to home, American narcotic exports to Canada showed a great increase after the Harrison Act. The consensus among the witnesses and the subcommittee was that most of the drugs illegally used in the United States were not of foreign origin but were domestic manufactures smuggled back after legal export.[46] The proposed act would plug this loophole and attempt to prevent transshipment of foreign products for the economic exploitation of China.

The health professions remained, however, the prime targets of reformers trying to diminish narcotic use in the United States. The renowned surgeon and gynecologist of Johns Hopkins Hospital, Dr. Howard Kelley, argued for stricter controls on narcotic exports to China on grounds of "an interest which is common to many of our citizens. I have investments there." But Dr. Kelly was a tireless reformer in many areas of human life, and his hatred of addiction arose from other considerations as well. Experience had taught him that physicians were largely responsible for the tremendous use of the drug in this country.

The culpability of another profession was pointed out by Henry N. Pringle, speaking for the International Reform Bureau. He maintained that "nine-tenths of the habit-forming drugs are sold by druggists or by persons who get their supply from druggists." The question of cure, which Dr. Kelley viewed so pessimistically, was raised again by Dr. Harvey Wiley, who favored the Lambert treatment as "a really rational treatment for the drug addict," and seconded Lambert's call for the outlawing of heroin. Representative Rainey was particularly incensed at heroin, "a German invention," which sentenced the addict to "sure death in less than ten years." [47]

Drug manufacturers opposed the total ban on exports but, as usual, approved the goal of the legislation to stop American compliance in the spread and sustenance of addiction abroad and at home. Open disagreement again arose between reformers and the drug trades. Representative Rainey in particular was angered by a suggestion from one pharmaceutical spokesman that his amendments to the Harrison Act in 1919 were put through in some dark fashion since no hearings had been held. Rainey replied that if the Act remained as Dr. Wright originally wrote it there would have been no adverse court decisions, "but after we had all these hearings with the representatives of the wholesale druggists and the retail druggists, clear down to the veterinary surgeons, the effect of all those amendments was to completely destroy the Act." Rainey went on to declare what numerous opponents of the Harrison Act had suspected, that the federal officials "charged with its enforcement were simply bluffing the thing through" until the 1919 amendments.[48]

When Nutt appeared at the hearings in the first week of 1921 he had almost no information that would be useful to the committee. He had no knowledge of the amount of opium smuggled into the United States, nor was he "in a position to say" that the use of narcotics had increased in America during the previous five or six years, but he was certain that the Harrison Act "is now being enforced better than it ever was." His most remarkable statement was that, in spite of not knowing the amount of narcotics smuggled into the nation, he estimated "we probably get half of it." He made no mention of the crackdown on ambulatory treatment or clinics which was well under way by the date of his testimony. Witnesses from the Public Health Service were in complete agreement with Dr. Kelley on the danger from the American medical profession which, according to one assistant surgeon general, "does not use narcotics in what might be regarded as a legitimate way." The witness who represented the "medical approach" was Dr. Charles Terry, who had established perhaps the earliest maintenance clinic under government authority in the United States. In the early years of his clinic he blamed physicians and druggists; even in 1921 he believed many addicts originated from professional malpractice but thought the number was decreasing. Dr. Terry pleaded for a moratorium on further legislation until a congressional investigation could look into the medical side of addiction. He hoped that the public and the majority of the medical profession could be persuaded that addiction was not a depravity or a vicious habit but rather a disease without moral stigma, at least when once contracted. He was heard politely by the Congress but without any sign of agreement. His notion for an investigation into the disease nature of addiction was opposed by Rainey as a duplication of the Secretary of the Treasury's committee, which had reported in spring 1919. But neither Terry nor Rainey had any word of hope for a cure.[49]

Dr. Terry's attitude toward addiction and its ease of treatment had been severely shaken in the early days of the Harrison Act. He felt he was responsible for the deaths of two children, one an infant who was addicted at birth. The baby died in a few days because Dr. Terry did not realize the need to provide the infant with narcotics. He believed he had also caused the death of an addict by using the Lambert method of withdrawal. The accepted "rational cure" so weakened the heart of a previously healthy woman that she died after several days of cathartics, hyoscine, and belladonna. His examples stressed the need to understand physiology, to move cautiously, and perhaps to maintain some addicts rather than kill by withdrawal.[50]

In February 1921, two weeks before the end of his term, Representative Rainey submitted a revision of the Jones-Miller proposal, which would permit narcotic exports, if approved by the Secretaries of State, Treasury, and Commerce, upon assurance that the nation to which the materials were exported would monitor the use and disposition of the drugs.[51] As finally adopted, the Narcotic Drugs Import and Export Act, approved 26 May 1922, led to the Federal Narcotics Control Board, composed of the Secretaries of State, Treasury, and Commerce to administer it.[52] The everyday details were left primarily to the Treasury Department's Narcotic Division. The Act was designed to limit exports to nations which had ratified the Hague Convention and which had an adequate license system; its provisions required proof from consigners that the purposes of the drugs were legitimate and guarantee that they would not be re-exported. The Act limited exports to areas where there was a proven opiate shortage.

The Secretary of the Treasury, Andrew Mellon, was the only official to oppose a key measure of the Act—the prohibition of in-transit shipments of narcotics—because, he pointed out, to police such a law effectively would require a greatly expanded customs service. Secretary Mellon also questioned the wisdom of restricting the importation of narcotic drugs since this would, in his view, stimulate smuggling. The customs service had an almost impossible task with smuggling as it was, its reports showing "conclusively that smuggling of narcotics into the United States is on the increase to such an extent that customs officers seem unable to suppress traffic to any appreciable extent." [53]

American Attempts to Regain International Leadership

After Rainey's defeat in 1920, congressional leadership in narcotic matters was assumed by Republican Representative Stephen G. Porter of Pittsburgh, chairman of the House Committee on Foreign Affairs.[54] Although Rainey was reelected in 1922 and eventually became Speaker of the House in 1933, he no longer took a leading role in narcotics legislation. Porter's national and international renown in narcotic control quickly exceeded that of Rainey. He sought in particular to revise the Hague Treaty which regulated world narcotic traffic and production. Although inexperienced as a diplomat, his chairmanship in the House caused the State Department to treat him with care. Perhaps his two years of medical training, taken before entering law school, gave him interest in and confidence about this medicolegal problem.

Porter became obsessed with the idea that the production of raw opium and coca leaves must be controlled before any other aspect of narcotic traffic was undertaken; without such basic restrictions, international regulation of pharmaceutical manufacturing, for example, or even such domestic laws as the Harrison Act in the United States, were "hopeless." The regrettable outcome of Porter's intransigent adherence to this priority was a curb on American involvement in international control until his death in June 1930.[55]

Porter's strategy called for Congress to endorse a specific antinarcotic position prior to international negotiations. He believed President Wilson's failure to obtain Senate approval to join the League of Nations might have misled foreign powers about the power of the executive branch.[56] He therefore sought to strengthen the American negotiators' hand by indicating that the American position had strong legislative support.

The State Department's suspicion of conspiracy to prevent the first Hague Conference in 1911 may have been well founded. When the League of Nations undertook to oversee narcotic control through the establishment in December 1920 of the Opium Advisory Committee, the League's custodianship of what had been an American program was closely watched. Within a year American leaders in the antinarcotic movement, such as Mrs. Wright, were extremely displeased by what they saw as obstruction by opium-producing nations, particularly India, represented by its British rulers.[57] India had crippled in the Assembly of the League of Nations an Advisory Committee resolution calling upon all nations to restrict the cultivation of poppies and production of opium to "strictly medicinal and scientific" purposes, by striking out the limiting words and substituting "legitimate." This made the resolution meaningless since legitimate would include, for example, smoking opium in India.[58]

Porter then framed a lengthy Joint Resolution (HJR 453) calling on certain nations to restrict their production. His resolution faulted Great Britain, the British government of India, and Persia and Turkey with regard to opium production; and Peru, Bolivia, and Java and the Netherlands with regard to coca. Heroin was specifically mentioned as a danger to the young within the United

States. The President of the United States was requested to ask these nations to restrict their production on humanitarian grounds and to report the result of his request by December 1923.[59]

Although the Resolution was aimed directly at the offending nations, not at a conference where a new treaty would be written, plans were begun by the League to call another opium meeting which would take up where the Hague Conference had ended. The plans were developed at a session of the Advisory Committee in May 1923 to which the United States sent Porter as chairman, with Bishop Brent, former Surgeon General Rupert Blue, and Edwin L. Neville of the State Department. Fortified by the Joint Resolution, Porter presented to the Advisory Committee the American program. In essence it was that the use of opiates for other than medical and scientific purposes was an abuse, and that control of production was necessary in order to curb it. The American delegation was prepared to return home should their program, presented as the "settled position" of the United States, fail. Following the presentation of their views the American delegates refused to discuss the issue any further. Apparently, the United States' attitude was that it was negotiating with a single international entity, the League of Nations. This would help explain a proposal by Porter to Secretary General Eric Drummond that a narcotic committee be established with ten members, five American and five from the League.

Although occasionally threatening to leave Geneva, the Americans finally did assist in drafting the Advisory Committee's final statement. This Resolution did not support the American position without reservation, but it did envisage a new world conference to look into the control of production and manufacture. The League Assembly adopted the Resolution in December 1923 and ordered the Secretary General to carry it into effect. As a result of Porter's participation, although he was opposed to American membership in the League, the United States was again taking an important position in the international antinarcotic campaign.[60]

Porter approached the Geneva Conference with as much care as Dr. Wright had used in planning his representation at Shanghai and The Hague. The strongest possible arguments and pressure had to be marshaled to persuade uninterested or dissembling nations to take action that would mean a financial loss and a difficult enforcement problem. To this end he planned two legislative actions. One would prohibit manufacture of heroin; the other would be a congressional resolution that would put in unmistakable language the American demands which, if accepted by the producing nations, would solve the American narcotic dilemma.

In March 1924 Porter proposed legislation to prohibit the import of crude opium for the manufacture of heroin. He realized that passage of this bill would not have a major effect on U.S. heroin consumption but, like Wright a decade earlier, he hoped other nations would be induced to pass similar legislation which he thought would solve this country's heroin problem by banning its manufacture all over the world.[61] In the exaggeration and staging which created one dominant and prohibitive attitude toward heroin, the hearing resembled the style and goal of the Marihuana Tax Act testimony thirteen years later.

Hearings were held on the bill on 3 April 1924. Testimony from a few witnesses and extracts from other hearings and letters to Representative Porter were all combined to show that heroin was the most dangerous of all habit-forming drugs. The various military services, the Public Health Service, and the AMA had already condemned its use, and many physicians believed it could be adequately replaced for medical purposes by morphine, codeine, or some other substance.[62] There were no witnesses in favor of retaining the legality of heroin, although some physicians believed it was useful in very persistent coughs and was less constipating and less nauseating than morphine. Testimony was also heard that heroin was a stimulus to crime as a result of its psychological effects, not just a crime-producer because addicts stole to get money to buy more. In Dr. Lambert's words, heroin "destroys the sense of responsibility to the herd." [63]

All witnesses agreed that most users of heroin were between 17 and 25 years of age. The most alarming indication of heroin's danger and attractiveness was that addicts were deserting morphine and cocaine for heroin in droves, and probably over 90 percent of addicts on the Atlantic Coast were now heroin addicts. The medical director of Sing Sing Prison reported that after the 1919 Supreme Court decision the number of addicts in the prison rose from 1 percent to 9 percent by the end of 1923. A representative of the New York City Department of Corrections linked heroin with cocaine, saying that many gunmen took one or the other to get up the courage to commit crimes. In the words of Dr. Charles Richardson, representing the AMA, "Heroin contains, physiologically, the double action of cocaine and morphine . . . more agreeable to take, not followed by nausea . . . nor marked depression afterwards." Although Dr. Richardson's statement linking cocaine with heroin was totally erroneous, it was consistent with the attitude most leading physicians held toward heroin. Later, in 1937, similar language associating the characteristic effects of cocaine with marihuana would be convincingly presented to Congress.

In spite of statements that "heroin addicts spring from sin and crime," Representative Porter repeatedly stated his sympathy with addicts. To Porter "viciousness seldom enters into the matter." He sought the establishment of two institutions for the care of addicts, one voluntary and one involuntary, where they could get the best treatment and, he stated, often be cured. In early 1924 a fairly knowledgeable and sympathetic legislator believed that institutional care, if comfortable, could effect a cure.[64]

Porter, in his desire to ban the domestic manufacture of heroin, was not oblivious of the smuggling which brought in a large amount of the heroin consumed in the United States. An American statute against heroin was only the first step; the goal was a worldwide halt of manufacture. The ultimate control he sought would include enforced quotas on the growing of poppies and coca bushes, which would necessarily limit manufacture of any opium or coca derivative. Porter summarized in a few optimistic sentences his plans for international control:

> *Mr. Porter:* The Resolution passed by Congress on February 26, 1923, HJR 453, declared that the true intent and meaning of the Hague Opium Convention was that the production of the raw materials should be limited to strictly medicinal and scientific needs. That had always been controverted by certain nations owning colonies in the Orient. At Geneva we got them to accept our construction. The Resolution passed in the last Congress is therefore the accepted construction. In November we return to Geneva with a plan to enforce the convention in accordance with this construction and interpretation.
>
> *Mr. Hawley* (Oregon): And the passage of the bill [to ban heroin manufacture in the United States] is an essential factor in connection with that plan?

Mr. Porter: Yes. In case this bill is passed the United States will be in a much stronger position to urge other nations to do likewise.[65]

Once again, as in the instance of the Harrison Act, the United States sought to enact domestically the strict legislation which required adoption by foreign nations to bring the desired result in America. But Porter was no more successful in obtaining effective international narcotic control than Wright.

THE SECOND GENEVA CONFERENCE, 1924–1925

Four days after the heroin hearings the House considered and overwhelmingly approved HJR 195. The Senate during consideration of the Resolution added the proviso that the American delegation not sign an agreement which did not contain the "conditions necessary for the suppression of the habit-forming narcotic drug traffic." In this form the Resolution was unanimously adopted by Congress in early May.[66] The American negotiating position was firm and left little opportunity for compromise. In many ways it resembled the unyielding Wilsonian position on Senate ratification of the Versailles Treaty, although the tactic was now adopted by a Republican Congress and administration. It was unusual for diplomatic strategy to be so explicitly defined by congressional action, but in Porter's view HJR 195 gave the strongest possible support to the only position that could effectively stop illicit traffic. Porter led the American delegation to the Second Geneva Conference, which began 17 November 1924. Bishop Brent accompanied him, along with Mrs. Wright, Dr. Blue, Edwin Neville, and William B. Morris, an assistant solicitor in the State Department and an expert on international law.

The opium-producing nations, with the exception of China and Egypt, were not inclined to agree with the American position. The exceptions were not significant: China had no effective control over its warring domestic factions, and therefore could do little to curb production; Egypt produced no opium for export. Moreover, the conference would not agree to ban the manufacture of heroin, lower the amount of narcotics in exempt preparations to ¼ grain per ounce, or take measures to stamp out opium smoking in the Far East. Some progress was made in the sharing of statistics and relevant administrative structures. International traffic in cannabis would be limited to "medicinal and scientific" consumption and use. A permanent central board was proposed to oversee the traffic and treaties with regard to narcotics.

Overall, the gains made in this conference were modest. Disgusted by the negotiations, and particularly by the British and Indian delegations, Porter walked out of the conference on 6 February 1925, after almost two months of discussion. Some Americans were proud of the delegation's walkout, for Porter's arduous negotiations had confirmed to the League's detractors that it was as hypocritical and useless as they had proclaimed. Pro-League papers and writers deplored the action. European observers disparaged the United States' abrupt and angry withdrawal from the conference in view of its high consumption of narcotics and particular need for cooperation. The remaining delegates stayed and produced the Convention which most experts, including later the U.S. State Department, agreed was an advance over the Hague Convention. But the United States refused to sign and even contemplated diplomatic pressure to prevent other nations from signing. Porter's reputation was at stake, and his congressional position enabled him to dissuade the State Department from any independent support of the Convention.[67]

By 1928 the State Department's internal opinion was that the Geneva Convention was better than the Hague Convention except for its "connection with the League of Nations and the substitution of a *recommendation* for an *obligation* to apply the restrictions of the Convention to dangerous new drugs." The United States, however, never signed. The League's Advisory Committee continued to meet periodically in Geneva, but the United States no longer sent consultants. The American consul at Geneva, an official inexperienced in narcotics, became an "unofficial spectator." The State Department maintained that the betterment of relations between the U.S. and the Advisory Committee awaited the committee's endorsement of the American position. In 1928 a more qualified observer was sent to Geneva, John T. Caldwell of the State Department's Division of Far Eastern Affairs, who continued as the chief American representative for several years.

The establishment of the Permanent Central Board also met with official silence from the State Department, although the League was anxious to have an American representative on it. Eventually an American national, Herbert L. May, a retired Pittsburgh manufacturer, was selected. He was not a representative of the American government, but he maintained informal contact with the appropriate federal agencies. To refrain from seeming to endorse the League, statistics requested by the Advisory Committee were sent by the United States to the Dutch government at The Hague, which the Dutch government then transmitted to the committee. May would then interpret the American statistics to the Permanent Central Board. Any messages for the League were sent to the American minister in Bern "for transmission in the usual informal manner." The effect of our nonrecognition of the League was to isolate the nation from the international narcotic movement which the U.S. had started in 1906. Subsequent American participation in an international conference to limit the manufacture of narcotics would not come until late in 1930, shortly after the death of Representative Porter.[68]

THE FEDERAL NARCOTIC FARMS

While waiting for the American display of pique at the Geneva Conference to have an effect, Porter began to move forward on the domestic front. As early as the heroin hearings in 1923 he had advocated federal narcotic hospitals. From other quarters came similar suggestions. As more and more addicts entered federal prisons, wardens complained of overcrowding and the unique difficulties of housing many drug-addicted prisoners. The Justice Department wanted something done about convictions under the Harrison Act— some alternative to traditional imprisonment which had led to more Harrison Act violators in prison than any other class of offender.[69]

The most concrete and impressive evidence of the need for more institutions in which to house convicted federal prisoners came from the wardens of the Atlanta and Leavenworth penitentiaries, who had urged such action for several years. Put simply, the three federal penitentiaries (including that on McNeil Island in Washington State) had a cell capacity of 3,738 while on the first of April 1928 they had a population of 7,598. Of the prisoners, about 2,300 were narcotic law violators, of whom 1,600 were addicted. The wardens did not like to care for addicts—prisons were not equipped to handle them, they smuggled drugs into the prison, and their association with other prisoners was bad for both groups. As far as cure went, the wardens had many stories about addict-prisoners who returned to drugs within a day of discharge from prison.[70]

Several congressional recommendations were made in late 1927 and early 1928 for alternative detention of convicted addicts. As usual in narcotic matters, no proposal carried much weight until Porter introduced a bill on 20 February 1928 which he had prepared in cooperation with the Justice Department.[71] Originally, final jurisdiction over the narcotic farms, as Porter called them, was vested in the Attorney General, but Porter later decided to shift control to the Secretary of the Treasury. The original mandate to the Attorney General was in keeping with what the narcotic farms were designed to be and became—separate prisons for addicts. The maximum security conditions and cells and bars were familiar to the wardens who transferred thousands of their prisoners; and the Public Health Service officers who were given the job of running the farms and treating the "patients" were not deceived. The two farms retained that name until the mid-1930s, when they were redesignated "hospitals."

The need for the farms was obvious to Congress. Representative John J. Cochran, who had earlier prepared a similar measure, told his colleagues on the day the Porter bill passed the House without opposition, "Notice has been served on the Congress that the great increase in the population at the Federal penitentiaries makes it imperative that either the Porter bill be enacted into law or two additional pentitentiaries constructed." Yet this practical reason was overcast with a humanitarian sentiment which had previously failed to persuade Congress to make federal provision for the general treatment of addicts: Representative Cochran went so far as to claim for the farms that "2,000 or 3,000 men and women, slaves to habit-forming drugs, will be placed on these farms and be subject to treatment and eventually cured." [72] Everyone associated with the narcotic farm proposal enthusiastically endorsed it—except the Surgeon General of the Public Health Service, who would have the responsibility to operate the institutions.

Porter took a moment in the hearings to rebut the "slander" made against the United States in the Second Geneva Conference, that the United States had an inordinate number of addicts and high opiate consumption.[73] The reason for the denial was quite frankly stated:

I say this because in these international conferences we are constantly faced with these exaggerated statements put out by various organizations which are quite embarrassing. In fact, it is a slander upon the American people.[74]

Nutt agreed with Representative Porter, averring that "these foreigners can not show us we are greater users than a good many of the foreign countries." Yet no evidence against a high opium consumption in America was presented to refute past studies of the State Department, the Public Health Service, and the Treasury Department report of 1919, or testimony before Congress until the Second Geneva Conference when the slanderous charge was thrown at Porter.[75]

The Porter Narcotic Farm bill became law on 19 January 1929, but the Lexington farm was not opened until 1935, and the Fort Worth farm not until 1938. The cure rate at these hospitals was not impressive, but there never had been a well-substantiated high cure rate from any form of treatment. Operation of the farms by the Public Health Service was under the eye of both the Justice Department and the Federal Bureau of Narcotics so that the physicians were often disaffected, feeling that they were doing the dirty work of the other agencies.[76] Research was performed with some interesting results, although no cure was found. One function the farms performed was to provide training for the later leadership of the National Institute of Mental Health. The conditions under which the psychiatrists worked helps explain their disenchantment with the Federal Bureau of Narcotics and the "legal approach" toward addiction. Not until the late 1960s were the bars removed from the Lexington facility and the cells turned into rooms. These farms had been exactly what the wardens envisioned in the mid-1920s—additional prison space for convicted addicts. The institutions provided segregation and the best in medical treatment, but they were by no means rural retreats for the unfortunate addict, supposedly to be restored to health and permanent abstinence through medical treatment.

ESTABLISHMENT OF THE FEDERAL BUREAU OF NARCOTICS, 1930

As soon as the farms were authorized, Porter began to work for the establishment of a separate government agency to enforce the Harrison Act and represent the nation in foreign conferences. Again part of his motivation seemed to be the creation of a model which he hoped foreign governments would follow. A separate agency with domestic and international responsibilities would mean better enforcement and better cooperation with other nations in the prevention of smuggling, and the nations could keep in constant communication instead of meeting at occasional conferences.[77]

The right moment for a separate agency came in 1929. Friends of the Harrison Act had long regretted the close association between narcotic and liquor law enforcement, the latter steadily declining in public esteem and respect during the decade. But Nutt had stayed on in narcotics through Democratic and Republican administrations, trying to catch erring physicians, peddlers, and smugglers; he was becoming a permanent bureaucratic fixture.

Then misconduct in the operation of the federal narcotics office in New York City and the questionable actions of members of Nutt's family led to his transfer from the Narcotic Division and his replacement by Harry J. Anslinger, then Assistant Commissioner of the Prohibition Bureau with responsibility for foreign control. Nutt's troubles began the night before the 1928 elections which brought Herbert Hoover into the White House. An unknown assailant shot Arnold Rothstein, the liquor, gambling, and narcotics racketeer. Rothstein died two days later, leaving voluminous records, letters, and other documents which were said to implicate a number of prominent citizens, including key members of the New York City government. The destruction of some of these incriminating papers and the secrecy thrown around them by legal agencies brought considerable popular criticism, but little action.[78] A grand jury investigation caused some of the names in the documents to filter out. One surprise was the discovery that among those employed by Rothstein were L. P. Mattingly and Rolland L. Nutt, son-in-law and son of the Deputy Commissioner of Prohibition. The former operated a law and accountancy business in New York and gave retainers to Rolland Nutt, a Washington attorney, to represent the firm before the Treasury Department in tax cases. In 1926 Nathan Rothstein had given his power of attorney to both Mattingly and Rolland Nutt to represent him when an additional tax assessment for the years 1919, 1920, and 1921 was lodged against him. The grand jury which investigated in 1929 and 1930 the enforcement of narcotic law in New York City looked into the matter and heard Rolland Nutt testify that he had never met Rothstein—he just represented him on behalf of L. P. Mattingly and Company. Rothstein's records revealed that Mattingly had borrowed from him "from time to time and for personal purposes" sums totaling $6,200. This had taken place while Rothstein was widely considered the organizer of a worldwide narcotics smuggling organization bringing drugs into the United States. Levi Nutt testified that he knew nothing of his relatives' association with Rothstein. The grand jury concluded that although the acts of Mattingly and Rolland Nutt might be "thought indiscreet, we find no evidence that the enforcement of the narcotic law was affected thereby." [79]

The grand jury also discovered "wholesale padding of the record of the local Federal narcotic office in New York" beginning in April 1929 under telephoned orders from the assistant deputy prohibition commissioner for narcotics, who testified that he did so on Mr. Nutt's verbal order. Nutt also denied these allegations. The jury asked the Secretary of the Treasury to take "severe action" against all those responsible for the misrepresentations in the records.

The conduct of federal narcotic agents in New York was also investigated, with the conclusion that there had been "gross dereliction and incompetence." The release of the man higher up, if he was caught, but the arrest of small offenders strongly indicated collusion between some of the agents and the important sellers of narcotics, but there was not enough evidence to indict for bribery. Other corrupt practices reported were agents' failures to inform the U.S. attorney of evidence important for a successful prosecution, and an agent's reversal of testimony after an indictment had been secured on his original testimony. One agent appeared to be a drug user himself, and even after evidence to this effect was given to the division in July 1929, he was still working in the New York office in February 1930. The task of the jury was incomplete, in its opinion, when its report was submitted on 19 February 1930.

Ten days later Levi Nutt was removed as the head of the Narcotics Division and Anslinger was appointed. Nutt became field supervisor of the Prohibition agents and then head of the Alcohol Tax Unit in Syracuse until his retirement. Anslinger became Acting Commissioner of Narcotics upon the creation of the Federal Bureau of Narcotics on 1 July 1930 and was appointed Commissioner of Narcotics by President Hoover on 25 September, serving until his retirement in 1962.

Anslinger's career had been in diplomacy after World War I, with no specific duties in the narcotics field. Yet this was excellent training for the new job, in Porter's opinion. Porter questioned "whether a medical officer would measure up to the requirements necessary in an international conference" and he believed the "international aspect . . . is really more important than the domestic." [80] The new commissioner could always get the opinion of the surgeon general when necessary but the man to lead the American battle for narcotic control would need to be versed in diplomatic wiles. Anslinger was untainted by scandal and he had a creditable record for achieving international agreement to hinder liquor smuggling. These factors, plus his patriotism and his belief in the menace of certain foreign ideologies such as Communism, gained not only Porter's support but also, in Anslinger's opinion, the crucial support of William Randolph Hearst.[81]

Porter had other reasons for preferring a separate bureau. The Federal Narcotic Control Board established by the Jones-Miller Act of 1922 was a cumbersome apparatus for making decisions on routine matters. It was doubtful that the Board had convened even once. A commissioner could be given the board's authority and would also be able to provide a continuity abroad at international conferences which the current arrangement could not provide. Nutt's role had been domestic; Representative Porter was a member of Congress; the State Department experts came and went; there was no one to take the international aspect of narcotic control as his concern and stay with it over the years. Porter complained: "In all of our conferences our Government has been represented by subordinates, and about the time I get one trained to help me he is shifted off to the Far East or some place else and we have to take up and train a new man." [82]

When his bill became law in spring 1930, Representative Porter had accomplished the separation of narcotic and liquor law enforcement (the latter went to the Justice Department when the FBN came into existence). He had obtained by the accident of public scandal a commissioner who had the kind of diplomatic training he believed necessary for the ultimate control of smuggling, and he had consolidated most of the scattered federal activities in narcotic control into the hands of one man and one agency. But on 27 June, before the FBN became a reality, Porter died in Pittsburgh at age 61. Anslinger would begin his career in the Federal Bureau of Narcotics with a determination not to repeat the unpopular enforcement procedures that were destroying the Bureau of Prohibition.

9 Marihuana and the Federal Bureau of Narcotics

Anslinger became the first Commissioner of Narcotics in 1930, although he had had only sporadic contact with narcotic control.[1] Nonetheless, his more than ten years of government experience affected his attitude toward law enforcement and addicts. Anslinger was born in 1892 in Altoona, Pennsylvania. His father worked for the Pennsylvania Railroad, and while Anslinger went to high school and then to Pennsylvania State College, he also worked for the railroad during the summers, doing maintenance and landscaping and occasionally investigating suspicious incidents for the railroad's captain of police. Later, when the police captain became the state fire marshal, he offered Anslinger a job compiling statistics and investigating instances of suspected arson. In 1917, after the United States declared war on Germany, Anslinger was employed in Washington in the Ordinance Division of the War Department, where his chief task was to oversee government contracts. Ordinance officers were unpopular in Washington; the public expected young men to fight abroad and, when the opportunity came, Anslinger volunteered to the State Department which was looking for reliable German-speaking employees to work in Holland. He recalls being assigned to "check up on . . . and straighten out" the indirect American contacts with the Kaiser in order to let the German ruler know that President Wilson wanted him to stay on after the war, but Anslinger failed, obtaining from the whole episode only the Kaiser's field utility kit which he later gave to the Smithsonian. In 1921 he took the necessary examinations and was appointed to the rank of vice-consul.

After the war, from posts in The Hague and in Hamburg, Anslinger sent many reports to the State Department warning them of trouble to come from Russia, but he was discouraged by the lack of interest in the State Department which, he concluded, considered the Bolshevik menace a myth. Almost no one believed his frequent reports, although he was able to get important information from an informer in the Third International, held in Amsterdam in 1920. Bolsheviks were being signed on as seamen on freighters and were spreading propaganda across the world. In Hamburg he learned that seamen on American-bound ships were being bribed to smuggle narcotics into the United States.

Much to his regret, and in spite of the anti-Bolshevik intelligence work which he believed was of great value, he was sent as consul to La Guaira, Venezuela, a hot and lazy place. He wondered whether he had been mistaken in choosing foreign service as a career. But two years later his interest and ability in intelligence work, now focused on rum-running in the Caribbean, was rewarded by a temporary assignment to the Bahamas where he was asked to find a way to stop the smuggling of liquor into the United States. He persuaded the British to establish landing certificates which would keep a record of all ship movements. The Treasury Department considered this a remarkable accomplishment and Anslinger was, at the Treasury's request, detailed temporarily to the Prohibition Unit, where he soon became chief of the Foreign Control Section.

In 1929, two years after the unit had achieved bureau status, Anslinger became an Assistant Commissioner of Prohibition. His field experience in enforcement was limited; most of his valued work was at a higher level, but he had definite views on how to repair the flagging effectiveness of a statute like the Volstead Act. In 1928 Anslinger had entered a national competition on how best to enforce the 18th Amendment and prepared a comprehensive program to resuscitate the drive against illicit alcohol.[2] Although by that time the object of Prohibition as well as its mode of enforcement had become unpopular, he believed that the right sort of remedy could save the situation.

He suggested ways in which smuggling could be prevented through international agreements. He recommended that Prohibition investigations be made by the Justice Department rather than the Treasury and that additional federal attorneys and judges be appointed to expedite prosecutions; and that a coordinating director be appointed with authority to demand cooperation from the various Prohibition enforcement agencies.

The most interesting feature of Anslinger's proposals relates to penalties. The federal Prohibition laws made it a crime to sell, manufacture, or transport liquor for sale, but purchase of liquor was not a crime. Anslinger would have made the purchase of alcohol for nonmedical consumption a violation, and for the first conviction would set a penalty of a fine of not less than $1,000 and imprisonment for not less than six months. For a second or subsequent offense the fine would be between $5,000 and $50,000 and imprisonment for two to five years. In his view these penalties would put teeth into the law and greatly discourage violations. President Hoover did increase the enforcement effectiveness, although not by prohibiting purchase, and a much higher conviction rate was achieved. If a law was wrong, Hoover said, its rigid enforcement was the surest guarantee of its repeal; if it was right, its enforcement was the quickest method of compelling respect.

When Levi Nutt's leadership became awkward for the Treasury, Anslinger was promoted to head temporarily the Narcotic Division. Within a few months he was appointed the first federal Commissioner of Narcotics. There is no evidence that during Anslinger's tenure as commissioner he ever changed his mind that the most effective way of gaining public compliance with a law regulating a dangerous drug was a policy of high fines and severe mandatory prison sentences for first convictions. While the public did not agree with this attitude for liquor prohibition, it did support the policy in regard to narcotic control, thanks in part to propaganda like that spread by Richmond Hobson.

In the Federal Bureau of Narcotics, Anslinger's opinions on how best to put teeth into the law met with almost no objection. He rarely found himself curbed by the administrations under which he worked; he was in fact encouraged not to deviate from stringent enforcement. Early in Roosevelt's first administration Anslinger recalls a visit from the President's close adviser Louis Howe, who made it clear to Anslinger that should he ever forward to the White House a recommendation for clemency for a drug pusher, he could attach his resignation to it. That intelligence, Howe said, "came from the Boss." In the late thirties when a congressman from Washington State, perhaps inspired by the White Cross, argued in the House of Representatives for an investigation into the FBN and its style of enforcement, he received no effective support from his congressional colleagues.[3] In 1951 a mandatory minimum two-year sentence for first convictions of narcotic possession became law. Five years later the federal penalty for the sale of heroin by someone over age 18 to a buyer under 18 was raised to death at the jury's discretion.[4] Given the prevalent attitude toward narcotic addiction and pushers, Anslinger's views were in harmony with most of those citizens who were responsible for legislation or executive action. Although his accession as commissioner in 1930 was accidental, and his views on control harsh, Anslinger's views were not unusual.

The consistency of Anslinger's position may seem to imply that his experience with Prohibition had created too rigid an attitude toward drug abusers but the failure and demise of Prohibition taught him lessons which he carefully followed in his long tenure in the Federal Bureau of Narcotics. Among the first was the risk to any agency that meddled with the personal lives of citizens. Interviews with former Prohibition officers revealed a fear of federal judges, particularly in the dry era, who were angered by the large numbers of "ordinary citizens" hauled into court on minor liquor violations. Anslinger realized that similar judicial displeasure might follow if too many marihuana possession cases were taken to federal courts. He much preferred to have violators brought before local courts by the local police. Naturally this desire to keep within the good graces of the courts caused the FBN to seek control of only the most obviously dangerous drugs—cocaine and opiates. Anslinger "put sandbags up against the door" whenever anyone suggested that the FBN police barbiturates and amphetamines, for example, because the gray areas meant trouble and perhaps bureaucratic suicide for an enforcement agency with a small budget and staff.

Since both liquor prohibition and narcotic controls were directed at medicinal substances, the AMA, after World War I, resented the curbs placed on physicians—the medical profession was no more trusted in the discharge of its responsibilities to the 18th Amendment than it was in regard to the Harrison Act. A specific law, the Willis-Campbell Act of November 1921, was enacted in order to limit the number of liquor prescriptions permitted each doctor. The similarity of the Willis-Campbell Act's restraints to the contemporary Court interpretation of the Harrison Act is obvious, and the physicians' response, led in the House of Representatives by Congressman Volk, became equally loud.[5] Yet large segments of the medical profession were in sympathy with Prohibition. An AMA poll in 1921 revealed that almost 60 percent of the thirty thousand respondents stated that physicians should be restricted in their alcohol prescriptions; among those wanting curbs, "a large majority favor such restrictions as . . . under the Harrison Narcotic Law."[6]

Sanitariums often treated both narcotic and alcohol addicts; Charles B. Towns was only one operator in the 1920s who claimed great success with both kinds of patients. Yet among most physicians there was little optimism for the cure of alcoholism by any means other than keeping alcohol away from consumers, which was exactly what Prohibition attempted to do. The same kind of interdiction was adopted against narcotic users by the federal government. If the claim was made that alcoholism and narcotism were diseases, the government could claim that neither could be "cured" except by keeping the substance away from the "patients."

One further lesson the FBN learned from the Prohibition era was the great assistance citizen groups could offer a federal enforcement agency. The Anti-Saloon League and the WCTU had lobbied effectively. Anslinger remembers these groups and others like them with appreciation, recalling that opposition to Narcotic Bureau policies would be effectively met at times by giving the word to the WCTU or the General Federation of Women's Clubs, who would then oppose election of public officials who criticized the bureau's enforcement measures. For example, a son of the friend of a Maryland state legislator was arrested in the 1930s for possession of marihuana and sentenced to several years in prison. The legislator attempted to lessen the state penalties against marihuana, but cued by a word of warning from the FBN, the WCTU and the Federation of Women's Clubs appeared at the committee hearing when the bill came up and killed it then and there. These aggressive lay groups had gained experience in political lobbying over other issues from women's suffrage to Prohibition. They were welcomed by the FBN and in the mid-1930s they eagerly took up the battle against marihuana, the new menace to America's schoolchildren.

Two years after the FBN achieved bureau status its development was arrested by the Depression. The FBN's appropriations were cut by Congress and at times the Administration held annual expenditures even below the sums appropriated. The House Appropriations Committee examined the most minute details of the FBN's annual appropriation request and the matter of a few thousand dollars often required careful documentation for approval. The number of agents began to decline, and the bureau entered a decade of low budgets, averaging 1.1 to 1.3 million dollars annually. This limitation obviously affected enforcement. Publicity and warnings became the methods of control, complementing careful examination of the thousands of physicians' and druggists' records.

INTERNATIONAL ANTI-NARCOTIC ACTIVITIES, 1930–1936

In late 1929 the League of Nations called for a new conference to consider how manufactured drugs might be better controlled.[7] The State Department wanted to participate but it faced Representative

Porter's objection that participation might imply that the United States had shifted its stand from demanding a limit on raw production to the secondary issue of manufacturing, the issue which had led to Porter's departure from Geneva in 1925. Finally, Porter was persuaded to permit John T. Caldwell of the Division of Far Eastern Affairs to be present at the Advisory Committee meetings in early 1930 which would consider a preliminary conference to be held in London later that year—provided that Caldwell took no part in the preparations.

At the preliminary conference in October and November eleven nations discussed a plan for estimating their requirements for manufactured narcotic drugs and a means by which the manufacturers could divide the market. Although agreement was not reached then, the following May, at the Geneva Conference on the Limitation of the Manufacture of Narcotic Drugs, fifty-seven nations agreed on a Convention. The American delegation consisted of Caldwell as chairman, two other federal officials—Anslinger and Dr. Walter L. Treadway, head of the Mental Hygiene Division of the Public Health Service—and Sanford Young of the California Legislature. No congressman was named to the group; the State Department took pains that no member of congress should again assume Porter's role.

The State Department and most other observers believed that the Narcotics Limitation Convention embodied a number of improvements over previous international agreements. Criticism came chiefly from the Hearst press which referred to the American delegation's use of quieter and more congenial diplomacy in such derogatory headlines as "Britain Leading America by the Nose," and "Caldwell Backed Down."

The Convention divided drugs into two schedules, according to the hazards attached to their use. An annual estimate for scientific and medical needs of manufactured drugs was required of each signatory, and the manufacturers of each nation agreed to keep within that quota, or less if some of the quota was imported. A supervisory body would examine the estimates and, for nations which did not comply, make an independent estimate. Heroin could not be exported except at the request of the importing nation. Careful recording and reporting of all raw materials would be required. One of Porter's goals, a separate narcotic agency in each government, was requested. The several administrations were not only intended to regulate the trade in drugs and apply the Convention but were also expected to organize campaigns against drug addiction. The United States strongly favored this agreement and the Senate unanimously approved it on 31 March 1932. The Convention came into effect on 9 July 1933.

One of the advantages to American ratification was that a legal basis now existed for American cooperation with the League. The United States took a more cooperative role in the opium affairs of the League and contributed funds to support the Opium Advisory Committee. By the beginning of World War II the United States was an advocate of the League's antiopium activities.

The last international meeting before the war, which had significance for the domestic control of narcotics, was held in June 1936, the Conference for the Suppression of the Illicit Traffic in Dangerous Drugs. Its purpose was to improve detection and provide for more certain punishment of narcotic law violators. The United States until the last moment maintained that prevailing conventions and its bilateral treaties with various nations were sufficient, and that an additional convention would not facilitate the location and conviction of violators. Yet when the conference was formally announced in February 1936, the United States decided to attend, a new motivation having arisen: the possibility of securing a convention that would mandate domestic control of marihuana and opium-poppy cultivation.

FEDERAL CONTROL OF CANNABIS, 1906–1920

Social reformers successfully initiated federal restrictions on cannabis along with alcohol, opiates, cocaine, and chloral hydrate in the first decade of this century. The Pure Food and Drug Act of 1906 required that any quantity of cannabis, as well as several other dangerous substances, be clearly marked on the label of any drug or food sold to the public.[8] Early drafts of federal antinarcotic legislation, which finally emerged as the Harrison Act in 1914, also repeatedly listed the drug along with opiates and cocaine. Cannabis, however, never survived the legislative gauntlet, probably because of the pharmaceutical industry's opposition. At that time, and for at least a decade longer, the drug trades saw no reason why a substance used chiefly in corn plasters, veterinary medicine, and nonintoxicating medicaments should be so severely restricted. Not even the reformers claimed, in the pre-World War I hearings and debates over a federal antinarcotic act, that cannabis was a problem of any major significance in the United States.

Congress rarely heard any witness defend opiates or cocaine, but during the January 1911 hearings on a federal antinarcotic law before the House Ways and Means Committee, the National Wholesale Druggists' Association's representative protested the inclusion of cannabis alongside opiates and cocaine. Charles A. West, chairman of the NWDA legislative committee, testified that cannabis was not what might be called a habit-forming drug. Albert Plaut, representing the New York City pharmaceutical firm of Lehn and Fink, also objected to the inclusion of cannabis: he attributed its reputation more to literary fiction, such as the description of hashish in the *Count of Monte Cristo,* than to informed opinion. When questioned whether cannabis might be taken by those whose regular supply of opiates or cocaine was restricted, Plaut responded that the effects of cannabis were so different from those of opiates and cocaine that he would not expect an addict to find cannabis attractive.[9]

The drug industry's complaints received stern rebuttals, but no one denied that cannabis then constituted a very small part of the drug abuse spectrum. Arguments for including it rested on the belief of such authorities as Lambert, Towns, and Wiley, that the drug was habit forming. One of the most stirring attacks on cannabis came from Towns:

To my mind it is inexcusable for a man to say that there is no habit from the use of that drug. There is no drug in the Pharmacopoeia today that would produce the pleasurable sensations you would get from cannabis, no not one—absolutely not a drug in the Pharmacopoeia today, and of all the drugs on earth I would certainly put that on the list.[10]

While most spokesmen for the drug trades opposed federal regulation of cannabis, one distinguished member favored its control and most of the other provisions of the new legislation: Dr. William Jay Schieffelin of New York, who moved with the progressive and reform spirit of the era and was therefore somewhat apart from the rank and file of his colleagues in the drug trade. Schieffelin believed that cannabis was "used only to a slight extent in this country," but he had heard that there was a demand for it in the Syrian colony in New York, where he thought it was smoked like prepared opium. He concluded that the evil was small but that cannabis ought to be included in the bill.[11]

But cannabis was not included finally, and except for the Pure Food and Drug Act's provision for labeling, no federal regulatory law was enacted until 1937. Meanwhile the two contrasting attitudes toward cannabis remained pretty much the same—the reformers feared its use; the drug industry felt less concern about possible misuse and opposed its regulation.

Still, complaints about cannabis continued to come to the attention of the federal government. One of the American delegates to the First Hague Conference, Henry Finger, drew particular attention: Californians, especially in San Francisco, were frightened by the "large influx of Hindoos . . . demanding *cannabis indica*," who were initiating "the whites into their habit." Finger wanted the world traffic in cannabis to be controlled.[12] The United States delegation gladly adopted Finger's goal but did not find the Hague Conference favorably disposed. The best the United States could accomplish was the adoption of a recommendation that other nations look into the character of the drug.[13] Agreement that international traffic in cannabis should be regulated did not come until the Second Geneva Convention in 1925.[14]

Domestic concern over cannabis seemed to originate in the Southwest and to begin increasing after World War I. John M. Parker, governor of Louisiana, and Dr. Oscar Dowling, president of Louisiana's Board of Health, argued that cannabis also ought to be controlled. Their reaction to marihuana had elements which would become familiar in the 1930s. A white, 21-year-old musician in New Orleans had been arrested for forging a physician's signature in order to get some "mariguana" imported from Mexico. The musician said the substance was taken to "make you feel good," but its dangers seemed clear to Dowling and Parker. Dowling warned the governor that marihuana was "a powerful narcotic, causing exhilaration, intoxication, delirious hallucinations, and its subsequent actions, drowsiness and stupor." He also urgently requested of the Surgeon General of the Public Health Service that the federal government take "some action" to control the traffic in marihuana.[15] On 26 November 1920 Governor Parker wrote to Prohibition Commissioner John F. Kramer that "two people were killed a few days ago by the smoking of this drug, which seems to make them go crazy and wild," and he expressed his surprise that there were no restrictions against marihuana. But the trouble the government was already having with enforcing the Harrison Act did not encourage the bureau to take on the policing of more drugs.

RISING DOMESTIC FEAR OF CANNABIS, 1920–1934

Fear of cannabis, or marihuana, as it was beginning to be known, was minimal throughout most of the nation in the 1920s. Nevertheless it still concerned the federal government. For example, in the January 1929 authorization of the two narcotic centers for the treatment of addicted federal prisoners, the law specifically defined "habit-forming narcotic drugs" to include "Indian hemp" and made habitual cannabis users, along with opium addicts, eligible for treatment.[16] Although there seem to have been few cannabis users transferred to Lexington and Fort Worth, it is significant that congressional worry about cannabis continued after passage of the Pure Food and Drug Act and clearly was present before the Bureau of Narcotics was established in 1930.

In areas with concentrations of Mexican immigrants, who tended to use marihuana as a drug of entertainment or relaxation, the fear of marihuana was intense. During the 1920s Mexican immigration, legal and illegal, rapidly increased into the region from Louisiana to California and up to Colorado and Utah. Mexicans were useful in the United States as farm laborers and, as the economic boom continued, they traveled to the Midwest and the North where jobs in factories and sugar-beet fields were available.[17]

Although employers welcomed them in the twenties, Mexicans were also feared as a source of crime and deviant social behavior. As early as 1919 federal officials were reporting that marihuana was a cause of violence among Mexican prisoners in the southwestern states.[18] By the mid-twenties horrible crimes were attributed to marihuana and its Mexican purveyors. Legal and medical officers in New Orleans began studies of the evil and within a few years published articles claiming that many of the region's crimes could be traced to marihuana, for they believed it was a sexual stimulant that removed civilized inhibitions.[19] As a result, requests were made to include marihuana in the Harrison Act.

When the Great Depression settled over America, the Mexicans, who had been welcomed by at least a fraction of the communities in which they lived, became an unwelcome surplus in regions devastated by unemployment. Cotton, fruit, and vegetable growers in the Southwest and sugar-beet farmers in Colorado, Michigan, Montana, and the Northwest favored further immigration, but the American Federation of Labor understandably sought strict barriers. Another group that worked energetically for an end to Mexican immigration did so for social reasons, afraid that mixture with an inferior race was causing race suicide. Citizens anxious to preserve what they believed valuable in American life banded together into "Allied Patriotic Societies," "Key Men of America," or the group which united many of these associations, the "American Coalition," whose goal was to keep America American.[20] One of the prominent members of the American Coalition, C. M. Goethe of Sacramento, saw marihuana and the problem of Mexican immigrants as closely connected:

> Marijuana, perhaps now the most insidious of our narcotics, is a direct by-product of unrestricted Mexican immigration. Easily grown, it has been asserted that it has recently been planted between rows in a California penitentiary garden. Mexican peddlers have been caught distributing sample marijuana cigarets to school children. Bills for our quota against Mexico have been blocked mysteriously in every Congress since the 1924 Quota Act. Our nation has more than enough laborers.[21]

Southwestern police and prosecuting attorneys likewise protested constantly to the federal government about the Mexicans' use of the weed.

In 1934 Dr. Walter Bromberg, a respected researcher, informed a meeting of the American Psychiatric Association that some authors had estimated the number of marihuana smokers in the southern states to be one out of four.[22] Dr. Bromberg, who did not subscribe to the alarm over marihuana displayed by some writers, nevertheless told of its spread from the South to New York and to other large cities. Although asserting that it was something like alcohol in its effect, nevertheless, on the basis of good physiological and psychological studies of cannabis, he was persuaded that it was "a primary stimulus to the impulsive life with direct expression in the motor field. [It] releases inhibitions and restraints imposed by society and allows individuals to act out their drives openly [and] acts as a sexual stimulant [particularly to] overt homosexuals."

Dr. Bromberg's description of marihuana in 1933 differed in quality from the writings, for example, of New Orleans' Prosecuting Attorney, who in 1931 fearfully portrayed marihuana leading to crime.[23] Neither the New Orleans studies, which began at least in the late 1920s, nor Dr. Bromberg's research can be ascribed to any campaign by the FBN for a federal marihuana law. It is reasonable to assume that in the first few years of the 1930s marihuana was known among police departments and civic leaders, particularly those in association with Mexican immigrants, and even among scientific investigators, as a drug with dangerous possibilities. This situation led naturally to pressure on the federal government to take some action. What was the attitude of the new Federal Bureau of Narcotics to the growing concern over marihuana?

PRELUDE TO FEDERAL MARIHUANA CONTROL, 1935–1937

During its first few years, the bureau, as judged from its annual reports, minimized the marihuana problem and felt that control should be vested in the state governments.[24] The report published in 1932 commented,

> This abuse of the drug is noted among the Latin-American or Spanish-speaking population. The sale of cannabis cigarettes occurs to a considerable degree in States along the Mexican border and in cities of the Southwest and West, as well as in New York City, and, in fact, wherever there are settlements of Latin Americans.
>
> A great deal of public interest has been aroused by newspaper articles appearing from time to time on the evils of the abuse of marijuana or Indian hemp, and more attention has been focused upon specific cases reported of the abuse of the drug than would otherwise have been the case. This publicity tends to magnify the extent of the evil and lends color to an inference that there is an alarming spread of the improper use of the drug, whereas the actual increase in such use may not have been inordinately large.

In 1932 the FBN strongly endorsed the new Uniform State Narcotic Act and repeatedly stressed that the problem could be brought under control if all the states adopted it.[25] As late as January 1937, Commissioner Anslinger was quoted as advising that the distribution

of marihuana was an intrastate problem and that hope for its ultimate control lay in adoption of uniform narcotic laws.[26] The annual
reports spent an increasing amount of space on marihuana-asso-
ciated crime after 1935, but the bureau continued to recommend
the uniform act. There seem to be several reasons why the FBN
delayed advocating a federal marihuana law.

Commissioner Anslinger recalled that marihuana caused few
problems except in the southwestern and western states, and there
the growing alarm was directed at the Mexicans who the "sheriffs
and local police departments claimed got loaded on the stuff and
caused a lot of trouble, stabbing, assaults, and so on." These states
were "the only ones then affected . . . we didn't see it here in the
East at all at that time." To Anslinger, the danger of marihuana did
not compare with that of heroin, and after the Act's passage in 1937
he warned his agents to keep their eyes on heroin; if an agent was
making arrests for marihuana possession, he was told to get back
to "the hard stuff."

In addition to questioning whether a federal law would significantly ameliorate the so-called marihuana problem, the commissioner also doubted the possibility of a law that would be constitutional. But enactment in 1934 of a "transfer tax" on certain firearms
gave the Treasury's General Counsel Herman Oliphant a constitutional solution. In an effort to reduce the use of machine guns
by gangsters, Congress decreed that such firearms could be transferred only upon payment of a transfer tax (National Firearms
Act). As peculiar as this tax may seem, it was held constitutional
by the Supreme Court in March 1937.[27] Oliphant, according to
Anslinger, decided that this model could be applied to the transfer
of marihuana, and within a month of the Supreme Court's decision
the Treasury Department appeared before Congress requesting
enactment of a marihuana transfer tax. When the idea of such a
tax was first broached to Anslinger by the General Counsel, he
thought the notion was "ridiculous." Even after the decision was
made to recommend it to Congress Anslinger did not believe it
would pass.

The Bureau had avoided control of barbiturates and amphetamines, which would be very difficult to implement. Such an attitude
was consistent with Anslinger's disinclination to take on marihuana,
which grew, as the Commissioner ruefully pointed out in 1936,
"like dandelions," and had a few legitimate uses.[28] It is significant

that when marihuana was finally controlled by the federal government, it was outlawed for almost every use except in birdseed, where it was permitted only if first sterilized. The regulations for its use by physicians were so complicated that they are not likely to have prescribed it since 1937.

The pressure for a federal antimarihuana law was political, Anslinger states, from local police forces in affected states to the governors; from the governors to Secretary of the Treasury Henry Morgenthau, Jr.; from Morgenthau to the Treasury's General Counsel; and finally to the Commissioner of Narcotics. Apparently the decision to seek a federal law was made in 1935, since by January 1936 Anslinger was holding conferences to that end. The bureau's search for grounds on which to base a federal law was almost unsuccessful. It first claimed that only the treaty-making power of the federal government could sustain an antimarihuana statute. Such a treaty was then attempted, but with an appeal to other nations which had almost no chance of success. The bureau had performed faithfully the task it had been given and the effort was about to fall short, when, Anslinger claims, the Treasury's General Counsel ingeniously applied the transfer tax.

The pressure on the Treasury could well have been sufficient to induce the ingenuity, as the following letter of 1936 from the editor of the Alamosa, Colorado, *Daily Courier* suggests:

Is there any assistance your Bureau can give us in handling this drug? Can you suggest campaigns? Can you enlarge your Department to deal with marijuana? Can you do anything to help us?

I wish I could show you what a small marijuana cigarette can do to one of our degenerate Spanish-speaking residents. That's why our problem is so great: the greatest percentage of our population is composed of Spanish-speaking persons, most of whom are low mentally, because of social and racial conditions.

While marijuana has figured in the greatest number of crimes in the past few years, officials fear it, not for what it has done, but for what it is capable of doing. They want to check it before an outbreak does occur.

Through representatives of civic leaders and law officers of the San Luis Valley, I have been asked to write to you for help.[29]

THE MARIHUANA TAX ACT

Anslinger went to New York in January 1936 to meet with a group of distinguished experts to try to hammer out a marihuana control bill; present were a representative of the Foreign Policy Association; Joseph Chamberlain, professor of law at Columbia; Herbert L. May, member of the Permanent Central [opium] Board of the League of Nations; and Stuart Fuller, assistant chief of the Division of Far Eastern Affairs of the State Department. Anslinger reported their conclusion to Assistant Secretary of the Treasury Stephen B. Gibbons in a confidential memorandum: "under the taxing power and regulation of interstate commerce it would be almost hopeless to expect any kind of adequate control." [30]

The Commissioner's recommendation for the marihuana legislation was to follow the example of the Migratory Bird Act, which had been declared constitutional, although it intruded into the police powers of the states, because it had been enacted as a requirement of treaties with Canada and Mexico (*Missouri* v. *Holland*, 252 U.S. 416). Anslinger suggested a similar treaty requiring the control of marihuana. Once the treaty was ratified by the Senate, a federal marihuana law would not meet the constitutional blocks he felt sure it would face if it were based on federal tax or commerce powers. Otherwise, the memorandum went on, the various details that imperiled simple prohibition of marihuana were nearing solution:

> The State Department has tentatively agreed to this proposition, but before action is taken we shall have to dispose of certain phases of legitimate traffic: for instance, the drug trade still has a small medical need for marijuana, but has agreed to eliminate it entirely. The only place it is used extensively is by the veterinarians, and we can satisfy them by importing their medical needs.
>
> We must also satisfy the canary bird seed trade, and the Sherwin Williams Paint Company, which uses hemp seed oil for drying purposes. We are now working with the Department of Commerce in finding substitutes for the legitimate trade, and after that is accomplished, the path will be cleared for the treaties and for federal law.

The commissioner was permitted to try his idea in June 1936, when he and Fuller represented the United States at the Conference for the Suppression of the Illicit Traffic in Dangerous Drugs, held in Geneva. The United States sought to incorporate a requirement for cannabis control in a treaty with twenty-six other nations. Perhaps to have additional leverage, or perhaps to dramatize the opposition of other governments, just before the conference opened the U.S. delegation asked for permission to abstain from participation if American proposals were turned down. Still recalling the regrettable isolation that followed American departure from a similar conference in 1925, the State Department refused permission. So, although cannabis was excluded, the delegation stayed but did not sign the Convention. The United States was the only nation represented which did not do so.[31]

In the summer of 1936 it therefore became obvious that there would be no law to placate the Southwest unless some federal legislation under traditional legal powers was enacted. The Treasury's General Counsel then suggested the marihuana transfer tax, about which the commissioner had strong doubts, but the bureau loyally went along with the plan and did its best to present a strong case to Congress. To Anslinger, Congress did not seem very concerned and "the only information they had was what we would give them in our hearings."

The Treasury Department collected and considered scientific and medical opinion prior to the Tax Act hearings, but the desire to present a solid front when the department appeared before the committees of Congress caused the officials to ignore anything that qualified or minimized the evils of marihuana. The political pressure to put "something on the books," and the doubt that it could be done, combined to make the marihuana hearings a classic example of bureaucratic overkill.

In the tradition of federal departments, everyone from the Treasury Department who appeared for the Tax Act gave it full support, while those who might have had more moderate views remained in the background. In particular, the Public Health Service was not represented, although the opinion of its Division of Mental Hygiene (now the National Institute of Mental Health) was available to the Treasury Department months before the hearings in April. Like other authorities, Dr. Walter L. Treadway, head of the Mental Hygiene Division, answered a series of questions about marihuana, probably in late 1936. To the question: "What are the proofs that the use of marihuana in any of its forms is habit-forming or addictive, and what are the indications and positive proofs that such addiction develops socially undesirable characteristics in the user?" Dr. Treadway replied in full:

Cannabis indica does not produce dependence as in opium addiction. In opium addiction there is a complete dependence and when it is withdrawn there is actual physical pain which is not the case with cannabis. Alcohol more nearly produces the same effect as cannabis in that there is an excitement or a general feeling of lifting of personality, followed by a delirious stage, and subsequent narcosis. There is no dependence or increased tolerance such as in opium addiction. As to the social or moral degradation associated with cannabis it probably belongs in the same category as alcohol. As with alcohol, it may be taken a relatively long time without social or emotional breakdown. Marijuana is habit-forming although not addicting in the same sense as alcohol might be with some people, or sugar, or coffee. Marijuana produces a delirium with a frenzy which might result in violence: but this is also true of alcohol.[32]

The department held a conference in the Treasury Building on 14 January 1937.[33] Attending were fourteen government officials and consultants, many of whom would testify a few months later before the congressional committees deliberating the Tax Act. The purpose of the conference was to prepare a satisfactory legal definition of marihuana for the proposed legislation and to make some final arrangements for the presentation to Congress. Dr. Treadway was not present, although Dr. Carl Voegtlin, chief of the Division of Pharmacology of the National Institute of Health, was there to assist, along with some chemists, pharmacologists, and Commissioner Anslinger. Two members of the Treasury's legal office and the FBN's general counsel were also present.

Fortunately, the conference was stenographically transcribed. Most of the conference was devoted to ascertaining which part of the marihuana plant was pharmacologically active and what should be the name of the soon-to-be-taxed substance. Conversation was chiefly between the scientists and the Treasury lawyers and reveals that the department did take into consideration scientific and medical opinion in the preparation of the legislation.

The participants knew that they would have to be prepared to rebut any suggested valid use or inclusion of marihuana through an exemption—the goal was full prohibition. Trade or medical exceptions would make enforcement considerably more expensive, and cost was a consideration. This factor and the lack of increased appropriations for several years after its enactment are consistent with Anslinger's claim that the Tax Act was no boon to his bureaucratic structure.

Alfred L. Tennyson, the bureau's counsel, emphasized to the group that every detail of the legislation would have to be worked out well ahead of the hearings. Perhaps a little defensively, the commissioner wanted the group to know that the conference was not "a fishing expedition"; 296 seizures of cannabis had been made in 1936 alone. He complained that illicit traffic showed up in almost every state.

With regard to the effects of marihuana on the personality, S. G. Tipton of the Treasury's legal staff asked the commissioner: "Have you lots of cases on this? Horror stories—that's what we want." Anslinger did indeed have a collection. Then in one of the most significant moments in the meeting, the commissioner asked Dr. Voegtlin whether marihuana actually produces insanity. The NIH pharmacology expert replied: "I think it is an established fact that prolonged use leads to insanity in certain cases, depending on the amount taken, of course. Many people take it and do not go insane, but many do." To which the Treasury's consulting chemist, H. J. Wollner, responded with a characteristic poke at foreign intransigence: "At the League of Nations they whitewashed the whole thing."

The hearings before the House were held in late April and early May.[34] The Treasury's presentation to Congress has been adequately described (although no retelling can equal a reading of the original transcript). As anticipated, the House Committee members accepted all the Treasury Department's testimony. The only witness to appear in opposition to the Administration's proposal, AMA spokesman William C. Woodward, was bombarded with hostile questions. Nevertheless, he was able to get his message across: there was no need to burden the health professions with the bill's restrictions, the states could handle the problem without any additional assistance from the federal bureaucracy, and the evidence against marihuana was incomplete. He pointedly asked where the Public Health Service and Children's Bureau experts were, if it was indeed true that the weed had horrible physiological effects and was wreaking havoc among America's schoolchildren. Dr. Woodward's arguments were ignored. One reason for this poor reception was that the AMA had aroused considerable hostility with its successful opposition of President Roosevelt's plan to include health insurance in the Social Security Act. Reminiscent of their position in the fight over the Harrison Act, the most "liberal" spokesmen were among the most eager to protect the public by prohibiting cannabis.

After the House and Senate hearings, the bill was passed by Congress with no difficulty and came into effect on 1 October 1937. One of the regrettable aspects of the Marihuana Tax Act was that anything less than total prohibition of marihuana would greatly diminish its value as a sop to aroused citizens and would make it enormously more difficult to control without additional appropriations. Enforcement continued to be primarily the responsibility of local police aided occasionally by FBN agents. Marihuana violators were not difficult to apprehend, and the Bureau was able to reassure the public by an impressive number of arrests.

After passage of the Act, the educational campaign of the bureau stepped up, but other publicity campaigns by lay organizations, which claimed that the menace was still out of hand, were muted by bureau opposition. For example, the creators of the often reprinted marihuana poster warning children of the "killer drug marihuana" were in fact put out of business by the bureau because their tactics were beginning to alarm the citizens of Chicago. The bureau attacked such apostles of fear and had only contempt for their profit motives.[35] One reason for the bureau's action may have been because of its policy of designing educational literature that would dissuade young people from trying the substance.[36] Another reason may have been that it reflected the commissioner's belief that the problem was under control in most of the nation's communities, and any assertion that it was out of control would only embarrass the Treasury Department.

On the other hand, the bureau resented later medical rebuttal of claims that marihuana was not an extreme danger, for example in the La Guardia Report of 1944.[37] These responses from the bureau—one a strong and publicly effective attack on the medical criticism of the bureau's action and the other the closing down of the Inter-State Narcotic Association for spreading disturbing scare stories—were designed to show that the bureau fought a great menace, and that the menace was under control.

Why the marihuana law was so eagerly desired by some and, when enacted, so effectively placating are fundamental questions. From the evidence examined, the FBN does not appear to have created the marihuana scare of the early 1930s. Such scapegoating offers no more than it did in the era when marihuana was blamed for almost any vicious crime. When viewed from the narrow goal of placating fears about an "alien minority," the Act was serviceable for more than a quarter of a century. For the broader significance of the marihuana law and an understanding of the dynamics involved in prohibitive legislation, the Tax Act must be placed in its cultural and institutional context.

10 Federal Support of the Medical Approach

The years between World War II and 1970 witnessed, first, enactment of maximum legal sanctions against narcotic drug use, and then a strong reaction that gave considerable responsibility for control to physicians and psychotherapists. Under an onslaught of increased drug abuse and addiction, rising crime against property, and a renewed faith in medicine and psychological treatment, federal drug-abuse statutes retreated from death penalties and mandatory minimum sentences to more reliance on treatment, flexible sentences, and even addiction maintenance, not only with methadone but perhaps even with heroin itself. During the same period the reputation of marihuana, which some considered as dangerous as heroin, changed significantly: in 1972 a Presidential Commission on Marihuana and Drug Abuse recommended elimination of criminal penalties for private use of marihuana.[1] Advocates of severe punishment for addicts found themselves unheeded.

World War II minimized the Federal Bureau of Narcotics' problems with smuggling and domestic addiction. Enforcement of the Marihuana Tax Act did not present much difficulty except for illicit use secondary to licensed hemp production to compensate for unavailable Far Eastern imports. In 1942 one more domestic loophole was plugged: legal cultivation of opium poppies in the United States for commercial purposes was regulated by the Opium Poppy Act.[2] Yet the FBN feared the war's ending, for recollections of what was thought to have happened after World War I were still vivid—when trade was reestablished, so was smuggling,[3] and returning soldiers might again be habituated through the devious methods of the enemy. A major deterrent favored by Anslinger, but not yet enacted, was imposition of mandatory minimum sentences on the first drug conviction.

Modification of the Uniform [state] Narcotic Drug Act by adding mandatory sentences was therefore sought when a reported rise in addiction between 1947 and 1950, particularly in black and Puerto Rican ghettos of northern cities, confirmed the FBN's fears.[4] The federal statute was dramatically strengthened in 1951 by making first convictions carry a mandatory minimum penalty of two years, and by omitting provision for either suspension of sentences or probation on second and subsequent convictions.[5]

Congress decreed mandatory minimum sentences for narcotic

offenders in an emotional atmosphere similar to the years of the first Red Scare. Hale Boggs's bill, which contained mandatory sentences, was passed in 1951 at the beginning of the McCarthy era and fears of Soviet aggression, the "betrayal" of China to the Communists, and suspicion of domestic groups and persons who seemed to threaten overthrow of the government. Narcotics were later associated directly with the Communist conspiracy: the Federal Bureau of Narcotics linked Red China's attempts to get hard cash, as well as to destroy Western society, to the clandestine sale of large amounts of heroin to drug pushers in the United States.[6] This fear was similar to Hobson's more general allegations against foreign nations in the 1920s.

Senate investigations led by Senator Estes Kefauver drew attention to narcotic traffic as an element in organized crime. The FBN also strongly suspected the circumstances under which some federal district judges only mildly reprimanded narcotic dealers. Representative Boggs enthusiastically supported mandatory sentencing as an effective and appropriate weapon against narcotic addiction and was pleased to have his name attached to the act which partially removed judicial discretion in sentencing narcotic offenders.

Before and after this signal victory, the bureau attempted to show that mandatory sentencing worked in those states where it had been tried and that the new federal law was a boon to enforcement. Opposition from within the American Bar Association, however, led to reexamination. A resolution calling for a congressional investigation of narcotics passed the ABA House of Delegates.[7] Unlike the disinterest shown Representative Coffee's similar request in 1938, Senate authorization for a subcommittee to evaluate the narcotic problem came only a month after the ABA resolution. The subcommittee, headed by Senator Price Daniel of Texas, did not question current policy, as apparently the Bar Association had hoped, but recommended penalties even more severe than those of 1951.[8] Sentences for some offenses were raised to five years on the first conviction, while a jury could impose the death penalty on anyone over age 18 who sold heroin to an individual under 18.[9] These two federal statutes of 1951 and 1956 represent the high point of federal punitive action against narcotics. Although some states had even more severe sentences for some offenses, no state law had the breadth of jurisdiction or the unified enforcement service of the Federal Bureau of Narcotics.

There is a noticeable parallel between the association of internal subversion in the postwar periods of both 1919–20 and 1951–55; both led to extremely punitive sanctions against addicts and those who catered to addicts. Toleration of addiction was attacked as a dangerous weakness of soft-hearted or ill-informed persons; at least some of them must harbor evil intentions. Public sympathy was up against a social fear of addiction that had almost no connection with physiology or pharmacology.

THE AMERICAN BAR ASSOCIATION

The ABA responded to sanctions like the Boggs Act by declaring that in their opinion a harsh approach was unjust and ineffective, that the answer must lie elsewhere. This professional reaction was reminiscent of the AMA and the Public Health Service which, just after World War I, remonstrated that medical treatment for addiction was much less effective than laymen believed it to be.

In 1951 the ABA House of Delegates condemned the imposition of mandatory first sentences in narcotics convictions and two years later established a Standing Committee on Narcotics and Alcohol in its Section of Criminal Law.[10] A trend toward more sociological and psychiatric analyses of crime and its treatment helped the ABA toward a serious reevaluation of the narcotics problem and laws. By 1955 the ABA was ready to join with the AMA in a study of narcotics, and the Joint Committee of the ABA and the AMA on Narcotic Drugs was appointed.

Now that respectable institutions of medicine and law were beginning to question the trend of narcotic control, the liberal medical wing, based principally in New York City, began to assert itself again. Rigid enforcement of the Harrison Act had caused more physicians to become disaffected with FBN policies, and eventually in 1955 the Academy of Medicine of New York, which had taken a more restrained view of addiction control in 1918, adopted a policy not dissimilar to that of the Medical Economic League in 1917: it supported maintenance clinics and suggested that the decision to undertake cure be voluntary.[11] This pronouncement represented an important but nevertheless peripheral group within organized medicine. The AMA's cooperation, and especially the ABA's questioning of increasingly severe legal penalties, were more significant with regard to eventual change in narcotic control.

The direction of the Joint Committee's *Interim Report* (1958), although carefully phrased and tentative, seemed clear enough to the FBN. It was another move to soften penalties and, worse, open the door to clinics. Restrictions on private physicians would become relaxed, and narcotics would be prescribed more widely and easily. The *Interim Report* was cautious about clinics, but did not preclude dispensing narcotics in an outpatient experimental clinic for the treatment of drug addicts.[12]

The report, however, had two appendixes of a different tone. One, by the chairman of the Joint Committee, praised the British method of dealing with addicts.[13] The other, by the Director of the Narcotics Control Study, described the narcotic laws, criticized federal agents who intimidated physicians, expressed the hope that clinical errors of the past could be rectified, and suggested that crime might be prevented by providing addicts with their drugs.[14]

The bureau's shrill counterattack, an ad hoc Advisory Committee report entitled *Comments on Narcotic Drugs: Interim Report of the Joint Committee of the ABA and AMA on Narcotic Drugs* (1959), characteristic of a passing era and style, was the high-water mark of its public expression. It placed the Joint Committee in the same category as Doctors Bishop and Volk, the White Cross, and a few "crackpot" doctors and sociologists. Already chafing under restrictions placed on its enforcement activities and various Supreme Court decisions that seemed to favor the criminal element in the United States, the bureau had to contend with members of the legal and health establishments. The FBN discerned a much more direct threat from the *Interim Report* of the Joint Committee of the ABA and the AMA, because the prestige of the two associations gave the clinic idea respectability, in spite of the AMA's previous disapproval of clinics (1957), the widely reported Daniel's hearings, which had resulted in the extremely severe penalties of the law enacted in 1956, and a heavily biased brochure against clinics published by the FBN in 1955.[15]

The brochure's description of the old narcotic clinics is important for the kinds of errors and truths it contained. It can be divided into two parts: a description of respectable medical opinion in 1920 and an analysis of the clinics' operations. The bureau correctly portrayed the opposition of medical and scientific opinion to treatment of addiction by private physicians on an outpatient basis or by narcotic-dispensing clinics and its own support of law enforcement and drying up of the narcotic supply as the best "cure" for addiction. But the FBN presented only the worst aspects of the clinics and must have ignored the available evidence to the contrary.

Maintenance clinics would threaten the delicate legal authority that enabled the FBN to check up on doctors and other registrants. By the 1950s few of the original clinic opponents were still alive. Anslinger, who had not been in the old Narcotics Division then, accepted as true the prevailing opposition to the federal clinic experiment.

The belief that neither a clinic nor a physician could be "licensed" to prescribe narcotics—that if one person were legally permitted to maintain addiction anyone else could do the same—resulted from narrow Supreme Court decisions that had raised this question in the Harrison Act. Anslinger apparently prided himself on rarely asking for higher appropriations, and so as late as 1967 the FBN had only three hundred agents. A clinic system would make surveillance much more difficult; increased appropriations would have to be requested or the entire national control system might collapse, causing a situation that could not be helped by any number of agents. The ABA–AMA report had not advocated a network of clinics, but an experimental clinic, and not necessarily one that gave out narcotics. The appendixes, however, did give a warm approval to the maintenance policies ascribed to the "British system."

The Joint Committee's *Interim Report* and appendixes, although repeating antibureau views, was not harsh or melodramatic. But the bureau's vituperative attack on the Joint Committee can be seen as a desperate response to the belief that, regardless of congressional support and official bureau statements, its control of narcotic enforcement in America was beginning to slip. In fact, the bureau's opponents had been rapidly gaining national power since the end of World War II.

RISE OF THE MENTAL HEALTH PROFESSIONS

After the war the government began to pour money into mental health training and research. By 1969, when the FBN annual budget was about $6 million—only twice the appropriation for 1932—the NIMH budget exceeded $250 million.[16]

Psychological and psychiatric studies, and therapies of various kinds, were to be President Kennedy's contribution to the mentally ill and retarded.[17] In spite of the most vigorous opposition of the AMA, which feared that the precedent of federally funded mental health centers might lead to enactment of some form of general health insurance, a gigantic program for mental health centers throughout the nation was adopted in 1963. This concrete expression of faith in the newer modality of deviance control and correction foreshadowed a decline in support for old-time law enforcement.

The leaders of the mental health establishment had an attitude toward addiction vastly different from that of the FBN, arguing anew that addiction was a psychological or physical disease and that the medical profession should therefore treat addicts. Their power and persuasiveness, now extensively funded and supported by congress, suggested that mandatory sentences and rigid control would be modified.

The directors of the Mental Hygiene Division (after 1946, the National Institute of Mental Health) had been either directors or trainees at the federal narcotic "farms." These psychiatrist–administrators had lost faith in policies that in effect turned the treatment centers into prisons; they had reluctantly done the bureau's dirty work since 1935. One of the NIMH's most symbolic actions in the late 1960s was to remove the steel bars from the cells at Lexington and to turn the facility into a recognizable hospital. Since Anslinger's retirement in 1962, support for the control in which he believed had gradually become less adamant and powerful. The NIMH attitude toward social dysfunction and individual behavior gradually replaced the bureau's approach, which on the New Frontier seemed crude.

Faith in the "British System" characterized the anti-FBN forces in the 1950s and 1960s. If in the United States the willing physician and addict were not kept apart by arbitrary rulings of the FBN and intimidation, America could, like Great Britain, solve the addiction problem.[18]

Although rival theories of deviance control were gaining credibility in the postwar period, the enforcement of narcotic laws did not become widely questioned and condemned until surveillance and penalties failed, even with mandatory minimum penalties and the death threat, to prevent a rapid rise in various forms of drug abuse in the 1960s. If the use of marihuana, which was more feared in the early 1960s because of a general lack of accurate medical information, was rapidly increasing among young people, and if heroin use was moving from the ghettos to the suburbs, then a new approach must be undertaken. If prohibitive enforcement had failed, perhaps the opposite would succeed. Commissions and public figures turned to answers consistent with current social science thinking: lesser penalties, medical treatment, and perhaps maintenance supplies to addicts at low cost.

In Great Britain, meanwhile, a similar rapid increase in drug use occurred in the 1960s. Heroin replaced morphine as the preferred drug; the number of addicts rose from a few hundred to several thousand. A black market developed, and youth seemed attracted to drugs regardless of the medical practitioners' availability and understanding. In Great Britain, also, the old form of control was criticized as inadequate. The Interdepartmental Commission on Drug Addiction recommended in 1965 more severe restrictions on physicians—limiting to a few the right to prescribe for addicts, setting penalties for prescribing too readily, and improving customs searches to prevent drug smuggling.[19] Eventually, addicts' clinics were established and operated under strict controls. The British were reacting to what they considered a new situation, never having had so large a narcotic problem in the twentieth century.[20]

Marihuana's increasing popularity in the U.S. created a gap between those who used it without becoming maniacs and the society that believed it had vicious effects. Youth, especially, grew doubtful that drug warnings had any credibility, since marihuana was being exposed after a quarter of a century as less than "the most dangerous habit-forming drug of them all." Perhaps as a result, more accurate information on other drugs, such as the amphetamines, was ignored. Long sentences for marihuana possession became examples to youth of an ignorant establishment's show of force. Confidence in the courts and fear as a deterrent to drug use declined. Sentiment began to favor a general reevaluation of drug laws to reflect both current medical and sociological information and beliefs.

Among the new insights gradually accepted by the informed public was an idea that the identification of crime and drug abuse with some ethnic minorities, such as blacks and Puerto Ricans, might have resulted from repressive and racist policies. Police collusion with drug suppliers in communities like Harlem, where such deals are common knowledge, gradually became known to the public. As this information spread, so did the suspicion that addiction was not necessarily associated with either crime or subgroups, at least not in any simple way.

The concept of "deviance" as a category, created by the majority in society to describe certain minorities on criteria perhaps unrelated to "justice," made perception of unusual or atypical behavior more relativistic. A deviant was not necessarily the product of a dangerous group nor attributable to the evil attraction of vicious activities. Thus the notion of addiction as a simple punishable vice increasingly shifted to a conviction that those who profited from addiction—corrupt police, the Mafia—were the criminals.

The evolution of this ameliorated view of the addict can be followed in court decisions. In 1962 the Supreme Court declared addiction to be a disease and not a crime. Courts became more critical of tracking down petty dealers who were also addicts. Mandatory penalties elicited opposition from judges, prosecutors, and the Federal Bureau of Prisons as well as the American Psychiatric Association. The rise in funds for research within and without the NIMH reflected a desire to find out what was the truth in a conflict of strong statements for and against drug use, particularly psychedelic drugs.

METHADONE AS A SUBSTITUTE FOR HEROIN

The example of institutions and outpatient clinics established in the mid-1960s for methadone maintenance helped create favor for "medical treatment" of heroin addiction. From the care with which it is dispensed, the public appears to believe that methadone is a medicine like an antibiotic rather than what it is—a synthetic and addictive morphine substitute discovered by German scientists in World War II. In the methadone maintenance program, various mental health services are also supplied. The knowledge that methadone substitutes one addiction for another and that only a minority of heroin addicts, very few under twenty-one, want to make the switch is rarely publicized.[21] Dr. Vincent Dole and Dr. Marie Nyswander, who established methadone maintenance as a result of their research at Rockefeller University, expressed the belief that opiate addiction creates a permanent biochemical change in physiology so that methadone maintenance might well be necessary for

the life of the addict. In their view, therefore, it is not an abstinence
cure, but it can be used to stabilize the life styles of those who will
cooperate in a treatment program.[22]

For a few enthusiasts methadone has become a panacea that will
solve the American addiction problem. It is, of course, diametrically
opposed to the earlier federal policy of keeping supplies of all
addicting drugs as scarce as possible. Every step toward respectability and public financing for methadone maintenance has frayed
the traditional view of opiate addiction as inherently perilous.

Property theft to obtain funds for opiates is claimed to cause
much property crime, estimated at more than 50 percent of all reported crimes in New York City. Therefore, if property crime is a
chief menace, and if addicts steal to pay for their supply, the argument goes, methadone maintenance—perhaps even heroin maintenance—is justified because it might cut the crime rate. Widening
acceptance of maintenance also indicates that certain medical facts
have filtered down to the public: the addict might steal to pay for
his habit but not because the drug stimulates him to steal—a notion
Richmond Hobson and his colleagues had sold to readily believing
audiences.

The election of John F. Kennedy to the presidency set in bolder
relief the decline of Anslinger's influence after thirty years of political and popular support. As Anslinger's retirement drew near, demands for a reevaluation of the drug policies increased. The final
ABA–AMA report was published in 1961. Then an outgrowth of the
ABA's study of narcotics, W. G. Eldridge's *Narcotics and the Law*
(1962), appeared; Anslinger retired; and the White House Conference on Drug Abuse met in September 1962.[23]

Anslinger's successor, Harry Giordano, a pharmacist, was considered much more reasonable. Perhaps Giordano lacked Anslinger's
drive and aggressiveness. In any case, during his tenure (1962–68)
groups like the NIMH made more effective challenges to older control styles.

To conclude what had started at the White House Conference,
the Presidential Commission on Narcotic and Drug Abuse was established. In 1963 the commission issued its report, recommending
relaxation of mandatory minimum sentences, increased appropriations for research into "all aspects of narcotic and drug abuse," and
the dismantling of the FBN and allocation of its functions to the
Justice and Health, Education and Welfare departments. The HEW

would assume responsibility for legitimate distribution and research; the Justice Department would be responsible for investigating illicit traffic. The medical profession would have the ultimate voice in saying what constitutes legitimate medical treatment and use of narcotic drugs. The Lexington and Fort Worth hospitals, rather than continuing as routine treatment facilities, would become centers of research operating with voluntary patients only. Localities would receive aid for establishing treatment centers. In accord with evidence that the best results in addiction treatment come from detention of a year or more in an institution, a federal civil commitment law was advocated as an alternative to prison for the federally convicted offender who was a "confirmed narcotic or marihuana abuser." [24]

The 1963 Commission report continued the policy of lumping together marihuana and narcotic offenders but suggested a policy that would shift the criteria for regulatory decisions regarding addicts and other drug users away from enforcement agencies to the health professions. The Drug Abuse Control amendments of 1965 established the Bureau of Drug Abuse Control within HEW and attempted to regulate hypnotics and stimulants such as barbiturates and amphetamines. In the 1965 Act, the constitutional basis for drug control shifted from taxing power to interstate and commerce powers, another recommendation of the 1963 Advisory Commission.[25] In 1966, the Narcotic Addict Rehabilitation Act (NARA) provided for civil commitment of some addicted federal prisoners and some categories of addicts before trial or before sentencing.[26] The faith in civil commitment, however, gradually faded as evidence of its success was less impressive than anticipated. Also, the estimated number of addicts was so large that adequate housing and care became problematical.

The NIMH, which in 1963 had succeeded in obtaining congressional approval for a program aimed at creating mental health centers throughout the nation, wished to set up in them the local treatment centers recommended by the 1963 Commission. The NIMH further wished to model addiction treatment along the lines of what was considered the latest and best in psychiatric therapy, the multimodality mental health center, and established several centers that were not committed to any one approach but to any combination of approaches that would process large numbers of drug abusers.

In 1967 the narcotic problem was examined again, this time by the Presidential Commission on Law Enforcement and Administration of Justice. The FBN still existed intact, but the Drug Abuse Control Amendments had presaged a new federal antinarcotic formula. Marihuana use was rapidly increasing, and the heroin epidemic had become a common issue in political campaigns and among enforcement personnel. Methadone therapy was now accepted in major centers of addiction. Drawing attention to the minuscule amount of narcotics seized annually compared to the minimum that had to be smuggled in to sustain addiction, the 1967 Commission recommended greatly increasing enforcement staffs of the Bureau of Customs and the FBN. The FBN's agents, spread over the nation and ten foreign countries, numbered about three hundred, not much higher than in the 1930s. The commission especially requested the FBN to institute long-range programs to attack "upper echelons of the drug traffic," and asked the states to cooperate, beginning with enactment of legislation complementary to the Drug Abuse Control Amendment Act.

By 1967 marihuana was clearly marked for attention as both medical information and use of the substance increased. Questioning its association with crime and its role as a prelude to addictive drugs, the Presidential Commission asked the NIMH to look into "all aspects of marihuana use." The commission commented impartially on various treatment programs for drug abuse, including methadone maintenance and drugless institutions like Daytop and Synanon. The strong recommendation for civil commitment by the 1963 Commission was not supported a few years later, by which time California and New York had had a fair amount of experience with it. Indeed, the 1967 Commission criticized civil commitment as denying freedom to an individual who was convicted of no crime but was merely suffering a diseased state—addiction. Its study found the California experience between 1961 and 1965 to be discouraging, with more than five thousand civilly committed addicts. Even if the objection to confinement for no crime could be answered by comparing addiction commitment to that for mental illness, the procedure would still have little chance of achieving the desired result, a "cure" for addiction.[27]

In 1968 the FBN was transferred to the Justice Department, joined with the Bureau of Drug Abuse Control of HEW, and became the Bureau of Narcotics and Dangerous Drugs. Increased appropriations, training of more agents, and the institution of a long-range program of enforcement and regulation including revived attempts to convince Turkey to stop growing opium poppies, fulfilled the expectations of past commissions. After lively controversies with health agencies and scientists, the Justice Department succeeded in framing the Drug Abuse Act of 1970.[28] In it the myriad regulations advanced during the Harrison Act's long evolution were brought into one statute, tempered now by a desire to have flexible penalties and to separate marihuana from addicting drugs. For both the 1965 Drug Abuse Control Amendments and the 1970 Act, jurisdiction was based on the interstate commerce powers of the Constitution, now greatly extended and strengthened by sixty years of constitutional development since Representative Mann and Dr. Wiley had attempted to use those powers in the first decade of the century.

THE CONTROL OF DEVIANCE BY LAW

Law enforcers and the mental health professions have at least one objective in common—effective and knowledgeable control of deviant behavior. Both may effect this control through custodial restraint (imprisonment in a penal institution or care in a mental hospital) or through relative nonrestraint (outpatient therapy or parole). Before World War I, physicians had the responsibility for treating addiction. Treatment, however, did not cure, and not all physicians used good judgment in prescribing and dispensing narcotics. The arrangement, therefore, did not work—it did not *eliminate* narcotic addiction.

By World War I the American addict was identified as a social menace and equated with the IWWs, Bolsheviks, anarchists, and other feared subgroups like the cocaine-using blacks and the opium-smoking Chinese. But these deviant subgroups that threatened the social fabric could still be considered subjects for psychotherapy or medical treatment.

In the post-World War I hysteria, however, attitudes changed. If outpatient treatment could not control deviance, if medical institutions like hospitals could not cure it, then police and jails were the last option.

That addiction rose spectacularly between 1915 and 1919—an assumption drawn to justify the repression of addicts after 1919—is not supported by evidence. On the other hand, any contention that this fact was deliberately constructed in order to permit the government to take dramatic action against a minimal threat is not supported by evidence either. Commissioner Roper, among others, seems to have honestly believed the drug problem was out of hand, and he was prepared for a serious national problem when the Supreme Court ruling and the Harrison Act Amendments of early 1919 were enforced.

Passage and enforcement of the 18th Amendment supported repression of addiction and dangerous drugs. Here again quarantine was adopted as the best solution for a social problem. The Harrison Act's interpretation in 1919 was aligned with social acceptance of repression, quarantine, prison, or fines for social danger whether political, bacteriological, or chemical. Congress continued to pass laws more severe until the ultimate in severity, the 1956 Narcotic Control Act, combined the threat of death with mandatory minimum sentences on the first conviction.

THE MEDICAL CONTROL OF DEVIANCE

Medical treatment for deviance is not an intentional penalty, although it may result in more "punishment" as measured by the kind and length of restraint than a sentence for a crime. Underlying medical therapy is the belief that behavior can be corrected through scientific treatment and that ascription of guilt and criminal sanctions are often inappropriate. Although the perfectibility of man is an old American belief, faith in treatment became extensively implemented only after World War II, with the entry of the federal government into national health and welfare areas. As elements in the medical quest for perfectibility, psychological and sociological insights strongly influenced sophisticated Americans, beginning with World War I.

The mental health center concept is a striking example of the acceptance by Congress of an attitude that had been accepted and promoted by mental health professionals for several decades. The mental health center program in 1963 envisioned a network of rather small community-based hospitals, about one for every two hundred thousand persons. These centers were proposed by President Kennedy in order to reduce the number of citizens under restraint in state mental hospitals by allowing them to be treated in their local communities. Presumably, admissions to state hospitals would also decline because the incipient mentally ill would be treated quickly and efficiently by the mental health center staff. If custodial care was necessary, even that could be accomplished through brief confinement in a mental health center rather than long stays in a far-off hospital. Hope existed also that the mental health centers scattered across the nation would treat sick communities as well as sick persons, and thereby lessen social disruption caused by the unhappy and maladjusted.

The development of a federal health establishment, phenomenal growth of the Public Health Service and its research body (the National Institutes of Health), and the rise of HEW provided Congress with new sources of help in social and health problems. Medical and scientific methods for the control of drug abuse are now under evaluation. The possibility exists that failure of such approaches to eliminate drug abuse may be interpreted, as in the period after World War I, to mean that they are worthless and should be abandoned.

11 The Dynamics of Narcotic Control

American concern with narcotics is more than a medical or legal problem—it is in the fullest sense a political problem. The energy that has given impetus to drug control and prohibition came from profound tensions among socio-economic groups, ethnic minorities, and generations—as well as the psychological attraction of certain drugs. The form of this control has been shaped by the gradual evolution of constitutional law and the lessening limitation of federal police powers. The bad results of drug use and the number of drug users have often been exaggerated for partisan advantage. Public demand for action against drug abuse has led to regulative decisions that lack a true regard for the reality of drug use. Relations with foreign nations, often the sources of the drugs, have been a theme in the domestic scene from the beginning of the American antinarcotic movement. Narcotics addiction has proven to be one of the most intractable medical inquiries ever faced by American clinicians and scientists. Disentangling the powerful factors which create the political issue of drug abuse may help put the problem in better perspective.

Fear of narcotics has grown with the awareness of their use. Dr. Holmes in 1860 and Dr. Beard in the 1870s and '80s warned that narcotics abuse was increasing. They based their attacks not only on direct observation but on the open record of import statistics. By 1900 restrictive laws on the state level had been enacted, and reformers began to look to the federal government for effective national regulation. Reform-minded leaders of the health professions agreed on the need to eliminate the nonmedical use of narcotics. Those seeking strict narcotic controls believed that either the need for money to buy drugs or a direct physiological incitement to violence led to crime and immoral behavior. Inordinate pleasure caused by drugs, moreover, was seen to provide youth with a poor foundation for character development, and a resulting loss of independence and productivity.

The most passionate support for legal prohibition of narcotics has been associated with fear of a given drug's effect on a specific minority. Certain drugs were dreaded because they seemed to undermine essential social restrictions which kept these groups under control: cocaine was supposed to enable blacks to withstand bullets which would kill normal persons and to stimulate sexual assault. Fear that smoking opium facilitated sexual contact between

Chinese and white Americans was also a factor in its total prohibition. Chicanos in the Southwest were believed to be incited to violence by smoking marihuana. Heroin was linked in the 1920s with a turbulent age-group: adolescents in reckless and promiscuous urban gangs. Alcohol was associated with immigrants crowding into large and corrupt cities. In each instance, use of a particular drug was attributed to an identifiable and threatening minority group.

The occasion for legal prohibition of drugs for nonmedical purposes appears to come at a time of social crisis between the drug-linked group and the rest of American society. At the turn of this century, when the battle for political control of freed blacks reached a peak (as shown by the extent of disenfranchisement, lynchings, and the success of segregation policies), cocaine, a drug popular among whites and blacks and in the North as well as the South, was associated with expression of black hostility toward whites. Chinese and opium smoking became linked in the depressions of the late 19th century, when Chinese were low-paid competitors for employment, and this connection intensified during the bitter discrimination shown Orientals in the first decade of this century. The attack on marihuana occurred in the 1930s when Chicanos became a distinct and visible unemployed minority. Heroin, claimed to be an important factor in the "crime wave" which followed World War I, was implicated in the 1950s as part of the Communist conspiracy against the United States. A youth culture which attacked traditional values became closely connected with marihuana smoking and the use of other psychedelics. Customary use of a certain drug came to symbolize the difference between that group and the rest of society; eliminating the drug might alleviate social disharmony and preserve old order.

The belief that drug use threatened to disrupt American social structures militated against moves toward drug toleration, such as legalizing drug use for adults, or permitting wide latitude in the prescribing practice of physicians. Even if informed students of drugs such as Dr. Lawrence Kolb, Sr., in the 1920s argued that heroin does not stimulate violence, guardians of public safety did not act upon that information. The convenience of believing that heroin stimulated violence made the conviction hard to abandon. Public response to these minority-linked drugs differed radically from attitudes toward other drugs with similar potential for harm, such as the barbiturates.

Narcotics are assumed to cause a large percentage of crime, but the political convenience of this allegation and the surrounding imagery suggest the fear of certain minorities, and make one suspicious of this popular assumption. During the last seventy-five years responsible officials have stated that narcotics caused between fifty and seventy-five percent of all crimes, especially in large cities like New York. Narcotics have been blamed for a variety of America's ills, from crime waves to social disharmony. Their bad effects have been given as the excuse for repressing certain minorities, as evidence for stopping legal heroin maintenance in 1919, and as evidence for starting legal heroin maintenance in 1972.

Like the speculated percentage of crimes caused by narcotic use and sales, the number of addicts estimated for the nation appears often to have been exaggerated. Peaks of overestimation have come before or at the time of the most repressive measures against narcotic use, as in 1919 when a million or more addicts and five million Parlor Reds were said to threaten the United States. Both groups were the object of severe penalties, although in retrospect both figures appear to have been enormously inflated. Still, the substantial number of addicts in the United States has presented one of the most enduringly difficult aspects of any proposed control program. The size of this population has made control of misuse in maintenance programs difficult. There has been a fair amount of diversion of drugs to the illicit market and some registration of nonaddicts.

In America, control of narcotics could take only a limited number of legislative forms. The lack of broad federal police powers inhibited the restriction of drug transactions. The division of federal and state powers in effect permitted widespread and unscrupulous dissemination of untested products and unsafe drugs. When the danger of narcotics came to the attention of popular reform movements and after carefully phrased federal legislation was at last enacted in 1914, it took the Supreme Court five years to overcome the apparent obstacle of states' rights. In 1919 the court permitted the federal government almost prohibitory power for prevention of most addiction maintenance. The court's majority affirmed the reformers' belief that simple addiction maintenance was intolerable.

Nevertheless, after 1919, severe constitutional strictures continued to mold enforcement of the Harrison Act. Because all professionals (unless convicted of a violation) had to be treated equally under a revenue statute, the federal government could not discriminate against careless or unscrupulous physicians and druggists by refusing them a tax stamp or by employing some other fair form of flexible administrative punishment. This lack of legal accommodation to circumstances, the small number of agents, and a bureaucratic reward system which favored a large number of prosecutions led to harassment and intimidation as a prominent mode of regulation. Because government agents feared that precedents might prevent indictment of "dope doctors," exceptions to the no-maintenance rule were few. The mutual suspicion which grew up between agents and physicians inhibited reasonable enforcement of the law. The manner of closing the Shreveport clinic illustrates the combination of suspicion and inflexibility.

The federal narcotic authorities never forgot that theirs was a narrow path between federal and states' rights. As late as 1937 the Treasury Department chose to prohibit marihuana by a separate law because it feared an attack on the constitutionality of the Harrison Act. In spite of organized medicine's opposition in the 1920s, and despite several close Supreme Court decisions, the extreme interpretation placed on the Harrison Act in 1919 continued to prevail. Why did the Supreme Court agree that a federal statute could outlaw narcotics, when the Constitution itself had to be amended to outlaw alcohol? One answer to this may be that in the case of narcotics the consensus was almost absolute; everyone appeared to agree on the evils of these drugs. For alcohol, there was no such agreement.

Foreign nations have played important roles in the American perception of its national drug problem. World War I is the watershed in national self-consciousness vis-à-vis foreign powers, dividing respectable opinion on the relative importance of domestic and international causes of narcotics use in the United States. In the prewar years the United States displayed confidence in traditional diplomatic methods and the efficacy of international treaties. Prior to the war and the immediate postwar security crisis, the usual explanation for the American drug appetite rested on characteristics of American culture—the pace of life, the effect of civilization, wealth which permitted indulgence, and inadequate state and federal laws which did not protect citizens from dangerous nostrums and incompetent health professionals.

After World War I, open official criticism of America's defects was no longer common. Whereas Hamilton Wright saw international control of narcotics as a solution to America's indigenous problem and recognized that this nation would benefit more than others from international altruism, Representative Porter in the 1920s denied any unusual appetite for narcotics in the United States, blaming our problem on the perfidy and greed of other nations. Richmond Hobson, equally as patriotic, claimed the country had an immense number of heroin addicts and consequent crime waves due to the evil influence of other nations. Hobson viewed America as surrounded by other dangerous continents—South America sent in cocaine; Europe contributed drugs like heroin and morphine; Asia was the source of crude opium and smoking opium; Africa produced hashish. Porter and Hobson sounded one theme: the American problem was caused by foreign nations. The spirit of national isolation which excluded participation in the League of Nations extended easily to international narcotic control. Americans were encouraged to condemn diplomacy as zealously as they had once sought conferences and commissions.

Projection of blame on foreign nations for domestic evils harmonized with the ascription of drug use to ethnic minorities. Both the external cause and the internal locus could be dismissed as un-American. This kind of analysis avoids the painful and awkward realization that the use of dangerous drugs may be an integral part of American society. Putting the blame on others also permits more punitive measures to be taken against certain of the culprits.

The history of American narcotic usage and control does not encourage belief in a simple solution to the long-standing problem. Reasonable regulation of drug use requires knowledge of physiological and psychological effects, an understanding of social causes of drug popularity, and an appreciation of how legal sanctions will actually effect the use and harmful results of drug ingestion. In the construction of such a policy, recognition of accidental and irrational factors in past drug legislation is essential, although no ideal program can be simply extrapolated from an historical study.

Political judgment and values have been paramount in the establishment of national drug policies. The commonsense conclusions reached by legislators, high-ranking government bureaucrats, and influential public figures, without any special or technical knowledge of drug abuse, are likely to gain acceptance from other national social and political institutions. Political judgments made in harmony with popular demands for narcotic control (or release from liquor control) have a proven longevity. Resisting insistent popular demands is unusual among public officials; considerable political acumen is required to modify prevailing fear and anger into constructive programs.

As the pressure for political action reaches a climax, policy options are almost imperceptibly reduced to the few which have current political viability. The rapid crystallization of public policy in 1919–20 illustrates how quickly this last stage of policy formulation may pass. Dissidents like Rep. Volk and Dr. Bishop continued to protest, to little effect. Once the national mood had been settled, any attempt to reopen the painful question met strong resistance. The 1919 formulation defined a broad range of issues in narcotic control, and yet the battle was waged on curiously narrow lines. In the medical profession, for example, both those for and against the "disease" concept of addiction carried on their dispute over the question of whether antibodies or antitoxins were produced by morphine administration. The lack of such substances seemed to prove that addiction must be a mere habit, and that those who held out for the "disease" concept had unworthy motives. In that period of crisis over narcotic policies fifty years ago each side was unwilling to compromise and sought to sweep the adversary from the field.

Today an issue like methadone maintenance may form the model on which a consensus is reached. This might lead toward simple toleration, or to prohibition of natural and synthetic opiates for nonmedical purposes (which would include "mere addiction"). As new generations confront the narcotic question, the same old fundamental issues continue to arise. Current debates over heroin maintenance focus on such basic questions as the effect of heroin on the body and personality. One almost hears the voice of Dr. Bishop arguing that if an addict is in heroin balance he is a normal person as regards the effect of the drug, and Captain Hobson warning that heroin use gradually destroys the brain's higher centers. After more than half a century since the Harrison Act's passage one of the few statements about narcotics on which there is general agreement is that there is no treatment of hard-core addiction which leads to abstinence in more than a fraction of attempts. The lack of agreement on other crucial questions and their relative importance is almost total.

Although social and cultural influences are essential elements in the creation of the American drug problem, it is quite possible to provide a viable political response to public outcry and at the same time avoid an objective examination of critical issues: the nature of American society; the psychological vulnerability of addicts; the physiological effects of drugs; the social impact of drug use. Our society's blindness to alcohol's destructive effects is an example of how denial of reality is compatible with a politically comfortable resolution of a controversial drug problem.

We are now at a time when the credibility of previous solutions is sufficiently low so that some of the unresolved questions can be raised and again discussed. Gradually, and not necessarily as the result of formal decisions, the scientific and political alternatives regarding drug abuse may, as they have in the past, diminish. As a new workable political solution evolves the controversy tends to narrow to a few issues. Ideally, public pressure for elimination of the drug problem should not be met with fewer options. Rather the effective translation of knowledge, scientific and historical, should enable the public to avoid over-simplification, and to exert influence based on more rational understanding. But only the most determined efforts can prevent closure on drug policy by those two most powerful forces: fatigue and frustration.

The Return of Drug Toleration, 1965 – 1985

12

Gradually, at times imperceptibly, in the years after World War I, use of narcotics in the United States declined. The nadir was reached during World War II; not only had usage gone down prior to those hostilities, but it declined even further as the disruption of international transportation cut down on supplies. From being easily available and commonly used, heroin, morphine and cocaine almost faded out of nonmedical situations: when someone was caught with drugs, the event elicited headlines and comment. Once commonplace, narcotics use waned into little more than rumors about this physician or that movie star. Personal knowledge of a "dope fiend" was unusual for the vast majority of Americans by the 1950s.

The consensus on drugs—intolerance toward the use or advocacy of narcotics—was well-setablished by the mid- or late 1920s. As a result, members of the generation born in the 1920s grew to maturity with diminishing direct knowledge of, but a great deal of animosity toward, the substances. Their parents had lived through the drawn-out, intense experience with drugs that marked the nation's first wave of narcotics use, peaking around the turn of the century. It was an experience not unlike that we have endured over the last twenty years. Not only could the parents convey their fear of drugs, but they had the advantage of direct knowledge, which sustained their conviction and helped instill it in their children. The next generation, the grandchildren or great-grandchildren of those who knew about drugs, carried into the 1960s no direct knowledge of narcotics but had heard exaggerations about them that were in fact minatory rather than informative. Indeed, new generations not only lacked information gained firsthand sixty years earlier, but by and large had little awareness that there had been an earlier, extensive experience with morphine, heroin, and cocaine.

As documented in earlier chapters, it was when drug intolerance increased that laws such as the Harrison Act (1914) were enacted and the Supreme Court outlawed addiction maintenance (1919). The public continued to support vigorous law enforcement against addicts and physicians, among others, and the laws themselves were made increasingly severe. During that climate of growing intolerance, the Marihuana Tax Act was easily passed in 1937 because the substance was linked to other alarming drugs such as cocaine and heroin. In contrast, when cocaine surfaced again in the mid-

1970s, at a peak of drug (especially marihuana) toleration, it was easily assimilated with the drive to legalize or at least "decriminalize" marihuana, and the decriminalization of cocaine was widely discussed.

Anti-drug laws increased in severity from the 1930s well into the 1950s. The peak was reached in 1956 when the death penalty was applied to the sale of heroin to minors. Draconian penalties against narcotics faced little opposition during this era of drug intolerance and growing unfamiliarity with the direct effects of drugs. The Federal Bureau of Narcotics had meagre resources, and the research effort on the scientific front was modest. The bulwark against drug use was popular imagery—the more fearful the better. Not much should be said, but what was said should depict drugs as so revolting and dangerous that no youngster would try a narcotic even once.

The portrayal of narcotics in motion pictures had been banned under the Production Code of the Motion Picture Association (1934) so that no major studio would touch the subject until a slight relaxation in 1948 allowed filming of *To the Ends of the Earth*, a dramatization of the worldwide efforts of the Federal Bureau of Narcotics (FBN) to stop drug smuggling into the United States.[1] In 1955 the film *Man with the Golden Arm* broke Hollywood's silence shortly before the death sentence for selling heroin to minors became law. Both the film and the law, the so-called Little Boggs Act, had been prompted by the first stirrings of a renewed heroin wave in the United States (see p. 230ff).

When I interviewed former Narcotics Commissioner Harry J. Anslinger in 1972, he described his astonishment at the explosion of drug use in the 1960s. He felt the FBN had reduced the level of addiction to a minimum, and the rise of heroin and marihuana usage in the late 1960s was a phenomenon he had never seen before nor expected.[2] Anslinger had counted on stiff mandatory sentences, negative drug imagery, and the consensus of national institutions against drug tolerance. The 1960s broke through that brittle shell of defense, behind which lay an ignorance of drugs, perceptions so extreme as to be laughable to the new drug users, and a prison system that would be overwhelmed by a small fraction of those breaking the drug laws. The renewed popularity of drugs, about a lifetime after the previous surge of interest and consumption, arrived in an atmosphere that indeed was unfamiliar to Anslinger and others of his generation who had devoted their lives to reinforcing the intolerance toward drugs that had emerged by the beginning of this century.

I am reminded of a conversation I had with a narcotics officer while researching the original edition of this book. He offered whatever help he could, for, he said, he was very troubled by the change in public attitude toward his job: "Years ago, when I started arresting possessors of narcotics, I was a hero; now the public thinks I'm a rat. Yet, I'm doing exactly the same thing I have always been doing. I don't understand it."

Almost three decades have passed since the 1960s began, and we have moved from a peak of toleration during the Carter administration to an opposition to drug use echoing, although not yet matching in severity, those decades of intolerance. The recent years have given us experiences that allow us to understand both points of view and to appreciate the recurrent quandary drug use presents to Americans.

RESPONSE TO THE RISE IN DRUG USE, 1968–1973

The use of illegal drugs increased astoundingly in the 1960s. Drugs thought safely interred with the past, marihuana and heroin, rapidly resurfaced at the same time that new drugs such as LSD materialized and attained tremendous popularity among young people. This rapid turnaround occurred amid massive changes in American society, which we must appreciate in order to understand the reactions drug use evoked.

The entire decade was a period of enormous growth in the wealth of the United States. The gross national product doubled from 1960 through 1970. Funds were available not only to wage a war in Vietnam but also to fight the War on Poverty. All this productivity and money created an unparalleled market for consumer goods and anything else that promised to make a person feel comfortable, including drugs.

At the same time, the generation of "baby boomers" entered that period of their lifespan in which they were most susceptible to drug use, violence, and crime—ages 15 through 24. Within the decade this age group had increased by 11 million, an astounding gain of nearly 50 percent and over twice the increase that would take place in the next 10 years.[3]

Furthermore, these many young people were stressed by the war in Vietnam, which relied on military draft for manpower, and were encouraged to attack traditional culture by such older, charismatic figures as Dr. Timothy Leary, who urged youth to "turn on, tune in, and drop out." Increasingly, young people gathered to celebrate their own culture, as at Woodstock in August 1969, or to protest the war, as in the march on Washington in November 1969; and drugs, particularly marihuana, pervaded the crowds. Older Americans, viewing these gatherings through the media, saw drug use as a symbol of rejection of traditional values and patriotism and a prime illustration of the frequently bemoaned generation gap.

We can gauge the response to marihuana use by the increase in arrests at the state level for marihuana possession, which rose from 18,000 in 1965 to 188,000 in 1970.[4] A national survey in 1971 estimated that 24 million Americans over the age of 11 had used marihuana at least once. The highest incidence was among 18- to 21-year-olds, of whom 40 percent had tried marihuana.[5] A reflection of the rise in drug use, chiefly heroin, by needle injection can be seen in the rapid rise in narcotic-related hepatitis cases from about 4,000 in 1966 to about 36,000 in 1971.[6] Never easy to estimate, the number of heroin users rose from about 50,000 in 1960 to roughly a half-million in 1970. This wave of drug use alarmed most of the public and their representatives in Congress.

In November 1968, when drug use and its social damage were both rapidly increasing, Richard Nixon was elected President on a platform of restoring law and order. No President has equalled Nixon's antagonism to drug abuse, and he took an active role in organizing the federal and state governments to fight the onslaught of substance abuse.

THE NIXON WAR ON DRUGS

One year prior to President Nixon's inauguration in January 1969, the drug enforcement agency in the Department of Health, Education, and Welfare (HEW) and the FBN had been united as the Bureau of Narcotics and Dangerous Drugs (BNDD). Within the National Institute of Mental Health (NIMH) a small Center for Studies of Narcotic and Drug Abuse had been established. The Customs Bureau chiefly guarded the border, and the BNDD dealt with domestic and foreign matters (although the division of responsibility had overlapping elements, which frustrated both agencies). The drug budget for fiscal year (FY) 1969 was $86 million and in FY 1970, the last Johnson budget, $101 million.[7]

Treatment for those with drug problems ranged from outpatient care based on traditional psychotherapy or counseling to inpatient care for detoxification from addictive drugs such as heroin or extended drug-free care in a therapeutic community such as Phoenix House in New York City. The appearance of methadone stimulated the creation of outpatient facilities where that drug, and nothing else in many instances, could be obtained. After an initial optimistic report in 1966, methadone's popularity quickly spread; it was hailed as one of the first new ideas to combat heroin addiction, the most feared form of drug abuse at the time. Methadone, a long-acting opioid taken by mouth, could substitute for shorter-acting heroin taken by needle. It thereby reduced the danger of needle-transmitted diseases such as hepatitis, gave the patient a better chance for employment, and ended the need to commit crimes to maintain the addiction. Curiously, though, for some years it seemed as if methadone was seen by the public as a cure for addiction, more like penicillin for pneumonia than like insulin for diabetes.

Methadone's appeal was in no small measure due to its reputed effectiveness in cutting into the crime attributed to drug use, especially heroin addiction.[8] The initial medical or therapeutic response to the rise in drug abuse was accelerated by methadone's reputation for achieving results. For decades critics of the law enforcement approach had pleaded for a more humane solution to dangerous drug use. Not only did methadone seem to answer that call, but it was a big step toward sanctioning the most extreme anti-enforcement style, the provision of heroin itself to heroin addicts.

Lifting restrictions on individual choice—even to permit the unhindered use of drugs most Americans considered dangerous—harmonized with broader efforts at social reform in the 1960s. Barriers to individual opportunity were under attack at every level of American life, and it should not be surprising that some observers would see drug use as an expression of personal choice that no other person or social institution had a right to obstruct. Advocates of drug use, such as Dr. Leary, specifically hailed drugs for promoting individual fulfillment. Commentators on youth described drug experimentation as an ordinary element in adolescent life— a natural, not a fearful, phenomenon.

Although the government did not legalize heroin maintenance, arguments to do so on libertarian grounds and as a practical mechanism to cut down on thefts performed to maintain illegal addiction were part of a growing toleration around 1970 for unrestricted drug availability.[9] In this context, methadone maintenance in the Nixon anti-drug program can be seen as a compromise between simple toleration of drug use and the public's demand that crime associated with heroin be curbed. Addicts got something to assuage their drug cravings, but not their first choice.

The final component of the Nixon administration's "war on drugs" was greater emphasis on law enforcement, although the budgetary support for treatment programs was even larger. The twin goals were to cut off the foreign supply of heroin and at the same time to increase drug treatment programs massively so that those in trouble with drugs could find help if they wanted it. Drug availability and consumer demand for drugs were to be attacked simultaneously.

CURBING TURKISH OPIUM PRODUCTION

To facilitate enforcement Nixon took the lead in demanding that the influx of drugs from Turkey be stopped in one way or another.[10] The federal government estimated that 80 percent of heroin reaching the United States came from Turkey. The significance of the president's determination lay in the almost invariable rule that the drug problem is a secondary concern to American foreign policy goals. As bad as drug trafficking might appear to Americans, when a decision involves dealing effectively with a drug-producing or -exporting nation while maintaining national security interests through friendly relations with that country, national security and good relations nearly always win out over the important but less crucial issue of drugs. This makes Nixon's personal insistence regarding Turkish opium unusual in the history of American drug policy.

While making strong diplomatic representations and threatening to cut off aid if Turkey did not squash the export of drugs to the United States, the Nixon administration also promised to reimburse

Turkey for subsequent losses resulting from reduced poppy cultivation. Turkey did in fact cease being a significant source of heroin on American streets. Accounts generally agree that the drug was more scarce in 1972 and 1973, although the degree to which the Turkish ban was responsible has been debated. At about this time a smuggling ring that transported morphine base from Turkey to France (where it was changed into heroin and sent on to America) was broken up.[11] Also, from 1971–73 methadone and other treatment centers aimed at reducing demand for heroin increased enormously. Whatever the reason, it is generally agreed that the heroin problem was briefly reduced. Soon, however, the slack in supply was taken up by Mexican production and other supplies from Southeast Asia's Golden Triangle, Afghanistan, Pakistan, and so on. Turkey resumed growing poppies in 1975 using a method of harvest that appears to make diversion from licit production much less likely.[12] However, because estimates are that the U.S. demand for heroin can be met by the amount of opium poppies growing on a ten- to twenty-square-mile patch of land, ending one country's excessive production does not eliminate the supply.[13]

In retrospect, one lesson of the Turkish opium ban is that the political determination to take such an action and the circumstances that give the United States sufficient leverage with the producing nations are rare. Dramatic reduction in total foreign production is not to be expected soon or broadly. Decreased domestic demand for drugs, such as occurred in the United States after World War I, appears the more likely course for improving the drug problem.

In addition to addressing the Turkish supply and the "French connection," the Nixon program rapidly expanded law enforcement agencies such as BNDD. The budget for enforcement rose in FY 1970 from $43 million to $292 million in FY 1974.[14] In January 1972 the Office of Drug Abuse Law Enforcement (ODALE) was established. A domestic strike-force operation employing the "no-knock" provisions that federal law had authorized in 1970, it garnered bad publicity with its assaults on some innocent families.[15] ODALE had been criticized as an election-year gambit to go after local drug offenders with great fanfare. John Ingersoll, Director of the BNDD, had refused White House pressure to become deeply involved with small-scale operations, preferring to concentrate on major dealers and international interdiction. This lack of cooperation led eventually to his leaving the government when ODALE was melded into the BNDD with the creation of the Drug Enforcement Administration (DEA) in 1973.[16] Shortly before, Myles J. Ambrose, head of ODALE and a former customs commissioner who was widely assumed to be the administration's choice to head DEA, also resigned.[17]

DEMAND REDUCTION

The other prong of the Nixon strategy was drug abuse prevention, which included research, education, training, rehabilitation, and treatment—efforts to reduce demand for drugs among the American public. Here the monies authorized by the federal government rose from $59 million in FY 1970 to $462 million in FY 1974.[18] Nixon established the Special Action Office for Drug Abuse Prevention (SAODAP) to coordinate the many government programs linked to the drug problem but especially to give leadership to a crash program of treatment services. To head this unparalleled elevation of drug abuse issues to national prominence, Nixon chose Dr. Jerome H. Jaffe, an academic researcher who was familiar with treatment programs, especially methadone maintenance. Dr. Jaffe, who came to be known as the "drug czar," was urged by the President to knock heads together to achieve the high priority of curbing the drug menace.[19]

VIETNAM AND HEROIN

Dr. Jaffe faced an urgent problem, all the more troublesome because of its connection with the unpopular Vietnam War. This was the imminent return of American servicemen, many of whom had been frequent users of marihuana and heroin. Estimates for the number of men using heroin were as large as 25 percent.[20] Would these drug users spur the domestic drug problem to an even higher level of social disorganization and violence? The similarity to the fear of returning veterans following World War I is evident.

Dr. Jaffe organized a urine-testing program that allowed those with negative tests to return to the United States without interference; those who tested positive for opiates would be remanded for a brief period of detoxification and further treatment, if necessary. One of the most interesting aspects of returning veterans who had tested positive for heroin was that very few continued using it once back home.[21] This suggested that the easy availability of heroin in South Vietnam led to increased use and also that different settings had a profound effect on the desire to use drugs. Dr. Jaffe was so impressed by the efficacy of urine testing for drugs that he thought it might eventually be considered in the same light as chest X-rays for tuberculosis.[22]

EXPANSION OF TREATMENT PROGRAMS

The early 1970s brought an explosion in treatment facilities. SAO-DAP stimulated an increase in the number of cities with federally funded programs from 54 to 214 in the first 18 months of operation. From 20,000 clients in these programs in October 1971, the number climbed to over 60,000 by December 1972. Programs for methadone clients, either funded federally or otherwise, were enrolling 80,000 persons by October 1973, just over two years after SAODAP's creation.[23]

While methadone treatment expanded, some communities grew suspicious that those administering the federal program had insidious motives and that the drug was actually extremely dangerous.[24] Over the years, methadone has not been found to have any significant long-term negative effects; but at the same time the public's hope and expectation that methadone would solve the drug problem has faded. Methadone has been useful for some clients, particularly when assisted by the client's motivation and expert clinical support.[25]

Drug-free clinics and inpatient programs have paralleled the rise of methadone clinics. In the early 1970s, adherents of these differing approaches often carried on antagonistic public debates. Drug-free proponents argued that only completely getting away from drugs would result in a curative outcome. To take methadone, according to this way of thinking, was to be still dependent on a drug. The methadone advocates argued that some of those addicted to opiates had created for themselves a lifelong need that required an opiate to feel normal. Yet another position was that methadone was required for a while, perhaps a year or two, for an addict to reestablish a stable life and employment. Once this productivity had been set on a solid foundation, the client could be detoxified from methadone.

Whatever their persuasion, most people have acknowledged that withdrawing from methadone might be as hard or harder than ending a dependence on heroin, but that the advantages of stopping the use of needles and involvement with illicit drugs outweighed the disadvantages. As the years have passed, the two ways of dealing with opiate addiction have learned to live in better harmony, although in the 1980s drug-free treatment more closely matches the public's growing desire for a drug-free society. Abusers of other drugs—marihuana, alcohol, LSD, and so on—have so far no substitutes like methadone for heroin or morphine available, and so drug-free therapy for them is less controversial.

RANKING DANGEROUS DRUGS

Dr. Jaffe and other experts called into government service to handle the rapid rise in drug use faced the intriguing problem of how to list drugs in order of dangerousness. The history of drug laws in the United States shows that the degree to which a drug has been outlawed or curbed has no direct relation to its inherent danger. With the prospect of billions to spend on fighting drug abuse, the federal policymakers tried to reorient anti-drug thinking so that it reflected actual dangerousness. They were burdened by the fact that negative characterizations that had developed during the concluding, intolerant phase of the previous wave of drug use were so extreme. Left over from the 1930s, for example, was an image of marihuana far worse than its acknowledged adverse health effects.

Establishing actual dangerousness sounds reasonable, but the process had its difficulties. If the dangers of drugs were to be ranked according to deaths linked to their use, tobacco and alcohol would head the list. These substances, however, had powerful economic and political interests behind them and moreover were not part of the public's fear over the drug crisis, which had led to the Nixon response. How could these be included in the anti-drug campaign? If not included, how credible would this new scientific approach toward drugs' dangers be?

The first Federal Strategy for Drug Abuse and Drug Traffic Prevention (1973) granted the problems caused by alcohol and tobacco but argued that the federal anti-drug effort was primarily intended to attack illicit drugs and, furthermore, that alcohol and tobacco are deeply ingrained in American "social rituals and customs." Chief responsibility for the two familiar drugs lay with the National

Institute on Alcohol Abuse and Alcoholism and the "overall mission of the Department of Health, Education and Welfare."[26] As the years have passed, tobacco and alcohol increasingly have been perceived by the American people as dangerous drugs.

COMPREHENSIVE DRUG ABUSE AND CONTROL ACT (1970)

An attempt to rank drugs by a common standard of dangerousness was written into legislation in 1970. Specific drugs could be assigned to categories with appropriate restrictions. Britain had tried this way of differentiating among drugs of varying danger through its Pharmacy Act of 1868. The system permitted changes among the categories by an administrative process, should a drug be shown to be more or less dangerous than its first assignment.[27] Generally, laws had been enacted to deal with one dangerous drug at a time: in 1909, smoking opium; in 1914, cocaine and the opiates; in 1924, heroin; in 1937, marihuana. Obviously, the attitude a drug provoked at the time of its restriction could be frozen into the law, and changes were difficult later on, for every change required another law formulated in a political atmosphere.

In 1970 the earlier laws were combined in the Comprehensive Drug Abuse Prevention and Control Act (Public Law 91-513) with the establishment of five schedules for drugs, depending on the potential for abuse and dependency and the accepted medical use of each drug. Schedule One is reserved for drugs that are not permitted to be used in medical practice, such as heroin and LSD. Schedule Two contains the most dangerous prescribable drugs, such as morphine and cocaine; Schedule Three is for those less dangerous, including most barbiturates; Schedule Four, for chloral hydrate and meprobamate; and Schedule Five, for mixtures of low levels of narcotics such as codeine in a cough syrup. Different degrees of control are applied to manufacturers, distributors, and prescribers, depending on the schedule in which a drug has been placed.

This law represents a transition between reliance on law enforcement with severe penalties and a therapeutic approach—even a tolerance for at lease some previously forbidden drug use. It established no minimum sentences. It did provide that someone charged with a first offense for possessing a small amount of marihuana be placed on probation for one year or less with the possibility that the record would be expunged if no further offense occurred during probation. Still, law enforcement was strengthened in an extraordinary manner by allowing "no-knock" searches of premises at any time of day or night.

COMMISSION ON MARIHUANA AND DRUG ABUSE (1972–1973)

Uncertainty in this period of rising drug use, and conflicts between the philosophy of enforcement and that of treatment or toleration, were indicated by the establishment of a Commission on Marihuana and Drug Abuse (NCMDA). The Commission was composed of thirteen persons chosen by the President, Speaker of the House, and president pro tem of the Senate. Its first task was to report in a year on marihuana, descriptions of which were the most upsetting example of older, disgusting images from the 1930s colliding with youthful enthusiasm and praise for the drug in 1970. The Commission was ordered to report in two years on drug abuse in general.

Composed largely of traditionally minded members, the Commission had a powerful effect on the movement to tolerate marihuana use when it concluded in its first report that possession of small amounts of marihuana should be "decriminalized"; that is, possession for personal use could be a finable offense, like a parking ticket, but should no longer subject the possessor to jail. Dealing for profit in large amounts would still be a felony.[28] The public did not always understand decriminalization in the way the Commission intended, but it did realize that it meant relaxation, not more severe penalties. President Nixon also understood the drift of the Commission and refused to receive the report in public from former Pennsylvania Governor Raymond Shafer, the Commission's chairman. The President made it clear that marihuana would not be decriminalized while he was in office.[29]

The final report appeared in March 1973 and reconfirmed its original recommendation about marihuana. In addition, the report called for a single federal agency to combine all drug efforts— enforcement, research, and treatment—for a period of several years. Possession laws should be interpreted as providing an opportunity not to punish but rather to direct users to treatment. The report suggested a moratorium on drug education efforts, including curricula, movies, and posters being spun off in all directions with a wide variety of warnings, philosophies, and other bits of information. Sentiment had been growing among drug experts that these efforts were a waste of federal money.[30] Both the first and the final report stressed the greater problems posed for American society by alcohol and tobacco and urged that action be taken against them as well as the more conventionally perceived "bad" drugs.

THE NATIONAL INSTITUTE ON DRUG ABUSE (1973)

Although no single federal agency has so far combined all anti-drug efforts, in 1973 many programs were consolidated into the DEA and the National Institute on Drug Abuse (NIDA). Most prevention programs funded by the government were gathered under NIDA, which also became the center for drug research.[31] The goal, however, was to decentralize programs into the states, and a first step toward that goal was the establishment of Single State Agencies. These would oversee treatment efforts and guide federal monies into local projects. SAODAP was mandated by law to end in mid-1975, and its central planning role was taken over by groups within the White House such as the Office of Drug Abuse Policy (ODAP) in the Carter administration. Over the course of several administrations, ODAP and similar groups enjoyed varying public visibility and influence with presidents who were also advised by even more obscure bureaucrats in the Office of Management and Budget, where great power is wielded over the funding of government programs.

THE FORD ADMINISTRATION, 1974-1977

The departure of President Nixon in August 1974 brought to the White House a man much more relaxed about recreational drug use. President Ford simply did not share Nixon's intense anger at drug users. Ford's attitude facilitated creation of a federal policy that openly acknowledged that drug abuse was here to stay and that hopes of elimination were illusory. His formal recognition of the limits of even the enormous federal effort during the Nixon years was contained in the *White Paper on Drug Abuse*, prepared by the Domestic Council Drug Abuse Task Force and published in September 1975, a year after Ford assumed the presidency. In a wide-ranging review of the anti-drug effort starting in 1969 (which managed never to mention the name of President Nixon), the White Paper drew conclusions marking official recognition of a painful truth: "Total elimination of drug abuse is unlikely, but governmental actions can contain the problem and limit its adverse effects." The White Paper also made a clear statement on the ranking of anti-drug priorities: "All drugs are not equally dangerous, and all drug use is not equally destructive." When a choice must be made, "priority in both supply and demand reduction should be directed toward those drugs which inherently pose a greater risk—heroin, amphetamines (particularly when used intravenously), and mixed barbiturates."[32]

MARIHUANA AND COCAINE

In the summary of this report, the words "marihuana" and "cocaine" do not appear in any of the seventy-seven specific recommendations covering the entire spectrum of federal drug activities. Both omissions are significant. Only five years earlier, Congress had insisted that the Commission on Marihuana and Drug Abuse give highest priority to a report on marihuana. The result was unfavorable to the Nixon attitude but more congenial to the experts he had assembled and who were freer to express their own opinions after his departure. Americans were increasingly using marihuana, and the belief that smoking it regularly was dangerous was rapidly fading. In 1975 only 43 percent of high school seniors thought so, and that figure continued to fall until it reached its lowest point in 1978 when only 35 percent would hold that cautious view. At the same time the use of marihuana by high school seniors rose steeply. In 1975, 15 percent reported use in the last 30 days; at its peak, in 1978, 24 percent similarly reported.[33] Clearly, a momentum was gaining in 1975 toward the acceptance of marihuana.

Cocaine, in contrast, was just coming into wide use. The final report of the NCMDA (1973) had suggested that the federal government might well end production of licit cocaine after a study to determine whether any need existed that could not be met by some other drug.[34] Then, just as had happened in the mid-1880s, cocaine gathered adherents who deemed it a remarkable drug, a tonic promoting cheerfulness and industry with no negative after-effects—at least not with "moderate consumption," to quote an advocate from 1877.[35]

As in the nineteenth century, initial experiences with cocaine were so positive that some experts wondered whether the severe penalties for its use were not parallel to what they saw as those stemming from the misguided fear of marihuana. A prominent drug expert, Dr. Peter G. Bourne, wrote in August 1974: "Cocaine . . . is probably the most benign of illicit drugs currently in widespread use. At least as strong a case could be made for legalizing it as for legalizing marijuana. Short acting—about 15 minutes—not physically addicting, and acutely pleasurable, cocaine has found increasing favor at all socioeconomic levels in the last year."[36]

During a period of drug intolerance in the 1930s, marihuana was quickly outlawed when it was compared, among other dangerous drugs, to cocaine. In the mid-1970s, at the peak of recent drug tolerance, the effect of comparing the two was to imply that possibly both should be legalized.[37] In each era a consensus developed on the way to handle new drug issues, a response any apparently reasonable person would accept. The problem with cocaine, demonstrated in the 1890s and again in the 1980s, is that the most severe effects do not become obvious and eventually notorious until the drug has been used for an extended period of time by many people. Then praise for a tonic changes to fear of a poison, and society desperately seeks ways to repress the substance.

The Ford administration faced a resurgence of heroin addiction, which was attributed to establishment of Mexican poppy fields and heroin coming now from the South rather than from Turkey.[38] The previous drop in heroin availability had led President Nixon to announce on 11 September 1973 that "we have turned the corner on drug addiction in the United States."[39] That heroin should now re-emerge as a problem was discouraging and convinced policymakers that they were dealing with a much longer time-line than they had hoped was the case. Perhaps drugs would escalate indefinitely; perhaps drugs such as marihuana, cocaine, and even heroin should simply be legalized so as to end the enormous government expenditures of money and time on a problem that only seemed to bring profits to drug dealers and elicit contempt for the law from an ever-growing body of drug users. The presidential election of 1976 would carry this tolerant attitude to its peak.

PRESIDENT CARTER AND DRUG TOLERATION

President Carter's image combined disparate elements. A stranger to Washington politics, he could accomplish great things in government; a fervent Christian, he also appeared to tolerate drug use, particularly marihuana. As Governor of Georgia he had appointed Dr. Bourne as an advisor and to head the state's drug program. In 1972 Bourne took a high post in SAODAP but left two years later to become a major figure in Carter's campaign. Carter's narrow victory in 1976 gave hope to those who wanted a more unequivocally tolerant approach to drugs, much as Nixon's close victory in 1968 buoyed those who wanted an assertion of "law and order." Bourne was promptly named Special Assistant for Health Issues to the President and began to reorganize the drug policy of the federal government. His direct and easy access to the President and his intimate familiarity with drugs and drug policy made him the government's highest ranking and most influential drug authority in the nation's history.

Carter favored decriminalizing the possession of a small amount of marihuana. One ounce was chosen as that small amount. Civil penalties—for example, a small fine—might still be imposed, but criminal sanctions, such as a jail sentence, would be removed. Oregon had decriminalized marihuana in 1973, and studies credible to Bourne and other advocates of decriminalization indicated no dire consequences.[40]

In March 1977, less than two months after Carter's inauguration and forty years after the Marihuana Tax Act Hearings, Bourne and high officials from DEA, the State Department, NIDA, NIMH, the Customs Service, and the Justice Department appeared before the House Select Committee on Narcotics Abuse and Control to argue for the decriminalization of marihuana. Bourne, acknowledging that marihuana could pose some of the same dangers as alcohol does when, for example, a driver is intoxicated by either drug, explained that marihuana "is not physically addicting and in infrequent or moderate use, probably does not pose an immediate substantial health hazard to the individual." He recommended that federal law be amended in this area so that the states would have the option to determine what penalty to apply to the possession of small amounts. He noted that federal law "is now rarely enforced with regard to simple possession." Legalization, Bourne argued, "would only serve to encourage the use of the drug when we seek to deter it," and furthermore, "legalization would violate the 1961 Single Convention of which the United States is a signatory."[41]

Five months later, President Carter followed up this campaign with his own message to Congress on drug abuse. The President repeated a familiar theme: "Penalties against possession of a drug should not be more damaging to an individual than the use of the drug itself; and where they are, they should be changed. Nowhere is this more clear than in the laws against possession of marihuana in private for personal use."[42] He called for decriminalization and asked that this 1972 NCMDA conclusion be implemented.

In February 1978, Bourne addressed the United Nations Commission on Narcotic Drugs regarding United States drug policy. He did not specifically mention decriminalization, a process that some nations either had difficulty understanding or frankly opposed, but he called attention to the fact that priority of attention would be given to those drugs that caused the greatest threat to life. Barbiturates, implicated in nearly 2,000 deaths in the United States in 1977, ranked high on the list. Both heroin and marihuana, he reported, were being investigated objectively for their possible therapeutic value regardless of their historic reputations.[43]

Bourne highlighted to this U.N. commission a success story in the drug war that would paradoxically lead to the end of his government career. The Carter administration was sensitive to charges that it was soft on drugs and looked to improvements in the heroin problem as both a refutation and as a real achievement. After Nixon ended the Turkish supply, heroin slumped in the United States but then rose again during Ford's administration when it started arriving from Mexico. Bourne reported that heroin-related deaths were now at the lowest level since they had begun to be officially reported in 1973. Furthermore, heroin purity at the retail level also had fallen. The decline in heroin-related deaths had begun precipitously over the last year of the Ford administration, from a rate of about 2,000 per year to 800, but the low point did not come until Carter was in office and Bourne was heading the anti-drug effort.[44] Bourne and other Carter drug experts felt that this important claim for success in the war against heroin was the result of Mexico's spraying of opium poppy fields with the herbicide 2-4-D, after Mexico had been urged as well as provided with financial aid by the United States to do so.[45]

Mexico's actual priority was to eradicate marihuana, which it saw as its major domestic drug problem, not opium poppies. Clearly, the Carter administration had worried less about Mexican marihuana entering the United States than about Mexican heroin. Subsequently, though, Mexican marihuana created a big problem for Carter and Bourne because the herbicide used by Mexico for this part of the eradication program was paraquat. As news of this spread, so did the fear that paraquat-laced marihuana was entering the United States and endangering the health of millions of marihuana smokers, a fear that was excitedly fanned by the National Organization for the Reform of Marijuana Laws (NORML) and its sympathizers. Pro-marihuana forces were outraged: here was their favorite administration contaminating marihuana with a deadly poison. They insisted that it had to stop.[46]

Bourne was now in a strange position. If he discouraged Mexico from spraying with paraquat by reducing aid, Mexico would still maintain its priority of spraying marihuana before poppies and the effect on the paraquat problem would be minimal. Furthermore, no one could (or ever has) come up with a single verified instance of a marihuana smoker who had been injured by the paraquat spraying, although the Center for Disease Control had been ordered to look everywhere for potential victims. Still, the furor over paraquat continued unabated. On 12 March 1978, the Secretary of HEW announced in a press release that a "preliminary report" indicated that if an individual smoked "three to five heavily contaminated marijuana cigarettes each day for several months, irreversible lung damage will result." Senator Charles Percy announced in May that he was considering an amendment to the Foreign Assistance Act that would curb eradication programs such as the spraying of paraquat on marihuana plants. All the while, Keith Stroup, founder of NORML in 1971 (and still its Executive Director) kept up a steady drumbeat of fear and anger directed especially against Bourne and the White House drug policy staff over the spraying of marihuana with paraquat.

THE DEPARTURE OF DR. BOURNE

Stroup's opportunity to end Bourne's White House career came suddenly.[47] In July Bourne wrote a prescription for fifteen methaqualone tablets for an aide who complained of nervousness and difficulty in sleeping. He wrote the prescription for a fictitious name in order, he said, to be sure she would have nothing in her record to indicate an emotional problem. Such cover for prominent persons is said not to be uncommon in Washington, but because of a series of surprising coincidences, within days of the attempt to fill the prescription, the issue had become a national scandal. Bourne therefore decided to take a leave of absence in order to deal with the controversy. Then, at the height of the commotion, Stroup conveyed to a *Washington Post* reporter that an allegation was true that Dr. Bourne had snorted cocaine at a party marking NORML's annual meeting the previous December.[48] When this was reported on television the morning of 20 July 1978, Bourne decided he had no choice but to resign from the government. Earlier in the Carter administration, allegations of financial irregularities against Bert Lance, Director of the Office of Management and Budget, had dragged on an embarrassingly long time. Bourne felt that the administration should be spared a repetition.

From the short-term perspective, the focusing of NORML's Executive Director on the paraquat issue had rid the government of the most influential person defending paraquat spraying. Soon Congress adopted the Percy amendment, which required an environmental impact statement for any U.S. funds that might support such activities as herbicide spraying in a foreign country.[49] Meanwhile, the proposal to decriminalize an ounce of marihuana for personal use was still wending its way through Congress.

This state of affairs appeared quite satisfactory for the goals of NORML and of others who favored a more tolerant attitude toward drug use, but eventually a strategic error revealed itself. After Bourne's departure, government agencies, which he had been able to coordinate through his personal style and the authority he enjoyed as a personal friend of the President, returned to their own agendas and business as usual. Furthermore, because of the context of Bourne's departure (the chief drug adviser writing a fictitious prescription and accused of taking cocaine at a party), the Carter White House was in no position to appear soft on the drug issue. No longer did presidential messages urge Congress to decriminalize marihuana. It may not have been apparent at the time, but the tide of toleration, which had been rising since the 1960s, had reached its high-water mark in government and public opinion and was set to recede. In terms of the goals NORML espoused, the departure of Dr. Bourne was a disaster. For all opposed to any use of marihuana and other drugs, particularly those in what would become the parents' movement, 1978 was the dawn of a better day.

THE REVIVAL OF ABSTINENCE: THE PARENTS' MOVEMENT

The year 1978 was a watershed in American attitudes toward drugs and drug use. As after the peaking of the first great wave of drug toleration a lifetime earlier, approval of drug use has declined gradually since 1978, and change in public toleration has been difficult to perceive in any one year. It is most easily seen in attitudes toward marihuana, the drug that led the demand for toleration.

Among high school seniors, the perception that smoking marihuana regularly is harmful hit a low point of 35 percent in 1978, rising steadily to 70 percent in the class of 1985.[50] That near-reversal of attitude indicators within seven years reflects an increased wariness over the effects of marihuana. These figures are reinforced by those for seniors using marihuana within the past month: hitting their peak in 1978 at 37 percent, the figures dropped to 23 percent for the class of 1986.[51] It is important to note that the decline in reported marihuana use has been accompanied by a parallel increase in concern over its effects. Decline in the use of drugs again appears to be associated, as it was in the 1920s and 1930s, not with indifference but with a positive antagonism to drugs, their effects, and (to some degree) those who use them. The extent to which current antagonism, often described as "intolerance" by opponents to drug use, will continue affecting public attitudes and policies will be of great interest. It has not yet reached the settled condemnation that marked national attitudes in the 1930s and 1940s.

Illustrating both the change in attitude itself and the social and political forces that have fought for that change from the earlier tolerance of drug use are the parents' groups, whose origin can be traced back to the years of peak acceptance. The parents' groups also illustrate how drugs are perceived by those who must deal with their effects on young users and their effects on the family. Regardless of studies that could not find anything seriously troublesome about the "moderate" use of marihuana, the parents' groups carried forth into battle an absolute conviction about the danger of drug tolerance based on their own experiences as parents. The targets of their outrage included the sophisticated notion that "some" drug use was all right: they insisted that not only children but all members of society were endangered by drugs, including alcohol.

Parental concern over childrens' drug use was widespread, but the energy and organizational skills needed to gather parents into an effective political force emanated from a much smaller number of persons who give similar accounts of how they were drawn into actively opposing drug tolerance. Their initial experiences have in common a sudden revelation that the drug culture had invaded deeply their world, followed by outrage and stern determination to fight this unexpected, intrusive menace.[52] A Silver Spring, Maryland, housewife named Joyce Nalepka, who later presided over the National Federation of Parents for Drug-Free Youth, attended a rock concert in 1978 with her two young children and discovered rampant drug use all around them. Her anger, shared by others she contacted, apparently was a major factor in the defeat of her Congressman, Newton Steers, who had co-sponsored a bill favoring the decriminalization of an ounce of marihuana. That a broad base of parents were antagonistic to drugs, and that they were now organizing their political power, had been demonstrated.

In Atlanta, Georgia, Marsha Manatt had discovered in 1977 that parties for young teenagers were starting to become drug parties. After organizing parents there, she came into contact with drug-abuse professionals but found them to be often hostile to her concerns and perceptions. She did receive encouragement from some experts, however, particularly Dr. Robert L. DuPont, then Director of NIDA, and her message spread. Under commission from NIDA she wrote a handbook for parents' organizations, *Parents, Peers and Pot,* of which a million copies were distributed after it appeared in 1979.[53] Dr. DuPont had previously been an advocate for decriminalization but changed his mind, and by the time of his departure from government in 1978, he firmly opposed marihuana and its decriminalization. He later stated that "it was parent power that changed my mind on marijuana." Marsha Manatt had pooled her efforts with those of other activist parents to form PRIDE (Parent Resources Institute on Drug Education) in 1978. Two years later they formed a national umbrella for these parents' groups, the National Federation of Parents for Drug-free Youth (NFP).

Another parent, Otto Moulton, was shocked to discover in 1977 that a local newspaper shop in Massachusetts was displaying *High Times* next to the children's magazine *Sesame Street.* He and other parents decided in the late 1970s that they had had enough. In particular, they were unimpressed by the received wisdom of the experts, who assured them that marihuana was not harmful unless

used to excess. As Mr. Moulton told a Senate committee on the
health consequences of marihuana use in January 1980, "For the
past 18 years I have coached youngsters in Little League and youth
hockey. I don't have to be a doctor or scientist to note over the years
the change in these youngsters."[54]

It is instructive to compare these examples of outrage and organizing zeal with another equally energetic outpouring of righteous
indignation in the late 1960s: that of the pro-marihuana campaign,
which culminated in the establishment of NORML in 1970. In the
1960s marihuana users were also outraged—by the lengthy prison
sentences meted out to possessors of small amounts of marihuana,
the dangers of which were grossly misunderstood by the enforcers
of state and federal laws. Keith Stroup led a forceful drive to help
those imprisoned for marihuana use which ranked in anger and
zeal with the parents' movement a decade later. The parents' dis-
dain for the "experts" who told them not to worry about marihuana
was comparable to the pro-marihuana activists' contempt for official
descriptions of the drug, which implied that it inevitably drove
users mad or to violent crime.

One of the goals of drug experts around 1970 was to replace
exaggerated descriptions of marihuana in official literature with
more accurate information. As the *White Paper* of 1975 put it,
"Federal media efforts [should] provide basic information about
drugs . . . rather than using scare tactics."[55] In a parallel effort,
parents groups around 1980 began to monitor federal publications
with the goal of weeding out comments favorable to drug use. As
one high-ranking NIDA official put it, "The NFP has reviewed most,
if not all, of the NIDA publications in order to spot ambiguous
messages that could be interpreted as being anything other than
firmly against drug use. As a result of these efforts, several NIDA
publications have been revised or removed from circulation."[56]

Just as those who favored a more relaxed attitude toward drugs
by and large had encountered a congenial administration with the
election of Carter in 1976, supporters of the parents' movement were
delighted with the election of Ronald Reagan four years later. This
group and others like it were warmly received by the Reagan administration, which was headed by a President who had grown to
maturity during the last era of drug intolerance.

Nancy Reagan began a personal campaign against drugs by
speaking to student groups, visiting drug treatment centers, draw-

ing media to oppose drug use, and otherwise rousing public sentiment against drug use in any form. Her message was simple and dramatic: "Each of us has a responsibility to be intolerant of drug use anywhere, any time, by anybody. . . . We must create an atmosphere of intolerance for drug use in this country."[57] Meanwhile, the Reagan administration's attitude toward drug use was uncompromising. To the important post of Administrator of the Alcohol, Drug Abuse and Mental Health Administration, the President appointed a Florida pediatrician who had been an outspoken member of the parents' movement, Dr. Ian MacDonald. Eventually, MacDonald rose to become the top spokesman on drug issues for the administration.

During the Reagan years, law enforcement received larger appropriations, but until 1986, funds for treatment and research fell in constant dollars. Many factors played a part in this decreased funding, including attempts to shift payments to third-party payers such as health insurance companies and to reduce the budget generally. Although interdiction was the most adequately funded federal effort, the street availability of interdicted drugs such as marihuana, cocaine, and heroin was not reduced. In 1986 a reawakened concern about drugs led to administration announcements that a new approach was to be taken against the drug menace: demand reduction.[58] As is evident from the history of the last twenty years, this is hardly a new approach, but the statement does indicate that the Reagan administration saw itself as having emphasized enforcement—the reduction of availability—rather than treatment and education about the danger of drugs.

For Ronald Reagan and his wife, to be against drugs was as natural a reaction as tolerance would be for some of the young Carter supporters who had battled against draconian laws and scare tactics in the 1960s. Influential elements on each side had a vision of America where every person could achieve his or her maximum potential, but one saw drugs as helping people enhance life, while the other saw ultimate personal achievement only reduced by drug use. Each side translated its vision for the nation into a political movement that profoundly affected elected representatives, laws, and policy regarding drugs.

COCAINE, "CRACK," AND AIDS

As during the last wave of cocaine use in America, from the 1880s to World War I, the perception of cocaine has changed from that of an apparently harmless, perhaps ideal, tonic for one's spirits or to get more work done, to that of a fearful substance whose seductiveness in its early stages of ingestion only heightens the necessity of denouncing it. The calm with which experts until the early 1980s viewed cocaine consumption was one more bit of evidence, to those alarmed by cocaine, that the authority of "experts" should not prevail against the evidence of a citizen's eyes and ears. Examples of tolerant statements in a standard psychiatry textbook published in 1980 have been cited: "Used no more than two or three times a weeks, cocaine creates no serious problems. . . . At present, chronic cocaine use does not usually present as a medical problem."[59]

In 1985 the appearance in several areas of the United States of "crack," a smokable form of cocaine, created a wave of fear that resulted in enormous media and public attention to the drug problem. Crack has several characteristics that make it appealing to users and frightening to observers. It is cheap: a single dose might cost only $10 or $15. It does not require needle injection, thereby avoiding a major route for hepatitis or AIDS infections. It also bypasses the danger of flammable liquids such as ether used to prepare another smokable form of cocaine, "freebase." Finally, smoking crack allows a large amount of cocaine to enter directly into the blood stream from the lungs and then to reach the brain quickly. (Snorting powdered cocaine through the nose limits its impact because cocaine constricts small blood vessels and slows absorption.) Thus, crack combines low cost with high absorption of the drug. Users often find this appeal irresistible and are unable to control their use. Violence and crimes, including murder, have been attributed to crack smoking, and thus an image of cocaine has been created that is close to the image common in the first decade of this century.

In the autumn of 1986, at the height of public furor over cocaine, Congress and the President vied with one another to show their hatred of drugs and to state how much money they were willing to pit against the drug issue. Shortly before the national elections that November, the President signed into law the Anti-Drug Abuse Act of 1986, which authorized nearly $4 billion for an intensified battle against drugs, most of which was destined for law enforcement activities.[60]

The law also promised some additional support for drug abuse research. Funding of research at NIDA has had ups and downs, which has created a field with an uncertain future in spite of advances in the knowledge about addiction over the past two decades.[61] Perhaps the most important discoveries have been that the brain has specialized receptors for opiates, and that the body itself produces opiate-like substances, enkephalins and endorphins, which appear to provide pain relief and pleasure.[62] Related to these findings is the discovery of a new opiate-antagonist, naltrexone, which blocks brain receptor sites and thereby nullifies the effects of opiates such as heroin.[63] A sign of the immense significance of opiate-receptor studies—widely thought to be of the Nobel Prize class—is a heated controversy among several claimants to the discovery of the receptors.[64] Other valuable advances include the finding that the drug clonidine, previously employed as an antihypertensive remedy, can relieve much of the distress of opiate withdrawal.[65] Unraveling the mechanism of cocaine's effect on the brain may also lead to drugs that relieve craving or block the effects of cocaine.

Acquired Immune Deficiency Syndrome (AIDS), a fatal disease that can be transmitted by contaminated needles used to inject drugs into the body, was described in 1981. Since then, the number of persons exposed to the virus and the percentage of those who then have contracted AIDS have rapidly increased. The intimate association of AIDS with drug users who share contaminated needles adds to the general and powerful disapproval of drug users, for they promote the spread of AIDS into the rest of the community. The specter of AIDS in fact has scared some casual as well as habitual needle users into quitting intravenous drug use. Some have switched to smoking crack, and others have entered methadone or drug-free treatment programs.

This growing intolerance now resembles in many ways the intolerance early in this century, which was associated with a reduction in drug use until the 1960s. Perhaps the explosion of fear regarding cocaine will lead the broad anti-drug effort as it apparently did in the first decade of this century. Some other anti-drug movements, though, such as the vigorous one against tobacco, may in the end form the model on which abstinence advocates will once again achieve substantial success.

People opposed to the use of dangerous substances have a new instrument in their arsenal: sensitive drug tests that are relatively cheap and capable of mass usage. Earlier we noted that urine tests were administered to returning Vietnam service personnel. The practical value of urine testing in this instance led observers to speculate that these drug tests would become a part of routine physical examinations—but that was in the 1970s, an era of drug tolerance and assumption of a right to bodily privacy with regard to drugs. In such an atmosphere, the tests did not become common. During the fifteen years since the Vietnam drug surveys, tests have been devised to be more accurate and feasible for even larger numbers. In the mid-1980s, with the dramatic alarm over crack and other forms of cocaine and the accompanying decline in drug tolerance, testing gained acceptance as a good way to discover drug use. The armed services used drug testing beginning in the late 1970s as part of an anti-drug program and have claimed considerable success in reducing the level of drug use.[66]

When President Reagan asked in 1986 that the workplace and schools be made "drug-free" and that government workers in crucial occupations be required to take random urine tests, the issue of drug testing aroused intensive debate across the nation. Several groups, including unions and the American Civil Liberties Union, have attacked drug testing as an unwarranted invasion of privacy for a person exhibiting no difficulty in school or work that would make testing reasonable.[67] Severe criticism has also been leveled at the accuracy of the tests and the ignorance that some who administer them show about the need to confirm results after a positive screening test.[68] Drug tests may be seen as an anti-drug program in themselves, without provision for treatment or counseling and where a positive test means dismissal, not referral to an employee assistance program. Taking the long view, those wielding this new instrument in an era of increasing drug intolerance might seek out drug users with a righteousness and vigor last witnessed in the 1920s and 1930s, without appreciating the likelihood of error and possible damage to lives and livelihoods. The legal limits of drug-testing programs are still vague and their future course unclear, although it appears that the evolution will occur in an environment favorable to drug testing as a method to root out drug users.

An additional factor that might ease the way for drug testing is the fear of AIDS, which could lead to general blood testing for antibodies to the AIDS virus. AIDS is so frightening that it makes extreme control measures seem reasonable. Under the umbrella of measures taken to combat this menace, testing for drugs might fit in easily.

Reflecting on the earlier wave of drug intolerance, one cannot help but be concerned that the fear of drugs will again translate into a simple fear of the drug user and will be accompanied by draconian sentences and specious links between certain drugs and distrusted groups within society, as was the case with cocaine and Southern blacks in the first decade of this century. Is there some sort of inherent symmetry between excessive praise of drugs in the phase of rising tolerance, and zealous and at times prejudiced denunciation of users in the decline phase? That aside, knowing about our earlier wave of drug use at the turn of the century offers us some assurance that the problem can recede; and perhaps this knowledge will allow a decline in consumption to proceed with a minimum of distortion. We are, however, an impatient people.

Notes

Chapter 1

1   Research and clinical papers on narcotics were many in the 19th century, but few current articles attempt to trace the evolution of medical opinion on these drugs. I am greatly indebted to Glenn Sonnedecker's "Emergence of the Concept of Opiate Addiction," *J. Mondial Pharmacie*, Sept.–Dec. 1962, pp. 275–90; Jan.–Mar. 1963, pp. 27–34. Another article of relevance is D. I. Macht, "The History of Opium and Some of Its Preparations and Alkaloids," *JAMA 64* : 477–81 (1915). Macht describes some of the history and composition, usually including opium, of the immemorial antidotes diascordium, mitradatium, theriaca, and philonium. *The Opium Problem,* by Charles E. Terry and Mildred Pellens (New York: Bureau of Social Hygiene, 1928; reprint ed., Montclair, N.J.: Patterson Smith, 1970), is a very useful anthology of articles published up to the mid-1920s.

2   Norman Howard-Jones, "A Critical Study of the Origins and Early Development of Hypodermic Medication," *J. Hist. Med. 2* : 201–49 (1947). Growth of addiction in the U.S. is commonly attributed to morphine injections or other opiates to lessen the pain of Civil War battle wounds; direct attribution is more common in the 20th century and after World War I. Earlier studies equally emphasized the emotional stress engendered by conflict. The lack of statistics on the number of Civil War veterans who became addicts in the service suggests that the war was a convenient event to blame for late 19th-century addiction. According to a recent study, morphine was usually dusted or rubbed into wounds and only sometimes injected (Stewart Brooks, *Civil War Medicine* [Springfield, Ill.: Thomas, 1966], pp. 65, 88). An extensive report on rising opium consumption in the U.S. published only seven years after the war makes no mention of the recent conflict as the cause of addiction, but rather places its beginnings in the rising teetotalism of the 1840s and 1850s (F. E. Oliver, "The Use and Abuse of Opium," Third Report of the Massachusetts Board of Health, 1872, pp. 162–77). So far no thorough study of morphine use in the Civil War has been located.

3   Excessive opiate use in the 19th century was not considered "un-American" but "peculiarly American" (Harvey Washington Wiley, "An Opium Bonfire," *Good Housekeeping*, August 1912, p. 252). An anonymous writer in 1861 bemoaned, "in no country in the world is quackery carried on to so enormous extent as it is in the United States" ("Quackery and the Quacked," *Nat. Quart. Rev. 2* : 354 [1861]). George Beard, a leading neurologist and psychiatrist of the latter half of the century, associated narcotic use with the frailty of advanced civilization and predicted a great increase in the 20th century (*American Nervousness: Its Causes and Consequences* [New York: Putnam, 1881], p. 64). This interpretation was common until World War I when "perfidious foreign nations" were usually held responsible for American drug taking.

4   Some opium was grown in the U.S. during the 19th century and perhaps

later (Terry and Pellens, *The Opium Problem,* p. 7). During the blockade the Confederacy attempted to grow opium to replenish its supplies
but found smuggling to be more certain (Norman H. Frank, *Pharmaceutical Conditions and Drug Supply in the Confederacy* [Madison, Wis.:
Institute of the History of Pharmacy, 1955]; *Memoranda on the Manufacture of and Traffic in Morphine in the U.S. . . . in Continuation of
Senate Doc.* 377, 61st Cong., 2nd Sess., 31 Oct. 1911, prepared for the
Secretary of State by Hamilton Wright; for cocaine exports see p. 12;
for morphine, p. 14).

5   Statistics on opium and morphine importation until the Harrison Act
(in effect after 1 March 1915) are among the best available for estimating the use of narcotics in the United States. The drugs were im-
portable without restriction and at modest or even at times, free duty.
Imports do not reveal what segment of the population might have been
addicted or how many, but they do reveal a remarkable increase in the
domestic demand for narcotics which began to rise at least in the 1840s
and continued until the 1890s, when average domestic consumption of
crude opium leveled off to about a half-million pounds each year, and
that of morphine and its salts to about 20,000 ounces annually. A convenient source of these figures for 1850–1926 is Terry and Pellen's *The
Opium Problem* (pp. 50–51) where the important distinction is made between total imports and that portion of imports "entered for consumption." Hamilton Wright provided statistics which extend the record back
to 1840 (ibid., "Report," Appendix IV, pp. 81–83).

6   M. I. Wilbert, "Sale and Use of Cocaine and Narcotics," *Publ. Health
Rep.* 29 : 3180–83 (1914); *Registration of Producers and Importers of
Opium, etc.,* Committee on Ways and Means, H. Rept. no. 23, 63rd
Cong., 2nd Sess., 24 June 1913, p. 3.

7   L. F. Kebler, *Habit Forming Agents: Their Indiscriminate Sale and Use,
a Menace to the Public Welfare,* Agriculture Dept., Farmer's Bulletin
no. 393 (April 1910), pp. 8–12, 15–18. William Hammond, "Dr. Hammond's Remarks on Coca," *Trans. Med. Soc. Virginia,* 1887, pp. 213–26,
esp. p. 226 for hay fever. Oscar E. Anderson, *The Health of a Nation:
Harvey W. Wiley and the Fight for Pure Food* (Chicago: Univ. of Chicago Press, 1958), p. 315.

8   To protect their formulas they did not patent their products; only the
names were legally protected by trademarks. But by 1905 the Proprietary
Association of America had endorsed a law to exempt small amounts of
narcotics, similar to Section 6 of the future Harrison Act. The PAA was
fighting for its life against disclosure laws affecting all proprietaries and
was burdened by the bad name some products were giving the industry.
Manufacturers whose medicines continued to contain excessive narcotics
(e.g. Dr. Tucker's Asthma Specific, which contained cocaine) were not
permitted to join the PAA. See J. H. Young, *The Toadstool Millionaires*
(Princeton Univ. Press, 1961), pp. 237 ff., and idem, *The Medical
Messiahs* (Princeton Univ. Press, 1967), p. 34; typed transcript of proceedings of 31st Annual Meeting of the PAA, 20–22 May 1913, Wash-

ington, D.C., pp. 14–15; editorial, *Amer. Druggist Pharmaceut. Rec.* 57 : 126 (1910). The model law prepared in 1905 by representatives of the PAA, NARD, NWDA, and the APhA is found in "Sale of Narcotics and Proprietary Medicines Containing Alcohol," *Am. J. Pharm.* 78 : 145–48 (1906).

9 See above (ch. 1, n. 5.), for source of statistics. Wright's "Report" describes manipulation of duty in an attempt to reduce the importation of smoking opium in the late 19th century (Hamilton Wright, "Report on the International Opium Commission and on the Opium Problem as Seen within the United States and Its Possessions," contained in *Opium Problem: Message from the President of the United States,* Sen. Doc. no. 377, 61st Cong., 2nd Sess., 21 Feb. 1910).

10 See, e.g., *General Laws of Texas, 1905,* ch. 35, sect. 2.

11 "Address before the Massachusetts Medical Society, 30 May 1860," in *The Works of Oliver Wendell Holmes* (Boston: Houghton Mifflin, 1892), 9 : 200–01.

12 See F. X. Dercum, "Relative Infrequency of the Drug Habit among the Middle and Upper Classes," *Penn. Med. J.* 20 : 362–64, n. 22 (1917). Some physicians did begin to sense the danger: in 1900 Dr. John Witherspoon, who was to become AMA president in 1913, delivered his "Oration on Medicine, A Protest against Some of the Evils in the Profession of Medicine" (*JAMA* 34 : 1591 [1900]):

> Ah Brothers! we, the representatives of the grandest and noblest profession in the world . . . must . . . warn and save our people from the clutches of this hydra-headed monster which stalks abroad throughout the civilized world, wrecking lives and happy homes, filling our jails and lunatic asylums, and taking from these unfortunates, the precious promises of eternal life. . . .
>
> The morphine habit is growing at an alarming rate, and we can not shift the responsibility, but must acknowledge that we are culpable in too often giving this seductive siren until the will-power is gone.

See also T. D. Crothers, "New Phase of Criminal Morphinomania," *J. Inebriety* 21 : 41–51 (1899).

13 The number of narcotic addicts in the U.S. is a very difficult figure to arrive at. One problem is in the definition of an addict, for there are at least two major categories among those who use narcotics in a regular fashion, the hard-core addict who requires daily opiates to hold off abstinence symptoms, and occasional users who can stop without any significant symptoms. There is another category of "addict," composed of individuals who are not taking enough opiates to create the possibility of an abstinence syndrome but who believe they are. These individuals are dependent on addict life style or even simple needle injections, although physiologically they could not be classified as addicts.

Given these qualifications, most authors who have closely studied the question of the addict-population in the past (Wilbert, Terry, Pellens, Kolb, DuMez, Lindesmith) tend to agree that there was a peak in addic-

tion around 1900 and that in the teens of this century this number began
to decrease and reached a relatively small number (about 100,000) in
the 1920s. The peak might be 200,000 to 400,000 in 1900. A peak of
drug use in 1919 reported by New York City and Federal officials which
estimated the total in the U.S. at about one million seems highly unlikely. It seems reasonable to maintain that the decline in opiate use
after 1900 probably continued. What actually increased was the fear
directed at addiction by officials and the public. By 1930 only the most
irresponsible spokesmen argued that addiction had not reached a low
figure and was represented chiefly in the largest urban centers. In general,
exaggerated figures of the number of narcotics addicts have reflected
public concern rather than actual numbers. Nevertheless, the number in
the U.S. seems to have exceeded in the 20th century the per capita rate
in other Western nations and without question was so perceived by the
federal government until the 1920s, when the admission became an
embarrassment.

14 E. C. Sandmeyer, *The Anti-Chinese Movement in California* (Urbana:
    Univ. of Illinois Press, 1939). Sandmeyer points out the similarity of
    complaints made against the Irish, who had preceded the Chinese as the
    lowest-paid workers in California (pp. 38–39). Anti-Chinese feeling was
    not confined to the West Coast; see e.g. John W. Foster, "The Chinese
    Boycott" (*Atlantic Monthly,* January 1906, pp. 118–27), for extralegal
    methods directed at Chinese, particularly in Boston; and Jacob Riis,
    How the Other Half Lives (New York: C. Scribner's Sons, 1890) for
    his prejudicial remarks about New York's Chinatown.

15 The association of cocaine with the southern Negro became a cliché a
    decade or more before the Harrison Act. See W. Scheppegrell, "The
    Abuse and Dangers of Cocaine," *Med. News* 73 : 417–22 (1898), esp.
    p. 421. In June 1900 the *JAMA* (34 : 1637) editorially reported that
    "the Negroes in some parts of the South are reported as being addicted
    to a new form of vice—that of 'cocaine sniffing' or the 'coke habit.' In
    February 1901 the *JAMA* (36 : 330) called attention again to this new
    vice. See also in the New York *Tribune,* 21 June 1903, an extended
    statement by Col. J. W. Watson of Georgia on how cocaine sniffing
    "threatens to depopulate the Southern States of their colored population."
    Atlanta seemed particularly affected, and legal action was urged against
    the sale "of a soda fountain drink manufactured in Atlanta and known
    as Coca-Cola." The Colonel was satisfied that "many of the horrible
    crimes committed in the Southern States by the colored people can be
    traced directly to the cocaine habit," and that the habit was also present
    among young whites. Examination of the Atlanta *Constitution* (27 Dec.
    1914) also reveals a frequently claimed association between cocaine use
    and the Negro; by 1914 the Atlanta police chief was blaming "70% of
    the crimes" on drug use. There is no indication in the *Constitution* of
    effective enforcement of drug laws; rather, narcotics appear to explain
    conveniently crime waves and other problems. In the District of Colum-
    bia the police chief considered cocaine the greatest menace of any drug.
    There it was peddled from door to door (*Report of the President's*

Homes Commission, S. Doc. no. 644, 60th Cong., 2nd Sess., 8 Jan. 1909 (GPO, 1909), pp. 254–55.

Philadelphia had a cocaine scare in 1910 which resulted in the arrest of several pharmacists, physicians, and policemen for sales to citizens, including school children. The leader of a drive against cocaine, Dr. Christopher Koch, of the State Pharmacy Board, testified before Congress on behalf of federal antinarcotic laws and drew attention to the dangers of the cocaine-crazed southern Negro. In 1914 Dr. Koch was quoted as asserting, "Most of the attacks upon white women of the South are the direct result of a cocaine-crazed Negro brain" (*Literary Digest*, 28 March 1914, p. 687). Dr. E. H. Williams portrayed in the N.Y. *Times* (8 Feb. 1914) a lurid and fearful picture of "the Negro cocaine fiends" who terrorized the South. Dr. Williams published a similar study, but with more statistics, in the *Medical Record* (85 : 247–49 [1914], "The Drug Habit Menace in the South"). There Dr. Williams attempted to answer a study from the Georgia State Asylum (see ch. 1, n. 20 below) which reported almost no Negro cocaine takers admitted in the years 1909–14. In his *Opiate Addiction: Its Handling and Treatment* (New York: Macmillan, 1922), Dr. Williams attributed popular agitation for antinarcotic laws to spectacular crimes, especially in the South. Also in 1914 Dr. Harvey Wiley referred to "old colored men" hiding cocaine under their pushcart wares and spreading the drugs throughout America's cities (H. W. Wiley and A. L. Pierce, "The Cocaine Crime," *Good Housekeeping*, March 1914, pp. 393–98). Thus the problem of cocaine proceeded from an association with Negroes in about 1900, when a massive repression and disenfranchisement were under way in the South, to a convenient explanation for crime waves, and eventually Northerners used it as an argument against Southern fear of infringement of states' rights. For example, Wright wrote the editor of the Louisville *Courier-Journal* that "a strong editorial from you on the abuse of cocaine in the South would do a great deal of good [but] do not quote me or the Department of State" (16 April 1910, WP, entry 36). In each instance there were ulterior motives to magnify the problem of cocaine among Negroes, and it was to almost no one's personal interest to minimize or portray it objectively. As a result, by 1910 it was not difficult to get legislation almost totally prohibiting the drug.

16 Perhaps it is impossible to describe accurately the distribution of morphine addiction or nonmedical use in the 19th century among the various social groups. It is reasonable, however, to assume that morphine's introduction as a replacement for opium meant a wide distribution among the middle class, which enjoyed professional medical care. But as fear of morphine grew, and the need for symptomatic relief declined, the middle class may have used morphine less often. (See F. X. Dercum, "Relative Infrequency of Drug Habit . . . ," *Penna. Med. J.* 20 : 362–64 [1917].)

17 G. Archie Stockwell, "Erythoxylon Coca," *Boston Med. Surg. J.* 96 : 402 (1877).

18 Freud's first and most comprehensive study, "Über Coca," was abstracted

in the *St. Louis Med. Surg. J. 47* : 502–05 (1884), the year of its publication in Vienna. Freud believed cocaine could cure morphinism and alcoholism through a ten-day course of hypodermic injections without recourse to an institution. The second paper, "Beitrag zur Kenntniss der Cocawirkung" (1885), continued the optimistic tone which was much muted in his last paper, "Bemerkungen über Cocaïnsucht und Cocaïnfurcht" (1887), a response to an attack on cocaine therapy by Erlenmeyer. The three papers are translated in S. A. Edminster et al., trans., *The Cocaine Papers* (Vienna: Dunquin Press, 1963). Two substantial and illuminating studies of Freud's interest in cocaine are Siegfried Bernfeld, "Freud's Studies on Cocaine, 1884–1887, *Yearbook of Psychoanalysis 10* : 9–38 (1954–55); and Hortense Koller Becker, "Carl Koller and Cocaine," *Psychoan. Quart. 32* : 309–73 (1963). Karl Koller, Freud's colleague, received from Freud the whimsical nickname Coca Koller.

19   N.Y. *Times,* 8 Feb. 1914; *Med. Record 85* : 247–49 (1914).

20   E. M. Green, "Psychoses Among Negroes: A Comparative Study," *J. Nerv. Ment. Dis. 41* : 697–708 (1914). Dr. E. H. Williams's reply that the cocainized Negroes were in jails and not insane asylums is found in the *Medical Record* (*85* : 247–49 [1914]), and also in *Everybody's Magazine* (August 1914, pp. 276–77). Williams in these writings does not seem so much anti-Negro as anti-Prohibition and uses the stories of cocainized Negroes to show what might happen if alcohol were not available.

21   Hamilton Wright, "Report International Opium," *Opium Problem: Message,* p. 49.

22   M. I. Wilbert, "Sale and Use of Cocaine," *Publ. Health Rep. 29,* 3180–83 (1914).

23   247 U.S. 251 (1918). For discussions of the complicated byways of the federal police powers involved in such attempts at federal regulation see B. F. Wright, *The Growth of American Constitutional Law* (New York: Holt, Rinehart and Winston, 1942).

24   According to a memorandum by Dr. Reid Hunt of the Public Health Service, Wiley and the drug trades—the retail interests especially (represented by the National Association of Retail Druggists)—cooperated to perfect an antinarcotic law based on the interstate commerce powers of the Constitution after it became apparent that pure food advocates feared any tampering with the Pure Food and Drug Act through amendment (*PHSR,* 2 Nov. 1908).

25   See statement of C. M. Hester, Assistant General Counsel of the Treasury Department, in *Taxation of Marihuana, Hearings before the Committee on Ways and Means of the House of Representatives on HR 6385,* 27–30 April and 4 May 1937, 75th Cong., 1st Sess. (GPO, 1937), pp. 7–13. Fear of a new attack on the Harrison Act's constitutionality led the treasury to model the Marihuana Tax Act after the National Firearms Act in which tax was levied on the transfer of certain firearms.

26   For recent comment on the interstate commerce powers and the resting of national restrictive drug laws on these powers, see M. P. Rosenthal, "Proposals for Dangerous Drug Legislation," in Appendix B of *Narcotics*

and Drug Abuse, Presidential Commission on Law Enforcement and the Administration of Justice (GPO, 1967), pp. 80–134, esp. p. 129 and n. 484.

27   Reprinted in book form by the AMA particularly for the reception rooms of physicians. Similar exposés of proprietary medicines made by the AMA appeared in three volumes, *Nostrums and Quackery,* in 1911, 1921, and 1936, the last entitled *Nostrums and Quackery and Pseudo Medicine.* Adams attacked such well-known proprietaries as Pe-ru-na which contained more than 25% alcohol, and Hostetter's Stomach Bitters which contained more than 40%; and those containing unlabeled narcotics, acetanalid, and other dangerous substances. He also attacked miracle workers who used such devices as magnetic belts to cure disease. He said they took in a quarter-billion dollars in annual sales, owing to their mass advertising, which he therefore sought to eliminate or regulate.

28   C. H. Brent to James F. Smith, Commissioner of Education, Manila, 6 July 1903 (BP, container 6).

29   Beal's model law and the New York State Whitney Acts (1917 and 1918) avoided prohibition but attempted to prevent new addicts and did permit maintenance of confirmed habitúes.

30   The standard biography of Wiley is Anderson's *The Health of a Nation.*

31   Ibid., pp. 210, 243 ff. Dr. Presley M. Rixey (1852–1928), Surgeon General of the Navy, was the President's official physician. Wiley resigned his post in 1912 after bitter and continual disputes with his superiors in the Department of Agriculture.

32   The history of the pharmaceutical profession and drug trades in America is outlined in *Kremer's and Urdang's History of Pharmacy,* 3rd edition, revised by Glenn Sonnedecker (Philadelphia: Lippincott, 1963), pp. 133–296. For the history of medicine in America see R. Shryock, *The Development of Modern Medicine* (Philadelphia: Univ. of Pa. Press, 1947); M. Fishbein, *A History of the American Medical Association, 1847–1947* (Philadelphia: Saunders, 1947); R. Stevens, *American Medicine and the Public Interest* (New Haven: Yale University Press, 1971). J. M. Burrow, *AMA: Voice of American Medicine* (Baltimore: Johns Hopkins Press, 1963), describes the weakness of the AMA before World War I (see pp. 27 ff. and his ch. 3, pp. 5 ff.).

33   The Flexner Report recommended closure of substandard medical schools in the United States and pointed to Johns Hopkins as the model for a modern medical school. (A. Flexner, *Medical Education in the United States and Canada,* Carnegie Foundation for the Advancement of Teaching, Bull. no. 4, New York, 1910.)

34   On the founding of the APhA see Glenn Sonnedecker, *History of Pharmacy,* 3rd ed. (Philadelphia: J. B. Lippincott Co., 1963), pp. 181 ff. Some of the important national drug trade organizations and their dates of founding are: Proprietary Association of America (PAA), 1881, composed of manufacturers of "patent medicines," and over-the-counter proprietaries; National Wholesale Druggists Association (NWDA), 1876, and National Association of Retail Druggists (NARD), 1898, for owners of pharmacies; American Pharmaceutical Manufacturers Association,

1908. The National Association of Manufacturers of Medicinal Products (1912), makers of prescription drugs, merged in 1958 with the PMA. See Sonnedecker, *History of Pharmacy,* pp. 188 ff.

35 The APhA's 1856 constitution listed one of the association's goals: "To as much as possible restrict the dispensing and sale of medicines to regularly educated druggists and apothecaries" (Sonnedecker, *History of Pharmacy,* p. 185). Although hampered in its attack on proprietaries, because they were profitable for retail druggists, the association was condemning proprietaries at the turn of the century and cooperating with the AMA's Council on Pharmacy and Chemistry, founded in 1905, to expose proprietary frauds and dangers.

36 J. H. Beal, "Report on Pharmacy Legislation," *Proc. APhA* 49 : 460–64 (1901), esp. pp. 460–61.

37 "Minutes of the Section on Education and Legislation," ibid., pp. 464–66. At about this time a bill was introduced into the Senate prohibiting opium imports except for medicinal purposes (*Chemist and Druggist* 60 : 224 [1900]).

38 E. G. Eberle, "Chairman's Address, Minutes of the Section on Education and Legislation," *Proc. APhA* 50 : 550–61 (1902), esp. p. 559.

39 "Report of Committee on Acquirement of the Drug Habit," *Proc. APhA* 50 : 567–73 (1902), esp. p. 569. Although the committee may have chosen the previous five-year statistics without propagandizing intent, the year of comparison, 1898, had had the lowest import of crude opium since 1865. The reason for the small importation was the imposition of the higher Dingley tariff that year and the importation of the largest amount ever recorded in 1897 in anticipation of the rise. Therefore the report that opium importations had risen 600% in five years was grossly misleading. Actually if 1898 and 1897 figures are averaged, the importation of opium had reached a plateau. George Beard had noted the increase in annual importations of opium as early as 1880 (*American Nervousness,* p. 308; see n. 3 above).

40 "Committee on Acquirement of the Drug Habit," *Proc. APhA* 50 : 570 (1902). In 1924 Lawrence Kolb, Sr., and A. G. DuMez estimated a maximum of 240,000 addicts of cocaine and opiates in the United States, in "The Prevalence and Trend of Drug Addiction in the United States and Factors Influencing It," *Pub. Health Rep.* 39 : 1179–1204 (May 1924).

41 *Proc. APhA* 50 : 570, 572–73 (1902).

42 J. H. Beal, "An Anti-Narcotic Law," *Proc. APhA* 51 : 478–82, 485–86 (1903).

43 "Draft of an Anti-Narcotic Law," *Proc. APhA* 51 : 486 (1903). This model law was substantially adopted by a conference in 1905 of the NARD, NWDA, PAA, and APhA and became the basis of the District of Columbia Pharmacy Act's provisions with regard to narcotics in 1906; it persisted as the exemption section of the Harrison Act. One of the purposes of the model act was to permit proprietaries to include some narcotics, but not the extremes that had aroused public furor.

44 "Report of Committee on the Acquirement of Drug Habits," *Proc. APhA* 51 : 466–77 (1903).

45 For the discovery and spread of heroin see "History of Heroin," *Bull. Narcotics* 5 : 3–16 (April–June 1953); W. Z. Guggenheim, "Heroin: History and Pharmacology," *Internat. J. Addiction* 2 : 328–30 (Fall 1967).

46 *Proc. APhA* 51 : 475 (1903). The army's Surgeon General reported that admissions to hospitals for "narcotic poisoning" were first noted in 1900 as 60; in 1901, 108; in 1902, 63; and in 1903, 194. In 1904 the annual report drops narcotic classification. The army declined between 1900 and 1904 from 100,000 to 60,000. Discharges for narcotic poisoning from 1900 to 1903 were, for each fiscal year, 7, 7, 10, and 22, respectively. These data are from *Report of the Surgeon-General of the Army to the Secretary of War,* fiscal years ending 30 June, War Department (GPO, 1898–1904).

47 *Proc. APhA* 51 : 477 (1903).

48 See ch. 1, n. 8 above.

49 District of Columbia Pharmacy Act, approved 7 May 1906, *Public Law No. 148.*

50 Ibid., sections 11, 12.

51 Philippine Tariff Revision Act, 3 March 1905, 33 *Stat. L.* 944; Sect. 11, Class III(b).

52 Hamilton Wright, "Report International Opium," *Opium Problem: Message,* p. 19. HWW to C. H. Brent, 22 Aug. 1908: "Almost unanimous opinion that there has been a decrease from 25% to 50% in the sales of patent medicines containing opiates since the Pure Food Law went into effect." Similarly, J. P. Street, "The Patent Medicine Situation," *Amer. J. Publ. Health* 7 : 1037–42 (1917).

53 HWW to Robert Bacon, 2 Jan. 1908, BCR. In this letter Wiley remonstrates that it would be unwise to put medical practitioners under the Bureau of Internal Revenue, the alternative to an interstate law based on the commerce powers, because of inconvenience and the uncertainty, if not impossibility, of constitutional regulation of the practice of medicine.

54 The need to put the American house in order by enactment of some federal statute regulating the importation of opium, especially smoking opium, was raised as early as 13 August 1907 by William Phillips, the Second Secretary of the Peking Legation in a memorandum to the State Department, "The Importation of Opium into the United States." A copy of Phillips's memorandum was sent to Wiley by Bacon as evidence for the need of some law (RB to HWW, 20 Dec. 1907, BCR).

55 RB to HWW, 4 Nov. 1908, BCR.

56 RB to HWW, 2 Oct. 1908, BCR.

Chapter 2

1 See C. Hoffman, "The Depression of the Nineties," *J. Economic Hist.* 16 : 137–64 (June 1956). The effects of the Depression, its frustrations,

both economic and psychological, supported the aggressions of the Spanish-American War.

2   The China market's attractions, which proved to be almost completely illusory, have been described recently in T. McCormick's *China Market* (Chicago: Quandrangle, 1967). Beyond the larger goal of increasing American trade, some attention was directed specifically at opium, a Chinese import by 1900 almost solely in the hands of Great Britain. Samuel Merwin in a series of articles in *Success* magazine (Oct. 1907–April 1908), later published as *Drugging a Nation: The Story of China and the Opium Curse* (New York: Revell, 1908), claimed that immense amounts of human energy and material resources in China were absorbed by the opium habit. R. P. Chiles in predicting "The Passing of the Opium Habit" (*The Forum,* July 1911, pp. 36–37) noted that opium took up 7.5% of Chinese imports. Arnold H. Taylor attributes a major role to missionaries for creating and sustaining the anti-opium movement at the turn of the century: "American missionaries in the Far East . . . played the greatest part in inducing the United States to take the lead in the movement against the traffic (*American Diplomacy and the Narcotics Traffic, 1900–1939,* Durham, N.C.: Duke Univ. Press, 1969, pp. 29–30).

3   G. E. Mowry, *The Era of Theodore Roosevelt and the Birth of Modern America, 1900–1912* (New York: Harper and Row, 1958), pp. 182, 186.

4   H. U. Faulkner, *Politics, Reform, and Expansion, 1890–1900* (New York: Harper and Row, 1959), p. 239.

5   F. P. Dunne, *Mr. Dooley in Peace and War* (Boston: Small, Maynard, 1898), p. 43.

6   Mowry, *Era,* pp. 125, 167–69.

7   The standard biography is A. C. Zabriskie's *Bishop Brent: Crusader for Christian Unity* (Philadelphia: Westminister, 1948).

8   CHB to Bishops Potter, Doane, Satterlee, and Leonard, 28 Oct. 1901 (BP, container 5). Bishop Brent saw himself in the tropics as a martyr, isolated from civilization, representing what was best in America in its most crucial sphere of activity. He insisted that the new diocese be properly outfitted, not for the bishop's vanity nor just for the Church's image, but for the good of the nation which he, in so many ways, represented. A cathedral, a substantial one, was needed because "hitherto the Filipino has estimated the value of the State through the Church." A committee of six laymen stepped forward to raise money for the Philippine Endowment Fund. J. Pierpont Morgan, whose banking services would receive the donations, headed the group which included the leading fund raiser of the Republican National Committee, Senator Marcus A. Hanna of Ohio. Morgan's committee informed potential donors that "American Christianity should be in a position to carry on such work among the natives as will convince them of the benevolent intention of the people of the United States." Other committee members were G. McC. Miller, J. I. Houghteling, W. H. Crocker, and S. Mather. The pamphlet distributed by the committee is dated March 1903 (BP, container 6).

9   The history of opium in the Philippines can be found in the *Report of the Committee Appointed by the Philippine Commission to Investigate the Use of Opium and the Traffic Therein* . . . , Bureau of Insular Affairs, War Dept., 1905, pp. 129–72 (hereafter cited as *Philippine Opium Investigation*); also see Arnold H. Taylor, *Narcotics Traffic*, pp. 31–45; P. D. Lowes, *The Genesis of International Narcotics Control* (Geneva: Librairie Droz, 1966), pp. 102–06.

10 L. P. Beth, *Development of the American Constitution, 1877–1917* (New York: Harper and Row, 1971), pp. 161–62.

11 A. H. Taylor, *Narcotics Traffic*, pp. 3–40.

12 Rev. W. F. Crafts, Superintendent of the International Reform Bureau, *Memorandum Concerning Concerted International Restraint of the Traffic in Intoxicants and Opium among Aboriginal Races*, a pamphlet dated 22 Feb. 1907 (BP, container 9), p. 2.

13 One letter of refusal is CHB to Juan Preysler, Manager, Manila Jockey Club, 1 July 1903; the letter of justification and self-assurance is CHB to Bishop Hall, 20 July 1903 (BP, container 9).

14 Elihu Root to WHT, 14 June 1903, (Library of Congress: Elihu Root Papers).

15 Act of the Philippine Commission no. 800, 23 July 1903; amended by Act 812, 31 July 1903. Letter commissioning Bishop Brent, A. W. Fergusson, Executive Secretary, Government of the Philippine Islands, to CHB, 31 July 1903 (BP, container 6).

16 CHB to WHT, 6 Feb. 1904 (BP, container 6).

17 *Philippine Opium Investigation*, pp. 45–49.

18 Philippine Tariff Revision Act, 3 March 1905, 33 *Stat. L.* 944.

19 *Philippine Opium Investigation*, p. 47.

20 The commission asked Congress to reconsider its imposition of absolute prohibition after 1 March 1908. The commission believed that simply restricting opium use to Chinese would, because of the Exclusion Act, end the abuse of opium gradually and easily as the smokers aged, returned to China, or reformed; but Congress did not modify its uncompromising stand (*Philippine Commission Seventh Annual Report, 1906*, Bureau of Insular Affairs, War Dept. [GPO, 1907], part 1, p. 62). To carry out Congressional intentions, the commission enacted a system of licenses for habitual users and dealers (Act 1461 of the Philippine Commission, 8 March 1906). About 12,700 habitual users were given licenses. To the surprise of the commission, a year's search for users who wished to be cured of their habit located only ten applicants (*Philippine Commission Eighth Annual Report, 1907*, Bureau of Insular Affairs, War Dept. [GPO, 1907], part 2, p. 18). In 1907, for gradual reduction in opium use the commission provided for licensed opium dispensaries, and a 15% reduction of the original maintenance amount each month beginning with November 1907; on 1 March 1908, dispensing would end (Act 1761 of the Philippine Commission, 12 Oct. 1907). Both Acts specifically prohibited physicians from dispensing any form of opium to habitual users unless for a physical condition requiring it. Thus were established the earliest federal narcotic clinics, and based on the same principle of anti-

maintenance as the New York City clinic of 1919. After Act 1761 the number of users volunteering or sent to hospitals for treatment increased but does not seem to have exceeded a thousand. The cure rate of opium smokers was reported as very high—"the admission of any patient a second time has been extremely unusual"—establishing, at least in print, the success of total narcotic prohibition (*Philippine Commission Tenth Annual Report, 1909*, Bureau of Insular Affairs, War Dept. [GPO, 1909], p. 102).

Bishop Brent proudly reported on the success of opium prohibition to the Shanghai Commission, in *Report on Opium, Its Derivatives and Preparations for Presentation to the International Opium Commission Assembled at Shanghai, China, February, 1909* (Shanghai: Methodist Publishing House, n.d.), pp. 51–55, (BP, container 37). See also Taylor, *Narcotics Traffic*, pp. 43–45.

21 Early in opium prohibition the revenue services complained of having only one outdated revenue cutter, few customs agents, and of encountering bribery and public disinterest. In the United States the experiment was viewed more enthusiastically. Rep. James Mann, chairman of the Interstate and Foreign Commerce Committee of the House, announced enforcement in the Islands a success. But as time passed the ineffectiveness of prohibition was more realistically faced. In 1926, H. L. May, the American on the Permanent Central (Opium) Board of the League of Nations inspected various opium-using areas, including the Philippines, for the U.S. Foreign Policy Association. May called attention in the Philippines to the easy availability and low price of opium, common allegations of collusion between smugglers and Island enforcement officials, low enforcement appropriations, and inadequate equipment. Other nations were becoming suspicious of American failure to provide statistics or other information, and May's frank disclosures did not allay doubts about the effectiveness of American narcotic prohibition in the site of its earliest enactment (*Survey of Smoking Opium Conditions in the Far East*, Opium Research Committee [New York: Foreign Policy Assoc., 1927], pp. 15, 21–23).

22 For a history of the Indian-Chinese opium trade see D. E. Owen, *British Opium Policy in China and India* (New Haven: Yale Univ. Press, 1934). Antagonism to the opium trade in the 19th century is described in Lowes, *International Control*, pp. 58–84. The *Report of the Royal Commission on Opium*, 7 vols., 1894–95, is analyzed by Owen, pp. 311–28.

23 See Lowes, *International Control*, pp. 76–78 for the debate in Commons: *Parliamentary Debates*, 4th ser., vol. 158, 30 May 1906, pp. 494–516.

24 Taylor, *Narcotics Traffic*, pp. 22–23.

25 Chester C. Tan, *The Boxer Catastrophe* (New York: Columbia Univ. Press, 1967).

26 For a recent analysis of the ruthlessness with which Chinese officials rooted out poppy cultivation and opium production see R. V. DesForges, "Hsi-liang: A Portrait of a Late Ch'ing Patriot" (Ph.D. diss., Yale Univ., 1971), pp. 252–81. Also see Meribeth E. Cameron, *The Reform Move-*

ment in China, 1898–1912, Stanford University Publications in History, Economics, and Political Science (Stanford, Calif.: Stanford Univ. Press, 1931), vol. 3, no. 1, pp. 136–59; E. J. M. Rhoads, "Nationalism and Xenophobia in Kwangtung (1905–1906): The Canton Anti-American Boycott and the Lienchow Anti-Missionary Uprising," *Papers on China* (East Asian Research Center, Harvard Univ., 1962–63), vol. 16–17, pp. 154–97.

27 President Roosevelt publically denounced unfair treatment of the Chinese in the U.S. when the embargo was threatened and in a private letter admitted even more clearly, "we have behaved scandalously toward Chinamen in this country. Some of the outrages by mobs which have resulted in the deaths of Chinamen were almost as bad as anything that occurred at the hands of the Chinamen themselves in the Boxer outbreak" (TR to Secretary of the Treasury Leslie M. Shaw, 2 Aug. 1905 quoted in H. K. Beale, *Theodore Roosevelt and the Rise of America to World Power* [Baltimore: Johns Hopkins Press, 1956], p. 230). Contemporary explanations of the Chinese boycott as the natural result of American treatment of the Chinese immigrant include Chester Holcombe, "Chinese Exclusion and the Boycott," *Outlook,* 30 Dec. 1905, pp. 1066–72; and John W. Foster, "The Chinese Boycott," *Atlantic Monthly,* January 1906, pp. 118–27.

28 Beale, in *Theodore Roosevelt,* has one of the best accounts of the embargo (pp. 191–223). Also see Mowry, *Era,* pp. 186–87; C. F. Remer, *A Study of Chinese Boycotts with Special Reference to Their Economic Effectiveness* (Baltimore: Johns Hopkins Press, 1933), ch. 6, "The Anti-American Boycott of 1905." Remer and Beale agree that the actual damage to American trade was modest but that American traders and manufacturers were greatly upset by the threat and put pressure on the American government to stop the boycott. A financial leader such as J. J. Hill called the boycott "the greatest commercial disaster America has ever suffered" (Charles Chailé-Long, "Why China Boycotts Us," *The World Today,* March 1906, p. 314).

29 As in the imbroglio (1904) over the American China Development Company, which failed to live up to its contract to build the Hankow-Canton railroad, Roosevelt intervened on the boycott issue not because the Chinese case was unjust but because the U.S. stood to lose face and aid its competitors by acceding to Chinese demands. As he explained to the American minister, William Rockhill, "Unless I misread them entirely [the Chinese] despise weakness even more than they prize justice" (TR to W. W. Rockhill, Minister to China, 22 Aug. 1905 in *Letters of Theodore Roosevelt,* Elting Morison, ed., [Cambridge: Harvard Univ. Press, 1951], 4: 1301). Taft and Root appeared before the Senate Finance Committee in early 1906 to request money for a Chinese expeditionary force to be housed in the Philippines (Washington *Post,* 10 and 11 Feb. 1906).

30 C. H. Brent to T. Roosevelt, 24 July 1906 (BP, container 6).

31 Taft enthusiastically supported Brent's proposal. He also had placed the blame for the boycott on the Chinese Exclusion Act, "an unjustly

severe law [which threatened] one of the greatest commercial prizes of the world . . . the trade with the 400,000,000 Chinese" (Beale, p. 197).

32   *Public Law 141* (1908); "International Investigation of the Opium Evil: Message from the President of the United States," House Doc. no. 926, 60th Cong., 1st Sess., 11 May 1908 (GPO, 1908).

33   See A. H. Taylor, *Narcotics Traffic,* pp. 54–56; *National Cyclopedia of American Biography* 9 : 430–31.

34   Taylor, *Narcotics Traffic,* pp. 302–05; Elizabeth was the daughter of industrialist William Drew Washburn of Minneapolis who had served in the House and Senate; his brothers Cadwallader, Israel, and Elihu also served in Congress. The brothers represented different states (Wisconsin, Maine, and Illinois). Elihu B. Washburne (as he spelled it) served as minister to France and remained in Paris during the German siege of 1870–71, publishing later his personal account. Mrs. Wright was said to be the first woman to receive plenipotentiary powers as a diplomat and at the time of her death in 1952 was still active in the fight against narcotics, having recently urged the passage of the antinarcotic bill known as the Boggs Act (1951) which mandated minimum sentences on first conviction of a narcotic offense (N.Y. *Times,* obit., 14 Feb. 1952).

35   Undated typewritten sheet signed Hamilton Wright, entitled "Memo in regard to White House letter April 30th 1908, signed Loeb to Root" (WP, entry 36).

36   Taylor, *Narcotics Traffic,* p. 54.

37   ER to William Loeb [Jr.], 7 Sept. 1908 (WP, entry 36).

38   Some of the returns from Wright's survey are contained in WP, entry 36. Those preserved reveal the spottiness and varied quality of the responses. The request to other nations to prepare a report on their domestic laws, opium production, and consumption was necessary if shipments to China from such nations as Turkey, Persia, and India were to be monitored. Lack of information or effective laws would also demonstrate the need for further international action. Turkey, as noted, did not attend the conference, and Persia made no survey. For a summary of the diplomatic correspondence, see Lowes, *International Control,* pp. 111–17.

39   Phillips's memorandum of 1907 (see above, ch. 1, n. 54).

40   Wright estimated that in the general population there were 0.18% opium addicts. In the professional classes, the rates were higher, as noted. Since the population was about ninety million in 1909, the number of addicts would be 175,000—not far different from the APhA committee's estimate in 1902 of about 200,000. See Hamilton Wright, "Report on the International Opium Commission and on the Opium Problem as Seen within the United States and Its Possessions," contained in *Opium Problem: Message from the President of the United States,* Senate Doc. no. 377, 61st Cong., 2nd Sess., 21 Feb. 1910, p. 47.

41   HW to CHB, 22 Aug. 1908 (WP, entry 51).

42   *Importation and Use of Opium,* Hearings before Committee on Ways and Means, House, 61st Cong., 3rd Sess., 14 Dec. 1910 (GPO, 1910), p. 32.

43   For decrease in patent medicine sales, see above, ch. 1, n. 52. The drop in narcotic-containing compounds occurred while proprietaries in general rose 60% in sales between 1902 and 1911, "a rate unparalleled in history," a claim made by the President Frank Cheney of the PAA in his address to the 35th Annual Meeting of the association in 1913 (stenographic typescript of proceedings, Archives of the Proprietary Association, Washington, D.C., pp. 31–32).

44   HW to CHB, 22 Aug. 1908 (WP, entry 51).

45   ER to Rep. James S. Sherman, 26 Dec. 1908 (WP, entry 36).

46   Ibid.; also see testimony of Hamilton Wright in *Importation and Use of Opium,* Hearings before the Committee on Ways and Means, House, 61st Cong., 2nd Sess., 31 May 1910 (GPO, 1910), pp. 502–03.

47   Congress was often reminded of the impressive effect the announcement that the U.S. had enacted the Smoking Opium Exclusion Act had on foreign delegates to the Shanghai Commission. For example, see Wright's testimony (ibid., p. 502). I have failed to locate any evidence in foreign accounts of the Act's psychological impact.

48   Robert Bacon to HWW, 2 Oct., and 20 Nov., 1908 (BCR).

49   HWW to Secretary of State, 29 Oct. 1908 (BCR). Wiley refers to provisions in Section 11 of the Pure Food and Drug Act which permitted the federal government to bar importation of harmful substances.

50   RB to HWW, 4 Nov. 1908 (BCR). Bacon referred to the proposed law as a "sentimental" help to delegates.

51   HW to Root, 30 Oct. 1908 (WP, entry 51).

52   Dean C. Worcester to HW, 9 and 11 Dec. 1908 (WP, entry 51).

53   For correspondence on the question of diplomatic status of the Shanghai meeting, see Lowes, *International Control,* pp. 112 ff. In Brent's opinion the downgrading of the meeting to a commission was at the request of Great Britain and led him to favor another meeting which would have treaty-making powers. CHB to Bishop Lawrence, 7 May 1909, to Bishop Hall, 2 July 1909 (BP, container 8).

54   In describing the American stance at Shanghai, Wright later wrote, "We believed in prohibition for ourselves in the use of opium—except for medicinal purposes, and for the principle of prohibition for all other nations as soon as it could be accomplished." "Report of Dr. Wright," in *Proc. Amer. Soc. Internat. Law* 3 : 89–94 (1909). To the other nations the American representatives declared that "there is no non-medical use of opium and its derivatives that is not fraught with grave dangers, if it is not actually vicious" *Report to the Department of State by the American Delegation to the International Opium Commission at Shanghai,* typescript signed by the delegates contained in WP, entry 33, p. 17.

55   Hamilton Wright, "Memorandum for the Committee on Ways and Means, the House of Representatives, on . . . Bills Intended to Redeem the Pledges of the United States," 10 Feb. 1913 (WP, entry 36).

56   Taylor states that this was the first international meeting dealing with Chinese problems in which China did not participate under threats (*Narcotic Traffic,* p. 79). See also Wright (ch. 2, n. 54 above), p. 94. The

Hague Convention is similarly described as the first conference and treaty in which China was accorded equality with other foreign states (Taylor, p. 109).

57   Wright, "Report International Opium," in *Opium Problem: Message,* p. 65.

58   For Wright's claims that it was difficult to adopt this resolution, see his description of his efforts (Wright, in *Proc. Amer. Soc. Internat. Law,* p. 92; see also Wright, "Report International Opium," in *Opium Problem: Message,* p. 70; for a discussion of both sides of the fight see Lowes, *International Control,* pp. 144–45.

59   A second meeting to conventionalize the Shanghai resolutions and consider other international drug issues seems not to have been adopted in advance by the State Department or the President. On his return, Wright sought the approval of the Secretary of State to urge continuation of the campaign as a responsibility of the U.S. to complete the work begun in Shanghai (CHB to WHT, 29 Dec. 1909, and CHB to P. C. Knox, 29 Dec. 1909, WP, entry 51). For the opposition of Huntington Wilson to Wright's plans for another conference and domestic legislation, see HW to C. Tenney, 1 July 1910 (WP, entry 51).

60   Taft and his Secretary of State embarked on a vigorous effort to increase American financial investment in various market areas, eventually known as "dollar diplomacy" and condemned as a form of economic imperialism, although there was nothing unique about such diplomatic efforts if compared to other major trading nations. See Mowry, *Era,* pp. 226 ff. A detailed account of foreign policy with regard to China may be found in *The United States and China, 1906–1913: A Study of Finance and Diplomacy,* by Charles Vevier (New Brunswick: Rutgers Univ. Press, 1955). A very helpful recent study which touches on many of the diplomatic and financial involvements with China by the Roosevelt and later administrations is Jerry Israel, *Progressivism and the Open Door: America and China, 1905–1921* (Univ. of Pittsburgh Press, 1971).

61   Acting Secretary of State to . . . Delegates of the United States to the International Opium Conference, 18 Oct. 1911 (WP, entry 38).

62   The winner of the contest for the Chinese ministry was Chicago plumbing magnate Charles Crane. For his selection among the various candidates, his embarrassing recall and resignation before reaching China, see Israel, *Progressivism,* pp. 60–82.

63   CHB to HW, 28 May, and 28 Sept. 1909 (WP, entry 51).

64   P. C. Knox to Chairman, Senate Committee on Appropriations, 28 July 1909, quoted in "Memorandum Relative to American Trade Possibilities on the Far East," prepared by J. B. Osborne, Bureau of Trade Relations, Department of State, 15 Sept. 1909 (Library of Congress: P. C. Knox Papers, Box 27).

65   HW to CHB, 29 Nov. 1909 (WP, entry 33).

66   U.S. Department of State, "The Acting Secretary of State to the Diplomatic Officers of the U.S. Accredited to the Governments Which Were Represented in the Shanghai International Opium Commission, 1 Sept.

1909," *Papers Relating to the Foreign Relations of the U.S. 1909* (GPO, 1914), pp. 107–11.

67 HW to CHB, 12 Nov. 1909 (WP, entry 33).

68 HW to CHB, 9 June 1909 (WP, entry 33); see also Wright, "Report International Opium," *Opium Problem: Message*, p. 74.

69 HW to Jeremiah Jenks, 18 March 1910 (WP, entry 51). Jenks was a leading authority on currency reform and trade in the Far East and one of the theoreticians of the Open Door policy of the State Department. Israel's study reveals the many contributions of Jenks to Far Eastern policy and the respect with which his views were held by the Taft and Roosevelt administrations.

70 HW to CHB, 12 Nov. 1909 (WP, entry 33). Wright made this estimate of the Secretary of State: "Knox who is a cold blooded little fellow is only now grasping the fact that in this opium business he has the oil to smooth any troubled waters he may meet with at Peking in his aggressive business enterprises there."

71 HW to CHB, 29 Nov. 1909 (WP, entry 33).

72 Wright quickly realized that the federal government's powers to restrict consumption of opium and other drugs were either accepted as limited or undesirable as a precedent. The intricacies of federal-state relationships were not so well perceived by other antidrug reformers such as Joseph Remington, an eminent leader of the pharmaceutical profession in America and dean of the Philadelphia College of Pharmacy; see HW to J. Remington, 26 April 1910 (WP, entry 51). Similarly, Wright had to defend his carefully framed bills against another reformer, Charles B. Towns, as late as 21 April 1914, on grounds that the federal government could enact an antinarcotic measure only in a tax guise in order to allay congressional fears of federal interference. The limitations of federal powers were also clearly spelled out in a letter to the Philadelphia *North American* (18 April 1910, entry 51). As an example of congressional doubt about federal police powers, the comment of Rep. J. H. Gaines might be adduced, made during the debate on the Smoking Opium Exclusion Act: "It takes plenary powers to stamp out [opium smoking]— if it can be suppressed at all—the full police power. Our federal government does not have it" (*Cong. Rec. 43* : 1683, 1 Feb. 1909, 60th Cong., 2nd Sess.). Wright complained, "it has been a difficult business. . . . The Constitution is constantly getting in the way" (Wright to Brent, 9 Feb. 1910, WP, entry 31).

73 James R. Mann to HW, 29 Dec. 1909 (WP, entry 51).

74 HW to David J. Foster, Chairman, House Committee on Foreign Affairs, 28 April 1910 (WP, entry 51). The bill, *HR 25, 241,* was introduced 30 April 1910 and referred to the Committee on Ways and Means. In the Senate the bill was introduced as *S 6810* by Senator Shelby M. Cullom on 28 Feb. 1910 and referred to the Finance Committee. There were, in fact, three Foster (and later Harrison) antinarcotic bills submitted to Congress, although only the one regulating domestic narcotic use kept the eponym. The other two antinarcotic bills were relatively uncontro-

versial and were enacted almost a year before the domestic antinarcotic bill. *Public Law no. 46*, 63rd Cong., was approved 17 Jan. 1914, and provided penalties for smuggling opiates and cocaine into or out of the U.S.; *Public Law no. 47* approved the same day, placed a prohibitive tax on any smoking opium produced in the U.S.

75   Wright always sought the prohibition of nonmedical drug use which he described as the American position in the Shanghai Commission (see above, ch. 2, n. 54). He soon discovered, however, that congressional leaders would not support a direct attack on the use of opiates and cocaine. Some thought such an approach unconstitutional; others feared it might be constitutional and could be broadened to include alcohol (see HW to A. A. Adee, Assistant Secretary of State, 2 Feb. 1911, WP, entry 51). The issue of an antinarcotic law was complicated because all sides admitted some legitimate use of the drugs proposed for control, which led to technical and intricate consultation with the many interests in the health professions. As a result, without almost unanimous support of the trades and professions the bill would probably never be brought to a vote. Balancing his way between ineffectiveness and apparently excessive police powers and unconstitutionality, Wright explained his thinking in 1914: "If I am correct in my opinion, the Courts will construe *HR 6282* [the future Harrison Act] not only as a Federal Statute but in the light of the terms of the International Opium Convention. If I am right in that opinion, the apparent defects in the Bill will not appear as defects at all except in the case of Section 6 [listing exempt amounts of narcotics in proprietaries]." HW to Charles B. Towns, 21 April 1914 (WP, entry 36).
      Another attempt for severe narcotic restriction without mentioning this as a goal in legislation would be the proposal to admit no exemptions, the promulgation of many regulations, a requirement for performance bonds for retailers, etc., thereby making trade in narcotics so cumbersome and dangerous that dealers would refuse to handle them. Such an approach was taken with the Marihuana Tax Act of 1937.

76   *Importation and Use of Opium*, Hearings before the House Committee on Ways and Means, 31 May 1910, 61st Cong., 2nd Sess. (GPO, 1910).

77   Wright, "Report on International Opium," in *Opium Problem: Message*.

78   Secretary of State to the President, 18 Feb. 1910, cited in *Opium Problem: Message*, p. 5.

79   Secretary of State to President, cited in *Opium Problem: Message*, p. 2; also *Importation and Use of Opium*, hearings, pp. 504, 509.

80   Wright, "Report International Opium," in *Opium Problem: Message*, pp. 59, 61; *Importation and Use of Opium*, 31 May 1910, p. 505.

81   Wright, "Report International Opium," in *Opium Problem: Message*, p. 44. This view contradicts that of the APhA committee which was disturbed by the increased use of opium by American servicemen (see above, ch. 1, n. 46) and represents an early refusal on the grounds of patriotism to criticize any American propensity to narcotics, a trend that became dominant after World War I.

82   Wright, "Report International Opium," in *Opium Problem: Message*,

p. 45; similarly Jacob Riis in *How the Other Half Lives* (New York: C. Scribner's Sons, 1890), pp. 72–76.

83 Wright, "Report International Opium," in *Opium Problem: Message*, p. 49; *Importation and Use of Opium*, 31 May 1910, p. 505.

84 See above, Chapter 1. Commenting on the fear of Negro cocaine users and the drive for a federal law, the *Chemist and Druggist* reported later that year from New Orleans: "The narcotic evil has become so pronounced in the city of New Orleans, where there is a large Negro population, that the police have undertaken a vigorous campaign of prosecution. . . . It is just this condition of things which has developed a demand during the last few years for the enactment of a federal law" (77 : 44, 31 Dec. 1910).

85 *Importation and Use of Opium*, 31 May 1910, p. 503.

86 Ibid., s.v. "retail pharmacists," pp. 507, 510.

87 *Importation and Use of Opium*, Hearings before the House Committee on Ways and Means, 14 Dec. 1910, 61st Cong., 3rd Sess. (GPO, 1910). Nonreform-minded members of the drug trades were "amazed" that representatives of such organizations as the NARD appeared in favor of the bill. See *Amer. Druggist Pharmaceut. Record 58* : 19 (1911).

88 William J. Schieffelin (1866–1955) was at this time chairman of the executive committee of the "Committee of One Hundred on National Health," an active group of leading educators, businessmen, and reformers. He also was prominent in political reform movements in New York City. He had sought strict antinarcotic laws at least as early as 1905 from the New York legislature. He held a doctorate in chemistry from the University of Munich, served as president of the NWDA in 1910–11, and was a model of the Progressive Era's public-spirited businessman.

89 *Amer. Druggist Pharmaceut. Record 58* : 2. "The Dangers of Enthusiasm" was an editorial warning of Dr. Wright's zeal. The *Record* wanted a bill similar to the District of Columbia Pharmacy Act (1906) with the familiar exemptions and no mention of cannabis and chloral hydrate, which roughly is what Congress enacted in 1914.

90 The "pressing necessity" of antinarcotic legislation was called to the attention of Congress by both President Taft and Secretary Knox in January 1911 (*Special Message of the President: The Opium Traffic*, Senate Doc. no. 736, 61st Cong., 3rd Sess., 11 Jan. 1911, pp. 2, 7). At the close of the year action to control opium in the U.S., "especially since the [Hague Opium] Conference is now in session," was urged on Congress in the "President's Message on Foreign Policy" (*Cong. Rec., Senate, 48* : 70–75, 62nd Cong., 7 Dec. 1911, esp. p. 74). This appeal was repeated a year later in the "President's Annual Message" (3 Dec. 1912) in which Taft characterized the failure to pass legislation approved by the appropriate federal departments and backed by the "moral sentiment of the country, [and] the practical support of all the legitimate trade interests likely to be affected" as most unfortunate. The U.S. had taken the initiative and then "failed to do its share in the great work" to correct the "deplorable narcotic evil in the United States as well as to redeem

international pledges" (p. 12, *Cong. Rec., 49* : 8–14, 3 Dec. 1912, 63rd Cong., 3rd Sess.).

91 *Importation and Use of Opium,* Hearings before the House Committee on Ways and Means, 11 Jan. 1911, 61st Cong., 3rd Sess. (GPO, 1911), pp. 49–84. Subsequent information and quotations are from the same source.

92 *Importation and Use of Opium,* 11 Jan. 1911, pp. 92–95; Dr. Kebler was also author of Farmer's Bulletin no. 393 on habit-forming drugs.

93 Sereno E. Payne, Chairman, House Committee on Ways and Means, to Huntington Wilson, Assistant Secretary of State, 28 Jan. 1911 (WP, entry 51).

94 Ambassador Bacon's warnings were relayed to Wright by F. Huidekoper of the Paris Embassy, 23 June 1911 (WP, entry 51).

95 E. Frank Baldwin to HW, 14 June 1911 (WP, entry 51).

96 Alexander Lambert to HW, 27 April 1911 (WP, entry 51).

97 Taylor, *Narcotics Traffic,* pp. 93–96.

98 CHB to HW, 24 Jan. 1911 (WP, entry 51).

99 Taylor, *Narcotics Traffic,* pp. 92–93; Lowes, *International Control,* pp. 166–67. Renewal of the ten-year treaty occurred on 8 May 1911.

100 Taylor, *Narcotics Traffic,* pp. 87–88.

101 *Amer. J. Internat. Law* 6 : 191 (Suppl., July 1912).

102 *International Opium Conference, The Hague, December 1, 1911–January 23, 1912.* Summary of the minutes (unofficial) (The Hague: National Printing Office, 1912), p. 105.

103 Bertil A. Renborg, *International Drug Control* (Washington, D.C.: Carnegie Endowment for International Peace, 1947), pp. 15 ff.

104 On 11 Feb. 1915, the U.S., China, and the Netherlands put the Convention into force among themselves. Norway and Honduras joined them later in 1915, but no other nations took action until after World War I. Ratifications (without implementation) continued at a modest pace, but not until the Convention was, in effect, made part of the Versailles Treaty in 1919, did almost all world governments enter into the constraints of the Hague Treaty.

Chapter 3

1 The first Harrison bill (*HR 1969*) was introduced in 1912.

2 For the rules under which the NDTC operated and its initial membership see *JAPhA* 2 : 238–39 (1913).

3 The PAA officials, who happened to be in the New Willard Hotel at the time of the meeting, assured the NDTC that they were "entirely satisfied with the provisions of the proposed legislation regarding narcotic drugs as it would not in any way affect the interests of the Proprietary Association" (*JAPhA* 2 : 236–37 [1913]). The PAA, having noted inclusion in the Harrison bill of the standard exemption dating back to the 1905 model law, was uninterested by other provisions of the bill which dealt with transactions of narcotics above the exempt amounts. Nevertheless, there were efforts made by proprietary interests to raise the exempt

amounts eventually adopted by the House the following June. The Harrison Act when approved in December 1914 had exemptions above those recommended by the NDTC and the House in June 1913. See also *NARD Notes* which described Wright's behavior as "distinctly antagonistic" toward the retailers (15 : 1004, 23 Jan. 1913).

4 *JAPhA* 2 : 247 (1913); J. H. Beal, editorial, *JAPhA* 2 : 737–40 (1913). The NDTC delegates visited Harrison's office and angrily denounced HR 1969 and demanded the changes which had been unanimously approved by the NDTC. Wright returned to negotiations and did not submit a revised bill to Harrison until differences were reconciled. Wright insisted that passage was important before the Second Hague Opium Conference met on 1 July.

5 At the next meeting of the NDTC, 10–11 April 1913, the executive committee met both before and after the plenary sessions. Of great significance in regard to the drug trades' view of federal police powers was an executive committee resolution, later adopted by the NDTC, that the proposed bill affected suppliers but not consumers (i.e. patients). Relationships between them and retailers and practitioners would be regulated as usual by state law (*JAPhA* 2 : 628–33 [1913]).

6 James G. Burrow, *AMA, Voice of American Medicine* (Baltimore: Johns Hopkins Press, 1963), pp. 51–52, 62 ff.

7 The issues of the *Medical Economist* (New York) and the *Illinois Medical Journal* (Chicago), two of the outspoken defenders of the "humble general practitioner," contain voluminous references to the elitist reform notions of national medical leadership prior to 1919–20. Fishbein's interview (ch. 3, n. 8 below) also provides evidence that "liberal" views predominated in the AMA's pre-World War I leadership, which included such men as Drs. George Simmons, Frederick Green, and Alexander Lambert.

8 "Report of the Judicial Council," *JAMA* 65 : 73–92 (1915); see Burrow, *AMA*, pp. 141–45; R. Stevens, *American Medicine and the Public Interest* (New Haven: Yale Univ. Press, 1971), pp. 136–39. George H. Simmons was a journalist who received a rather sketchy medical training at Rush Medical School in Chicago, obtaining his degree in 1882. He eventually entered obstetrical and gynecological practice in about 1885 in Lincoln, Nebraska, where he established a hospital. Dr. Simmons aroused a furor over alleged abortions, and he quit practice to become in 1899 the first full-time executive secretary of the AMA and editor of the *JAMA*. His remarkable organizational abilities assisted the rapid growth of the association after 1900 and his editorial talents raised its journal to a respected and powerful status as the leading voice of medical opinion. In 1911 he relinquished the post of executive secretary, but remained the single dominant figure in the AMA until his retirement in 1924. He was succeeded by Dr. Morris Fishbein who had been assistant to Dr. Simmons since 1913; upon retirement Dr. Simmons burned his personal papers (my interview with Dr. Morris Fishbein, 13 Jan. 1972, New York); *Morris Fishbein, M.D., An Autobiography* (Garden City, N.Y.: Doubleday, 1969), pp. 36–38, 93; Burrow, *AMA*, pp. 28 ff., 51.

9 Burrow provides evidence in many areas of the growing conservatism of the AMA after 1918 (*AMA,* pp. 146 ff.).

10 "An Act Supplemental to the National Prohibition Act," 23 Nov. 1921, 42 *Stat. L.* 222.

11 Like other medical journals, the *JAMA,* under Simmons's leadership, condemned simple maintenance of addiction: "merely to satisfy the cravings of the victims of the drug habit . . . would clearly appear [to be] an offense against the welfare of the community . . . much more serious than the mere infraction of a revenue law of the United States" ("State Rights, State Duties, and the Harrison Narcotic Law," *JAMA* 67 : 37–38 [1916]).

12 "Protection against Dangerous Drugs," *JAMA 46* : 1208–09 (1906).

13 One of the reasons the APhA originally saw some merit in the British health insurance scheme was that it clearly spelled out the relationship between pharmacists and physicians. See *JAPhA 6* : 314–17 (1917). Like the AMA, the APhA soon turned against federal and state control of the health professions. See Burrow, *AMA,* p. 146 n.

14 The NARD under the leadership of Frank Freericks led the battle for equality in the onerous burden of recording retail narcotic transactions. By making dispensing for the doctor as cumbersome as for the pharmacist, it was hoped that the dispensing physicians would revert to prescribing ("The Harrison Conference Bill," *JNARD 17* : 134–35 [1913]). Pharmacists also resented the massive public relations and lobbying tactics of the AMA (editorial, "Legislative Organization: Have a Laugh with Us," *JNARD 17* : 73–74 [1913]).

15 Physicians were pictured by pharmacists as well as by many reformers as the leading culprits in the creation of addicts. To omit physicians from strict record keeping, claimed an editorial of the *JNARD,* would leave "a loophole through which dispensing physicians if so disposed may continue to cart wagon-loads of narcotics for improper purposes" (*17* : 965 [1914]). The NARD created a scare among proponents of the Harrison bill in the summer of 1914 when it reopened the question of equalizing burdens among physicians and pharmacists. The NARD explained that it merely wished to suggest changes, not demand revision, but the telegram sent by the Philadelphia Convention to Treasury Secretary McAdoo did not seem very conciliatory (18 Aug. 1914, PHSR).

16 HW to Lloyd Bryce, Minister, The Hague, 18 March 1913 (WP, entry 36); HW to WJB, 31 May 1913 (WP, entry 36).

17 In formulation of the opium bills in 1912 and 1913, Wright mentions a joint committee of the State and Treasury Departments. During the Taft Administration the bills were examined by Treasury Assistant Secretary James F. Curtis and Commissioner of Internal Revenue Royal E. Cabell. The Commerce Department was also involved, but in a less intensive way because the burden of enforcement would be in the Treasury (see HW to Francis W. Taylor, private secretary to the Secretary of the Treasury, 27 Nov. 1912; HW to Francis Burton Harrison, 10 Feb. 1913; HW to WJB, 31 May 1913, WP, entry 36). Wright, therefore, mediated between the interdepartmental committee and the NDTC in formulation

of the final form of the Harrison bill, *HR 6282*, introduced 10 June
1913. The President assisted momentum for the bill by strongly urging
its passage in a message asking for an appropriation to cover participation in the forthcoming Second Hague Conference. Wilson termed failure
to take the few final steps in the worldwide movement "unthinkable"
(*Cong. Rec., Senate 50* : 265, 21 April 1913, 63rd Cong. Special Sess.).

18 For the debate in the House see *Cong. Rec., House, 50, pt. 3* : 2191–
2211, 63rd Cong., 1st Sess., 26 June 1913 (GPO 1913); for the committee report see "Registration of Producers and Importers of Opium,"
etc., House Rept. no. 23, 24 June 1913, 63rd Cong., 1st Sess. (GPO,
1913). President Wilson urged the Senate to adopt the legislation "recently passed by the House of Representatives without a dissenting vote
[to which] this government is now pledged . . . as soon as possible
during the present session of Congress." This request accompanied
Wright's report on the Second Hague Conference, *Second International
Opium Conference,* Senate Doc. no. 157, 63rd Cong., 1st Sess. (GPO,
1913).

19 For changes see Senate Finance Committee's "Registration of Persons
Dealing in Opium," Senate Report no. 258, 18 Feb. 1914, 63rd Cong.,
2nd Sess. (GPO, 1914). Among other changes, the committee added
hypodermic syringes and needles to the list of controlled items.

20 [J. H. Beal], "The Senate Amendments to the Harrison Bill," *JAPhA
3* : 479–81 (1914). The report of the President's Homes Commission
stated that a course of the Tucker Asthma Cure cost $12.50 [Report of
the President's Homes Commission, Senate Doc. no. 644, 8 Jan. 1909,
60th Cong., 2nd Sess. (GPO, 1909), pp. 269–70].

21 *Cong. Rec., Senate, 51, pt. 10* : 760, 20 June 1914, 63rd Cong., 2nd
Sess. In later withdrawing his amendment, Senator Atlee Pomerene
claimed it was prompted by an overly strict recording requirement
directed at physicians by Senator Knute Nelson. When the Nelson threat
passed, Senator Pomerene dropped his opposing amendment (*Cong.
Rec., Senate, 51, pt. 13* : 579, 15 Aug. 1914, 63rd Cong., 2nd Sess.).

22 "Conference Report and Statement," *Cong. Rec., House, 51, pt. 16* : 16,
818–19 submitted 20 Oct. 1914, 63rd Cong., 2nd Sess.

23 Bryan reported to President Wilson shortly after the Second Hague
Conference that "some of the members of the [House Appropriations]
Committee even objected to Wright's being continued at any price." At
the time Wright was being paid out of the Secretary's emergency fund
(WJB to WW, 22 Aug. 1913). In May 1913 Bryan penned a personal
note to the President that "the doctor looks like a drinking man" (WJB
to WW, 24 May 1913, Library of Congress: Woodrow Wilson Papers,
ser. 4, box 93, case file 77, "Opium").

24 WJB to WW, 12 Aug., and 16 Aug. 1913 (LC, Woodrow Wilson
Papers, "Opium").

25 The Appropriations Committee had remained hostile to Wright, but the
State Department needed to send a representative to the Third Hague
Conference, preferably Wright because of his long association with the
work. The need became more urgent, although by spring 1914 Bryan

wished he did not have to deal with Wright. He was, however, the acknowledged expert in the legislative negotiations and was brought back to the State Department early in the year to coordinate both domestic and foreign aspects of the antiopium campaign. In March Secretary Bryan wrote the President that "Mr. [William] Phillips [Assistant Secretary of State] also notes what I have reported on former occasions, viz., that Dr. Wright's breath smelt of liquor" (21 March 1914, Woodrow Wilson Papers, "Opium"). The demand that Wright "take the pledge" came on the 6th or 7th of June. Wright's lengthy memorandum to the President giving his side and the pressing need to leave on the 9th if he was to get to The Hague on time, is dated 7 June 1914 (WP, entry 36). President Wilson's affirmation of Bryan's dismissal of Wright is dated 17 June 1914 (Woodrow Wilson Papers, "Opium," and WP, entry 36).

26 "Free for some large affair," HW to William H. Welch, Professor of Pathology, Johns Hopkins Medical School, 26 Oct. 1914 (WP, entry 36). See also E. G. Adami, McGill Univ., to HW, 22 Sept. 1914; William Loeb, Jr., Guggenheim Exploration Co. to HW, 8 Dec. 1914; George Wickersham to HW, 19 Sept. 1914 (WP, entry 36).

27 HW to Andrew J. Peters, Asst. Secretary of the Treasury, 16 Jan. 1915; A. J. Peters to HW, 20 Jan. 1915 (WP, entry 36). At about this time Wright was preparing an article which for his career had a prophetic title: "The End of the Opium Question," *American Review of Reviews*, April 1915, pp. 464–66.

28 "I have no sympathy with these proprietary or patent medicine people. I would like to exclude the use of narcotics entirely from every one of these patent medicines if I thought we could do it," declared Rep. Harrison during the House debate, in opposing an amendment to *HR 6282* which would have cut in half the permissible limits for exempt preparations in Section 6 (*Cong. Rec., House, 50, pt. 3* : 2211, 26 June 1913, 63rd Cong., 1st Sess.). The amendment was defeated on a voice vote. In arguing against reduction in the exemption limits Rep. A. P. Gardner of Massachusetts predicted that unless the section was approved as negotiated with the drug trades, "interminable delay is in store for this bill" (p. 2210). Similarly, Rep. James Mann of Illinois: "Unfortunately I am forced to believe that if we should attempt in this way to attack all the proprietary medicines which contain opium, the bill would have a rocky road to travel, and would be consigned to oblivion. That may not be a very good excuse, but, after all, it is practical" (p. 2210).

29 241 US 401 (1916). HW to Charles Evans Hughes, 28 June 1916 (WP, entry 36). Wright was unaware that Hughes did not wish to stand alone in dissent against the Holmes decision, and voted against it only after Justice Pitney determined to take exception. Neither explained the grounds for his dissent. See Merlo J. Pusey, *Charles Evans Hughes*, 2 vols. (New York: Macmillan, 1952), 1 : 286–87.

30 "More about the Harrison Bill," *JAPhA* 3 : 1–4 (1914).

31 Beal had introduced the resolution to the NDTC in April 1913 that the Harrison bill would not affect the consumer (see above, ch. 3, n. 5).

32 Editorial *JAPhA* 4 : 4–8 (1914).

33 The Public Health Service followed a consistent policy toward the many requests for aid directed its way after March 1915. The service could legally care only for merchant seamen and a few other small groups such as some Indians, and made this very clear to importunate local officials and distressed individuals (Asst. Surgeon General to H. L. Lea, 24 March 1915, PHSR). There was also a request from Shreveport, Louisiana, that a hospital be established there to care for drug addicts because "a large number of helpless people are becoming mentally deranged on account of the enforcement of this law" (Rep. J. T. Watkins, 4th Louisiana District, to the SG, 11 May 1915, PHSR). This request is of interest since Shreveport was the site of the still controversial narcotic clinic operated by Dr. Willis P. Butler from 1919 to 1923 (see ch. 7).

34 The attitude of the Bureau of Internal Revenue is clearly revealed in its immediate steps to indict "dope doctors" and unscrupulous pharmacists. That such a disparity should exist within two branches of the same department (the PHS was at this time part of the Treasury) is partly a reflection of the peripheral place the PHS held in social policy planning of the federal government.

35 Considerable evidence was submitted, without effective rebuttal, that the percentage of physicians addicted was very high. In 1899, Dr. T. D. Crothers reported on a nine-year study involving 3,244 physicians and warned that 6% or more used morphine or opium regularly. He was convinced that 8–10% of physicians were secret or open drug and morphine habitués ("Morphinism among Physicians," *Med. Record* 55 : 784–86 [1899]). When the *Medical Economist* of New York opposed a state legislative proposal which would rescind the licenses of physician-addicts, their response did not deny that there were a sizable number of addicts, but recommended that the economic conditions of physicians should be improved so that a "great many of the gifted members of the profession [would not need] to seek relief in narcotics" (2 : 52 [1914]). See S. Garb, "Drug Addiction in Physicians," *Anesthesia and Analgesia* 48 : 128–33 (1969); R. B. Little, "Hazards of Drug Dependency among Physicians," *JAMA* 218 : 1533–35 (1971).

36 The Prohibitionist rarely belittled the narcotic problem, since he was opposed to the use of both drugs and liquor. Narcotics have been perceived as so mysteriously evil that few antinarcotic reformers ever felt the propriety of showing the often greater damage done to the physique and to society by alcoholism. One of the authorities in America who consistently tried to put narcotics and alcohol into perspective was Dr. Lawrence Kolb, Sr., of the Public Health Service. He liked to quote the British writer on inebriety Norman Kerr, who said in the late 19th century, "Whisky maddens man, while opium soothes him." Kolb had his own saying that there was more violence in a gallon of alcohol

than in a ton of opium (*Use of Narcotics in the United States,* Hearing before the Committee on Printing, 3 June 1924, 68th Cong., 1st Sess. [GPO, 1924], p. 27).

37 That narcotics use was spreading into the higher classes was, although without any specific evidence, the theme of the APhA studies in 1901–03 (*Proc. APhA 49* [1901]–*51* [1903]); Hamilton Wright's "Report on the International Opium Commission and on the Opium Problem as Seen Within the United States and Its Possessions" (contained in *Opium Problem: Message from the President of the United States,* Senate Doc. no. 377, 61st Cong., 2nd Sess., 21 Feb. 1910); the Special Committee of the Secretary of the Treasury (1919); Richmond Hobson's crusade against narcotics in the 1920s and 1930s; the campaign against marihuana in the 1930s, and so on. In other words dangerous drugs have been believed to be spreading into the middle and upper classes for almost a century at an alarming rate. This must be balanced against the claim, such as that made by Dr. George Beard in *American Nervousness: Its Causes and Consequences* (New York: Putnam, 1881), that America is generally an avid drug-using country, and the statement in "Quackery and the Quacked," *Nat. Quart. Rev. 2* : 354 (1861), that there is a national penchant for drugs and drug use.

38 Andrew Sinclair, *Prohibition: The Era of Excess* (Boston: Little, Brown, 1962), p. 154; Peter Odegard, *Pressure Politics: The Story of the Anti-Saloon League* (New York: Columbia Univ. Press, 1928), pp. 139–48.

39 The N.Y. *Times* noted the passage of the Harrison Act on 2 Jan. 1915.

40 See Odegard, *Pressure Politics,* pp. 151–59; Sinclair, *Era of Excess,* pp. 155–56; for the House debate, see *Cong. Rec., House, 52, pt. 1* : 495–616, 63rd Cong., 3rd Sess., 22 Dec. 1914.

41 Richmond Pearson Hobson (1870–1937) became one of the heroes of the Spanish-American War. For this he was eventually awarded (1933) the Congressional Medal of Honor and much sooner became "the most kissed man in America" as he took to the speaking circuits to describe his exploits. A confection was even named after him, "Hobson's kisses." He moved from his personal adventures to warning of the "yellow peril," particularly the Japanese. He served from 1906 to 1915 in Congress, from his native Alabama, and became one of the leading Prohibitionists. Defeated in 1914 in a Senate race against the powerful Oscar W. Underwood, he still had time to introduce the Hobson Resolution on Prohibition which foreshadowed the eventual defeat of the wet forces. In 1922 he progressed from liquor prohibition to narcotic prohibition with the zeal, platform style, exaggerated fears, and pseudoscientific warnings which had marked his liquor speeches. In 1933 he published *Drug Addiction: A Malignant Racial Cancer;* the following year Congress approved his promotion on the retired list to rear admiral. He died in 1937.

42 Odegard, *Pressure Politics,* p. 569.

43 Oscar W. Underwood (1862–1929) was a representative from Alabama from 1895 to 1915, when he entered the Senate. He was House Majority Leader from 1911 to 1915, and in 1912 a candidate for the Democratic presidential nomination. His outstanding legislative achievement was the

Underwood Tariff Act of October 1913 which lowered and reformed
tariff in a manner generally applauded (Arthur S. Link, *Woodrow Wilson and the Progressive Era, 1910–1917* [New York: Harper and Row,
1954], pp. 35–43).

44 Underwood quoted an editorial in the Louisville *Courier-Journal* (*Cong.
Rec., House, 52, pt. 1* : 520, 63rd Cong., 3rd Sess., 22 Dec. 1914). When
Harrison was appointed governor-general of the Philippines, Underwood
took over from his colleague the responsibility of seeing the Harrison bill
through the House. Mention of narcotics in the Hobson debate occurred
when Prohibitionists pointed out that the federal government had taken
steps against the narcotic evils and should not hesitate to take a similar
stand against alcohol (p. 513). But when Rep. Hobson linked the two
by claiming in the preamble to the original *HR 168* that "exact scientific
research has demonstrated that alcohol is a narcotic poison," he was
rebutted by Rep. Andrew Barchfeld, a physician from Pittsburgh, who
called the statement "either a play on words or an outright misstatement.
In either event it is misleading, and flies in the face of medical practice
and physiological science" (p. 555). In his major speech of the debate,
Hobson frequently refers to alcohol as a "habit-forming drug," as well
as by standard epithets, "a protoplasmic poison," and the "loathsome
excretion of a living organism." As he would say of heroin in the 1920s,
alcohol attacked the "top part of the brain," the location of man's higher
instincts (pp. 602–09). But opponents of Prohibition also used the specter of narcotics to support their arguments, as when Rep. James Gallivan
of Boston warned that drug use would increase if national Prohibition
were instituted (p. 581). It appears from the debate that a strong concern of the opponents to the constitutional amendment was the precedent of invading traditional states' rights. The South clearly expressed
its fear that Congress in the future would force upon that region voting
rights for Negroes, destruction of its segregation laws, etc. (see statement by Rep. R. L. Henry of Texas, p. 542). Rep. Edward Pou of North
Carolina explained that voting rights had been taken away from Negroes
not in anger or with malice but "as the adult takes the pistol from the
hand of the child." He feared that three-fourths of the states might approve an amendment requiring universal male suffrage if one were submitted (p. 597). Hobson attempted to assuage some of the fears of the
South by claiming that liquor makes the Negro a brute, causing him
"to commit unnatural crimes." The white man has the same tendency
except that "being further evolved it takes longer to reduce him to the
same level" (p. 605). And for all who revered medical progress and
efficiency, he called national Prohibition "scientific treatment for a deep
organic disease" (p. 504).

45 In 1913 the argument for the Webb-Kenyon Act had been that the
federal government should take this last step, the ultimate in helping the
states that so wished to maintain Prohibition. The government was declared not to have the power to enforce it by federal constitutional powers. But the overwhelming congressional support given to the Webb-
Kenyon Act, and its passage over Taft's veto, encouraged a growing

sentiment among dry forces to campaign for national Prohibition by a constitutional amendment. See Odegard, *Pressure Politics,* pp. 149 ff; also Charles Merz, *The Dry Decade,* reprint of 1931 ed. (Seattle: Univ. of Washington Press, 1970), pp. 14–17.

46   I interviewed Dr. Victor Heiser, 25 March 1970 in New York City. Dr. Heiser was Health Commissioner under Governor-General Harrison. In Dr. Heiser's opinion, Governor Harrison's tenure was marked by personal scandal which brought the American government into disrepute.

Chapter 4

1   Glenn Sonnedecker, *History of Pharmacy,* 3rd ed. (Philadelphia: J. B. Lippincott Co., 1963), pp. 278 ff.; D. I. Macht, "The History of Opium and Some of Its Preparations and Alkaloids," *JAMA 64* : 477–81 (1915); P. G. Kritikos and S. N. Papadaki, "The History of the Poppy and Opium," *Bull. Narcotics 19* : 17–37 (1966); S. Hamarneh, "Pharmacy in Medieval Islam and the History of Drug Addiction," *Medical History 16* : 226–37 (1972); A. Hayter, *Opium and the Romantic Imagination* (London: Faber and Faber, 1968).

2   H. E. Sigerist, "Laudanum in the Works of Paracelsus," *Bull. Hist. Med. 9* : 530–44 (1941).

3   John Jones, *The Mysteries of Opium Revealed* (London: Richard Smith, 1700), p. 32.

4   Samuel Crumpe, *An Inquiry into the Nature and Properties of Opium* (London: G. G. and J. Robinson, 1793), p. 177.

5   Glenn Sonnedecker, "Emergence of the Concept of Opiate Addiction," *J. Mondial Pharmacie,* Sept.–Dec. 1962, pp. 286–87; Jones denied any difference in reaction among nationalities (*Mysteries,* p. 307).

6   Crumpe, *Inquiry,* p. 177; Jones, *Mysteries,* p. 306.

7   Jonathan Pereira, *The Elements of Materia Medica and Therapeutics,* 3rd American ed., edited by Joseph Carson, 2 vols. (Philadelphia: Blanchard and Lea, 1854) 2 : 1039–46 passim.

8   Robert Christison, *A Treatise on Poisons,* 1st American ed., from the 4th Edinburgh ed. (Philadelphia: Barrington and Haswell, 1845), pp. 552 ff.

9   George B. Wood, *A Treatise on Therapeutics and Pharmacology or Materia Medica,* 3rd ed., 2 vols. (Philadelphia: Lippincott, 1868), 1 : 712–13, 1 : 725–28.

10   Wood, *Treatise,* 1 : 761; also see Christison (*Poisons,* p. 558), who is inclined to agree that morphine "in medicinal doses does not produce either the disagreeable subsequent or idiosyncratic effects of opium."

11   For example, Freud's "Über Coca;" see above, ch. 1, n. 18.

12   Clifford Allbutt, "On the Abuse of Hypodermic Injections of Morphia," *Practitioner 3* : 327 (1870).

13   B. F. Von Niemayer, *A Textbook of Practical Medicine,* trans. from 7th German ed. by G. H. Humphreys and C. E. Ackley, 2 vols. (New York: Appleton, 1869), 2 : 291.

14 Eduard Levinstein, *Morbid Craving for Morphia,* trans. by C. Harrer (London: Smith, Elder, 1878), pp. 6 ff.

15 E. Levinstein, "Die Morphiumsucht," *Berliner klin. Wochschr.* 12 : 646–49 (1875), esp. p. 647. Also see *Morbid Craving,* p. 109, where Levinstein comments on the extremely easy relapse after withdrawal.

16 Levinstein, *Morbid Craving,* pp. 109–18. Levinstein described the morphine abstinence syndrome and stated that it lasted about 48 hours, did not result in death, and improved if morphine were administered; he distinguished it from delirium tremens in chronic alcoholism. Morphine, unlike alcohol, produced no bodily deterioration, according to Levinstein.

17 Ibid. See also William Osler, *The Principles and Practice of Medicine* (New York: Appleton, 1894), p. 1006: "Persons addicted to morphia are inveterate liars, and no reliance can be placed upon their statements."

18 Although narcotic and alcohol reform movements and research can be distinguished, similar factors caused them to be often considered together. Many of the "cures" or treatments for one were also recommended for the other. The Towns-Lambert treatment was considered efficacious by its proponents for both habits. The chain of cure establishments, e.g. the Keeley, Oppenheimer, and Neal sanitaria scattered across the nation, treated both kinds of patients. Alcohol was often called a "narcotic" and the American Medical Society for the Study of Alcohol and Narcotics was established in the 19th century to pursue research in both. The *Journal of Inebriety,* edited by Dr. Crothers of a Hartford sanitarium (which cared for both classes), published articles mostly on alcohol but did not neglect opium and cocaine habitués. Various reform organizations, the WCTU, the International Reform Bureau, missionary societies, etc., opposed both habits. Richmond P. Hobson moved smoothly from his role as a leading antiliquor spokesman to head of an antinarcotic association in 1923. Distinctions between drugs were not clear to the public, and in the 19th century opiates occasionally were falsely considered to provoke violence whereas cocaine produced passivity (as in Sherlock Holmes), but the violence of alcohol intoxication was fairly frequently exhibited in all communities. Alcohol was hated as an old, familiar enemy; narcotics continued to have an aura of mystery.

19 W. Marmé, "Untersuchungen zur acuten und chronischen Morphinvergiftung," *Deutsch. med. Wochschr.* 9 : 197–98 (1883).

20 A. G. DuMez, "Increased Tolerance and Withdrawal Phenomena in Chronic Morphinism," *JAMA* 72 : 1069 (1919).

21 C. Gioffredi, "L'Immunité artificielle par les alcaloides," *Arch. Ital. de Biol.* 28 : 402–07 (1897); "Récherches ultérieures sur l'immunisation pour la morphine," ibid. 31 : 398–411 (1899).

22 See Leo Hirschlaff, "Ein Heilserum zur Bekampfung der Morphiumvergiftung und ähnlicher Intoxicationen," *Berliner klin. Wochschr.* 34 : 1149–52, 1174–77 (1902).

23 Ernest Simons Bishop (1876–1927) became one of the best known and most zealous American advocates of the antidote-antitoxin hypothesis of

opiate addiction. He received his M.D. from Cornell in 1908, interned and was a resident at Bellevue until 1912. He became particularly attracted to the medical treatment of addiction as resident physician in charge of the alcoholic and prison wards at Bellevue. In his first paper on the subject he praised the methods of his teacher, Dr. Lambert ("Morphinism and Its Treatment," *JAMA* 58 : 1499–1504 [1912]). The following year he announced his adherence to the antitoxin-antidote hypothesis and argued that this explanation removed the "stigma of mental and moral taint" from addiction. He claimed that the addict was wrongly "held by all of us in despite and disgust, and regarded as so depraved that their rescue is impossible and they unworthy of its attempt." Dr. Bishop now made no mention of the Lambert method and seemed under the influence of the hypothesis popularized by Dr. George Pettey, that morphine in the body stimulates antitoxin formation (see below, ch. 4, n. 24), although he does not mention Pettey's work in "Narcotic Addiction—A Systemic Disease Condition," *JAMA* 60 : 431–34 (1913). In the ensuing years Dr. Bishop increasingly emphasized that addiction was not the "popular and generally accepted" result of weakness of willpower leading to degeneration of the physical, mental, and moral being lost in "degrading thralldom," but that the addict was a sick man. The antidotal toxic substance manufactured by the body to protect it from the chronic opiate use could "be measured with mathematical exactness" and the addict could be adjusted to a precise amount of morphine so that he would appear and feel a well man. He credits Pettey with having independently come to this conclusion in "An Analysis of Narcotic Drug Addiction," *N.Y. Med. J.* 101 : 399–403 (1915). Dr. Bishop now became more confident and enthusiastic, claiming in 1915, that "without restraint, without specific remedies, without special methods, without routine medication, simply on the basis of an understanding of disease fundamentals and the application of rational therapeutics" he could treat the narcotic drug addict in the majority of cases purely on the basis of what he knew of his disease, and could restore him to health and competence. He opposed any restraint on the prescribing of opiates and denounced gradual reduction in most cases as "harmful, barbarous and futile" ("Some Fundamental Considerations of the Problem of Drug Addiction," *Amer. Med.* 21 : 807–16 [1915]).

Dr. Bishop decried the ignorance of the average physician in the treatment of addiction, which he attributed to lack of experience and training, and he favored the establishment of a legal and cheap supply of drugs for addicts until cure was available ("The Narcotic Addict, the Physician and the Law," *Med. Economist* 4 : 121–28 [1916]).

Bishop's various articles, published between 1912 and 1919, were the basis of his book, *The Narcotic Drug Problem* (New York: Macmillan, 1920), which appeared just as the New York City clinic was beginning to shatter the enthusiasm of the Health Department, and the Narcotic Division of the Prohibition Unit was deciding to close all clinics and prevent almost all maintenance. Even more coincidental was the indict-

ment of Dr. Bishop in January 1920 for violation of the Harrison Act;
he had still not been brought to trial in late 1922. The Treasury Department was accused of attempting to silence his strong stand against
the current interpretation of the Harrison Act (see "Resolution Relative
to Dr. Ernest S. Bishop," American Medical Editor's Association, 53rd
Annual Meeting, in *Amer. Med. 28* : 720–21 [1922]). The antimaintenance interpretations of the Harrison Act made Dr. Bishop's activities
futile, but in his peak years, 1912 to 1922, he was an opponent of specific cures and any laws that would restrict addicts from receiving medically supervised maintenance. He and Dr. Pettey were the chief experts
arrayed against Dr. Lambert and the Narcotic Division. His claim to be
the first proponent of the "antitoxin" hypothesis irritated other authorities (see J. McIver and G. E. Price, "Drug Addiction," *JAMA 66* : 478
[1916]) as well as the fact, probably, that he announced his "expert"
status the year he finished his residency.

24   Dr. George E. Pettey, *The Narcotic Drug Diseases and Allied Ailments*
     (Philadelphia: Davis, 1913), pp. 12–27. Dr. Pettey, prior to Dr. Bishop,
     proposed that addiction disease can be explained through formation of
     an antitoxin in reaction to the harmful effects of morphine. This hy-
     pothesis would make complete elimination of all morphine from the body
     the chief goal of treatment and make less important such "morphine-
     antagonists" as the belladonna group which figured so largely in the
     Towns-Lambert treatment. His major work, *Narcotic Drug Diseases and
     Allied Ailments*, was often quoted until the mid-1920s, and he was a
     featured speaker at New York Medical Society meetings and before the
     Whitney Committee. For a later modification of Pettey's method, em-
     ploying "catharsis of the blood stream" by means of intravenous in-
     fusions of isotonic saline, see C. S. Bluemel, "A New Treatment for the
     Morphine Habit," *JAMA 72* : 552–56 [1919]).

25   Metchnikoff (1845–1916) received the Nobel Prize in 1908. One of his
     most influential suggestions concerned the morbid effect of "intestinal
     autointoxication," which was applied to almost any disease—in this in-
     stance, addiction. The weight of his views and their reasonableness made
     autointoxication popular among physicians and the lay public; his belief
     that changing the intestinal flora could counteract the intestinal "poisons"
     and prolong life led to the fad for yogurt which still continues, although
     Metchnikoff's theoretical inspiration is forgotten.

26   Pettey, *Narcotic Drug Diseases,* pp. 58 ff.

27   A. Valenti, "Experimentelle Untersuchungen über den chronischen Mor-
     phinismus," *Arch. exper. Path. Pharmakol. 75* : 437–62 (1914); this re-
     search was among the most disputed in the debate over the "disease" of
     addiction. It was cited by Rep. Lester Volk, M.D., in his attack against
     opiate restriction to ordinary addicts (Appendix to *Cong. Rec., House, 62,
     pt. 13* : 13,340–13,345, 13 Jan. 1922, 67th Cong., 2nd Sess.). It was
     first accepted by DuMez (*JAMA 72* [1919]) and then attacked by the
     AMA Narcotic Committee of 1920 ("Report of the Committee on the
     Narcotic Drug Situation in the United States," *JAMA 74* : 1326 [1920]).

Eventually, Valenti's work was disproved to everyone's satisfaction (ch. 4, n. 40 below), but in 1918–22 each side of the disease controversy rested much of its credibility on this one line of research.

28 P. Sollier, "La Démorphinisation. Mécanisme Physiologique. Conséquences au point de vue thérapeutique," *Presse Méd.*, 23 April 1898, vol. 1, no. 34, pp. 201–02, and 6 July 1898, vol. 2, no. 56, pp. 9–10. See abstract in *Journal of Inebriety 20* : 436–40 (1898); E. S. Faust, "Über die Ursachen der Gewöhnung an Morphin," *Arch. exper. Path. Pharmakol. 44* : 217–38 (1900); M. Cloetta, "Über das Verhalten des Morphins im Organismus und die Ursachen der Angewöhnung an dasselbe," *Arch. exper. Path. Pharmakol. 50* : 453–80 (1903). W. H. Willcox, "Norman Kerr Memorial Lecture on Drug Addiction," *Brit. Med. J.*, 1 Dec. 1923, pp. 1013–18; A. Fauser and B. Ottenstein, "Chemisches und Physikalisch-Chemisches zum Problem der 'Süchten' und 'Entziehungserscheinungen,' insbesonders des Morphinismus und Cocainismus," *Ztsch. Neurol. Psychiat. 88* : 128–33 (1924).

29 Levinstein (see above, ch. 4, n. 14). Reported cure rates vary widely, but usually settle down to a rather low rate. If cure means abstinence, the rate is very low, perhaps 10%, but if cure means ability to return to a job then perhaps 30% could be considered cured, even if they did occasionally relapse. In many ways the argument over cure is similar to that in the treatment of neuroses and psychoses—"adjustment" to life often being the criterion employed, not attainment of perfect health.

In the era of therapeutic optimism, say 1905 to 1915, cure rates were estimated as high as 90% or 99%; but both before and after the decade, when the answer to "How many can be cured?" was less politically and emotionally charged, 25% was a rough approximation for treatment programs. Methadone maintenance, of course, is an "adjustment" cure, for the patient is not drug-free, and the goal is return to the community, optimally with a job. Hope for a cure is usually associated with a naïve belief that addiction is something like a cold or appendicitis and not like more frustrating chronic ailments. In each period, respected journals and scientists have swung with social attitudes and either entertained the possibility of a high cure rate or looked skeptically on such claims. Alexander Lambert is one of the highly respected clinicians who lived through pre-World War I optimism, and his publications trace his own raised and then dashed expectation for simple cures.

Some of the many papers written after the period of optimism based their studies on hospitalized patients, often those cared for in the Public Health Service Hospitals at Lexington and Fort Worth. Two papers that illustrate the epoch preceding the new forms of treatment popularized in the 1960s are: M. J. Pescor, "Prognosis in Drug Addiction" (*Amer. J. Psychiat. 97* : 1419–33 [1941]), which suggests that about 30% of addicts treated at Lexington were abstinent about three years after release, mostly according to the patients' own reports; and R. G. Knight and C. T. Prout, "A Study of Results in Hospital Treatment of Drug Addictions" (*Amer. J. Psychiat. 108* : 303–08 [1951]), based on information collected on the 75 consecutive admissions to New York Hospital, Westchester Division, between 1930 and 1950, in which barbiturates and other drugs were used as well as morphine and heroin: "36% seems to have been benefited," of which about half were abstinent "following hospitalization for one to fourteen years." In 1962 more than 90% of the addicts treated at Lexington who returned to New York became readdicted within six months according to G. H. Hunt and M. E. Odoroff, "Follow-up Study of Narcotic Drug Addicts after Hospitalization," *Pub. Health Reports* 77 : 41–54 (1962). A study of addicts released in Kentucky suggested that if the criterion of successful treatment were revised to include "some period of complete abstinence during the follow-up period," 76% of male addicts would be considered aided by treatment (J. A. O'Donnel, "A Follow-up of Narcotic Addicts: Mortality, Relapse and Abstinence," *Amer. J. Orthopsychiatry* 34 : 948–54 [1964]). For a recent survey of treatment success which concludes that "none of the presently available approaches to treatment of drug abuse can be expected to be successful with more than a small percentage of the drug-abusing population, and all approaches combined will have an undoubtedly limited effect," see R. M. Glasscote, J. Jaffe, J. N. Sussex, J. Ball, and L. Brill, *The Treatment of Drug Abuse: Programs, Problems and Prospects* (Washington, D.C.: Joint Information Service of the American Psychiatric Association and the National Association for Mental Health, 1972).

30   T. D. Crothers, *Morphinism and Narcomanias from Other Drugs* (Philadelphia: Saunders, 1902), p. 150; see also T. D. Crothers, "Drug Addictions and Their Treatment," *Med. Record* 90 : 238–41 (1916). Thomas Davidson Crothers (1842–1918) received the M.D. degree from Albany Medical College in 1865 and in 1881 organized the Walnut Lodge Hospital in Hartford, Conn., for the treatment of alcohol and opiate inebriates. He edited the *Journal of Inebriety* from 1876 to 1918. He was also a professor in the Boston College of Physicians and Surgeons and its dean in 1908. This medical school is described by Abraham Flexner after a visit in 1909 as a private institution which depended on tuition fees for its existence. The entrance requirements were called "vague," the facilities "wretched," clinical resources "dubious," and the dispensary "miserable" (A. Flexner, *Medical Education in the United States and Canada* [New York: Carnegie Foundation for the Advancement of Teaching, Bulletin no. 4, 1910], p. 242).

31   C. B. Pearson, "The Treatment of Morphinism," *Med. Times* 42 : 245–46 (1914). Pearson, like Bishop, wrote on behalf of the addict's personal worth, as in "A Plea for Greater Consideration for the Opium Addict" (*Med. Record* 83 : 342–43 [1913]), reacting against the more general depreciation of the addict among physicians as well as laymen.

32   Pearson, "Treatment of Morphinism," p. 246. Pearson's optimism was matched by C. J. Douglas, superintendent of the Douglas Sanitarium in Dorchester, Mass., who claimed in 1908 that he had yet to meet with his first failure. Douglas put his patients to sleep during withdrawal ("Narcotic Method of Treating Morphinism," *Med. Record* 74 : 404–05 [1908]).

33   Biographical sketches of Towns are found in two articles: Samuel Mer-

win, "Fighting the Deadly Habits: The Story of Charles B. Towns," *American Magazine,* Oct. 1912, pp. 708–17; and Peter Clark MacFarland, "The 'White Hope' of Drug Victims: An Everyday American Fighter," *Collier's,* 29 Nov. 1913, pp. 16–17. My description of Towns's life and progress up to the Shanghai Commission is largely taken from these articles, which were based upon interviews with Towns; there is no evidence that he was displeased with their adulatory tone or the outline of his life. In the years of his greatest credibility, 1908–20, magazines that featured articles by him included *Survey,* the highly respected journal of social welfare, *The Literary Digest, The Century Magazine, American Review of Reviews,* and *The Medical Review of Reviews.* At the height of his career he published *Habits That Handicap: The Menace of Opium, Alcohol, and Tobacco, and the Remedy* (New York: Century, 1915), with a preface by Dr. Richard C. Cabot of Harvard, one of America's most eminent physicians and social reformers, who described Towns as knowing "more about the alleviation and cure of drug addictions than any doctor that I have ever seen" (p. viii) and an appendix by Dr. Alexander Lambert, "The Relation of Alcohol to Disease." The mind reels at the thought of how magnificently Towns could have promoted an effective cure.

Towns was so prominent an authority on addiction that some newspapers and nonmedical periodicals occasionally referred to him as "Dr." Towns, an understandable error, and as recently as 1972 he appeared as "Dr. Towne" in Norman Zinberg and J. A. Robertson, *Drugs and the Public* (New York: Simon and Schuster, 1972), p. 59, and in E. M. Brecher, *Licit and Illicit Drugs* (Boston: Little Brown, 1972), pp. 46 passim. Towns's nonexistent doctorate seems to date from an earlier claim that he was one of the first "physicians" to recognize the addictive "triad" of compulsive need for an opiate, tolerance, and withdrawal signs upon abrupt withdrawal. See Marie Nyswander, *The Drug Addict as a Patient* (New York: Grune, 1956), pp. 1–13. In a recent study by Rufus King, *The Drug Hang-up: America's Fifty Year Folly* (New York: W. W. Norton, 1972, p. 24), Towns shifts occupations and becomes a New York State Senator.

34 9 Jan. 1908 (WP, entry 51).

35 See above, ch. 2, n. 4; I have not been able to identify Dr. Thomas. Perhaps he was Dr. Henry M. Thomas, at that time clinical professor of nervous diseases at Johns Hopkins. Towns later claimed that Dr. Victor Heiser, Commissioner of Health in the Philippines, said that he had treated 700 cases of addiction "with highly satisfactory results" (Charles B. Towns to Dr. Hamilton Wright, 13 June 1911 (WP, entry 36). Dr. Heiser recalled that Towns had an effective treatment of alcoholism at his hospital (My interview with Dr. Victor Heiser, in New York City, 25 March 1970).

36 Acting Secretary of State to Delegates of the United States to the International Opium Conference, 18 Oct. 1911 (WP, entry 38).

37 Alexander Lambert, "Obliteration of the Craving for Narcotics," *JAMA* 53 : 985–89 (1909), esp. p. 986. The Towns-Lambert method was criticized by Pettey (*Narcotic Drug Diseases,* pp. 401–24) for, among

other defects, being too brief, approaching the disease as a "vice," and using too drastic medication. Another criticism of the shortness of the treatment came from C. C. Wholey, a Pittsburgh psychiatrist, who also found it of little value in alcoholism and found that the "typical stool" was not a useful sign ("Dangers and Inconsistencies in Some Notable Short-Time Treatments for Drug Addictions," *JAMA* 64 : 390–92 [1915]). Lambert's association with the Towns Hospital, even if he did not personally profit from the highly successful operation, was another source of attack, for example from the *Medical Economist* of New York, and from other physicians who felt economically threatened by the lay-operated hospital.

Shortly after his initial article, Lambert's recommendations were evaluated in an unsigned review article (*JAMA* 54 : 794–95 [1910]) which generally praised the treatment but cast some doubt on the high percentage of cures claimed, suggesting that probably little more than half remained cured. Yet Lambert's approach was the dominant "respectable" specific treatment among physicians for about a decade. In 1913 he again described his treatment ("The Treatment of Narcotic Addiction," *JAMA* 60 : 1933–36 [1913]) with about the same enthusiasm. Sir William Osler, the most eminent physician in the English-speaking world, chose Lambert to write the chapter "Alcohol, Opium, Morphinism, Cocaine" in the 1914 edition of *Modern Medicine,* edited by William Osler and T. McCrae, 2nd rev. ed., 2 vols. (Philadelphia: Lea and Febiger, 1914), 2 : 396–499. Lambert was even more confident in this text than in the *JAMA.* He claimed that "this [Towns] treatment in my hands in some 800 patients has proved so successful that 80 per cent have remained well" (p. 445). In the pre-Harrison Act description, Lambert calls attention to the "perfect egotism" of morphinism, which is "often given to explosions of intense rage" making the addict destructive and dangerous (p. 439).

Lambert's conversion to psychological factors as the determinant in addiction was reflected in January 1920 in *Modern Medicine,* a new journal devoted to industrial and social medicine, of which he was one of the editors. Later, of course, he was attracted to Narcosan, and by the time of his death at the age of 78 in 1939, he may have been disillusioned about narcotic treatments.

38 Alexander Lambert, "Obliteration of the Craving for Narcotics," *JAMA* 53 : 985 (1909).

39 E. J. Pellini, "Report of the Special Committee on Public Health of the Greater City of New York to the House of Delegates of the New York State Medical Society," *N.Y. State J. Med.* 20 : 117 (1920).

40 By 1919 the crucial difference of opinion among medical authorities was whether there existed in the body a chemical produced in response to the presence of morphine and directly related to "addiction disease." Advocating a substance in the blood were Drs. E. S. Bishop, L. D. Volk, C. F. J. Laase, and the occasional visitor from Memphis, Dr. Pettey; opposed were Drs. Lambert, Hubbard, and A. C. Prentice. By at least the fall of 1919, Dr. E. J. Pellini, Assistant City Chemist, was conducting

experiments at Bellevue Hospital to locate the toxin in the blood claimed by Gioffredi, or the protective substance claimed by Valenti. Pellini was supported by Dr. Lambert; his papers, which sought to disprove either contention, had an unusual co-author, Arthur D. Greenfield, a New York attorney who had made a special study of addiction and the laws affecting it.

Dr. Pellini's research, which still stands fifty years later, was a major victory for the antimaintenance forces. At last it was possible to discredit the antibody doctors as unscientific, the very charge they had made against the antimaintainers. The Internal Revenue Bureau looked upon the antibody theorists as their special enemies. In a report on the New York situation made to the Assistant Commissioner of Internal Revenue, Thomas Cooper described his meeting with Dr. Pellini and his search for "the elusive antibody" expressing disbelief in such a theory (T. A. Cooper to H. M. Gaylord, 22 Oct. 1919, RPU). He also prepared a memorandum of a conversation with Major D. L. Porter, Revenue Agent in Charge, who told of difficulties being given the law enforcers by promoters of the antibody theory. Major Porter said that Dr. Bishop was under suspicion and that Dr. C. F. J. Laase, "his chief lieutenant in self-advertising propaganda," was under indictment for writing 13,000 prescriptions for addicts. Although his fellow "conspirators" pleaded guilty, Dr. Laase was acquitted after trial in federal district court July 1920 and died, apparently of a heart attack, the following month (N.Y. Times, 22 Aug. 1920). "These physicians," Cooper commented, "assume the attitude of being above and beyond the law" (Thomas A. Cooper, "Visit to New York City in Connection with the Narcotic Situation in That City," 21 Oct. 1919, RPU).

The Bureau of Internal Revenue sent a questionnaire on the antibody theory to leading clinicians and scientists in the U.S. apparently in the second half of 1919; 3 replies endorsed the theory, 27 rejected it, and 12 were noncommittal. The chief reason for rejecting the theory was that the experiments of Valenti and Gioffredi were not reproducible and that since morphine was not a protein, it could not stimulate antibody formation (*Digest of Replies: Antibody Questionnaire*, RPU; the exact date of the replies cannot be determined, but from internal evidence the digest seems to have been prepared in 1919 or very early 1920. For further details see below, ch. 6, n. 72).

When Dr. Pellini and colleagues believed they had proof of the non-existence of antibodies, they concluded that there was no organic basis for the abstinence syndrome, that abstinence had a "functional" or "psychological" cause (see above, ch. 4, n. 39). Their opponents, such as Rep. Volk, ignored the evidence and expressed confidence in Valenti and Gioffredi. That is, both sides appear to have decided to fight the battle of addiction's possible organic basis on the question of antibodies, and the Pellini advocates seemed to assume that if there were no antibodies, there was no organic basis for addiction. The intransigence in both camps led to the ferocity and hostility which now motivated much of the debate.

Pellini's refutation of Gioffredi is found in E. J. Pellini and A. D. Greenfield, "Narcotic Drug Addiction: I. The Formation of Protective Substances against Morphine," *Arch. Internal Med.* 26 : 279–92 (1920), his refutation of Valenti's research in "II. The Presence of Toxic Substances in the Serum in Morphine Addiction," ibid. 33 : 547–65 (1924). When A. G. DuMez of the PHS appeared to accept Valenti's contentions in a review article of 1919 (*JAMA 72* [1919]), he was criticized by the AMA Narcotic Committee which elicited a degree of retraction from him. DuMez replied to the committee's request for clarification (letter dated 17 March 1920, *JAMA 74* : 1326 [1920]), that Valenti's research "has not been conclusively proven." For later research in the 1920s which also questioned the existence of a detectable substance in the bodies of addicts caused by the use of opiates, see below, ch. 4, nn. 45, 47.

41 With the demise of specific treatments and immunological mechanisms, the AMA Narcotic Committee report of 8 May 1920 ("Report of the Committee on the Narcotic Drug Situation in the United States," *JAMA 74* : 1326 [1920]) sought answers in social science, psychotherapy, vocational rehabilitation, aptitude tests, "careful follow-up," a wise probation system, and in particular the "new psychology"—psychoanalysis. In advice which echoes the style of Shaw's Sir Ralph Bloomfield Bonington's admonition to "stimulate the phagocytes!", the AMA committee advocated a program to "irradiate and sublimate" the libido. Interestingly, the medical background of *The Doctor's Dilemma* (1913) is almost identical with that of the antibody craze in the treatment of addiction in the U.S. The great discovery in Shaw's play is an amazing vaccine which cured tuberculosis according to immunological theories of Metchnikoff, who, in addition to postulating the dire effects of intestinal autointoxication, described the phagocytosis of bacteria by white corpuscles.

42 Cf. Pellini, *N.Y. State J. Med.* 20 : 119 (1920). Lambert recalled in 1920 how some years earlier he had checked on 200 cases he had treated about 1909 and found to his regret that only 4% or 5% had remained abstinent. This revealed to him the essential place of aftercare in addiction treatment.

43 The disinterest of physicians in treating addicts does not seem to be explained by the threat of enforcement agencies in the period before 1919 or 1915. Although police and narcotic agents did use threats and intimidation as well as arrest, particularly after 1919, lack of knowledge or interest, or the unwillingness of most general physicians to treat addicts, was a source of comment well before the legal repression of addiction maintenance. Even a few addicts could disrupt a respectable physician's waiting room, particularly if they were lower class. The effect of an addict's abstinence syndrome on other waiting-room patients, lack of effective treatment reflecting on the physician's competence, and perhaps primarily, the typical physician's attitude toward the addict as a moral reprobate, which Dr. Bishop himself so eloquently described in 1912 (see above, ch. 4, n. 23), made the physician hesitate to treat addicts. Therefore when enforcement agents began to try to stop the

activities of addiction maintainers, they acted with the support of many in the medical profession.

44   L. Kolb, "Pleasure and Deterioration from Narcotic Addiction," *Mental Hygiene* 9 : 699–724 (1925), esp. p. 723. Dr. Lawrence Kolb, Sr. (1881–1972), entered the Public Health Service in 1909 and retired in 1944, as an assistant surgeon general. He served as head of the Mental Hygiene Division (now the National Institute of Mental Health). His career in the PHS bridges the era from Martin I. Wilbert and A. G. DuMez to that of contemporary medical experts. In the 1920s Dr. Kolb supported strict interpretation of the Harrison Act and believed that restraint had a very marked effect on reducing the number of addicts in the nation. In 1935 he became the first medical director of the Lexington Narcotic Farm. There he grew increasingly doubtful of the efficacy of jailing addicts and enforcing treatment. He has been critical of the former Federal Bureau of Narcotics and Commissioner Harry J. Anslinger for inculcating a fearsome picture of opiate addiction. In 1956 Kolb supported an experimental maintenance plan proposed by the New York Academy of Medicine and strongly opposed in 1951 and 1955 severe federal laws against opiate, marihuana, and cocaine use.

45   Research in Philadelphia was subsidized by funds from the Committee on Drug Addictions of which Dr. Terry was the executive secretary. The Philadelphia Committee for the Clinical Study of Opium Addiction was organized in 1925, conducted most of its research in Philadelphia General Hospital, and published its results in the *Archives of Internal Medicine* in 1929 and 1930. The papers were collected with an introduction and summary and published as *Opium Addiction* (1930) by the AMA. Internist in Charge was Dr. Arthur B. Light; Dr. E. G. Torrance and others were associates. The major topics included physical condition of the opiate addict, presence of any characteristic substance in the blood during morphine administration and after abrupt withdrawal, effect of scopolamine on addiction, and the excretion of morphine.

46   Alexander Lambert and F. Tilney, "The Treatment of Narcotic Addiction by Narcosan," *Med. J. Record* 124 : 764 (1926). By 1928, New York City was spending $25,000 to $50,000 annually on Narcosan treatment (R. C. Patterson, New York City Commissioner of Correction, to Rep. Stephen Porter, 15 May 1928, printed in *Establishment of Two Federal Narcotic Farms, Hearings before the House Judiciary Committee on HR 12, 781 and HR 13, 645*, 26–28 April 1928, 70th Cong., 1st Sess., rev. print., 1928, p. 132). The next year Lambert declared Narcosan to have "no merit" as a result of more careful clinical studies (*JAMA* 92 : 147 [1929]).

47   "Report of the Mayor's Committee on Drug Addiction," *Amer. J. Psychiat.* 10 : 433–538 (1930), esp. pp. 534–35. That current addiction theories and treatments based on them are inadequate is also concluded in L. Kolb and C. K. Himmelsbach, "Clinical Studies of Drug Addiction: III. A Critical Review of the Withdrawal Treatments with a Method of Evaluating Abstinence Syndromes," Suppl. 128 to *Public Health Reports* (GPO, 1938).

48 Statement of Rep. Stephen G. Porter, *Establishment of Two Federal Narcotic Farms,* hearings, p. 19; Rep. John J. Cochran, *Cong. Rec., House,* 69 : 9413, 21 May 1928, 70th Cong., 1st Sess. (GPO, 1928).

49 Recent standard descriptions of the effects of narcotics and summary of research findings include: J. Jaffe, "Narcotic Analgesics" and "Drug Addiction and Drug Abuse," in L. Goodman and A. Gilman, eds., *The Pharmacological Basis of Therapeutics,* 4th ed. (New York: Macmillan, 1970), pp. 237–313; and A. Wikler, "Opioid Addiction," in A. M. Freedman and H. I. Kaplan, eds., *Comprehensive Textbook of Psychiatry* (Baltimore: Williams and Wilkins, 1967), pp. 989–1003.

50 A. Wikler, "Opioid Addiction," pp. 996 ff., slightly rephrased.

51 Charles B. Towns, *Drugs and Alcohol Sickness* (New York: M. M. Barbour, 1932), pp. 15–16.

52 Charles B. Towns, *The Physician's Guide for the Treatment of the Drug Habit and Alcoholism* (n.p., n.d.), p. 7. This pamphlet of 8 pages appears to have been published about 1914, for the *Medical Economist* begins quoting from it then. It reveals that the charge in advance for a 5-day treatment varied from $200 to $350, depending on accommodations in the more expensive main building; in the Annex, "for patients of moderate means" willing to share a room with one or two other patients, the charge was $75.

53 Alexander Lambert, "The Treatment of Narcotic Addiction," *JAMA 60* : 1933–36 (1913).

54 See ch. 4, n. 42.

55 Towns, *Physicians' Guide,* pp. 6–7; Charles B. Towns, *Reclaiming the Drinker* (New York: Barnes, 1931), pp. 75–76.

56 Richard C. Cabot, "The Towns-Lambert Treatment for Morphinism and Alcoholism," *Boston Med. Surg. J. 164* : 676–77 (1911), p. 676. Cabot was a consultant to a Brookline sanitarium, founded in November 1910, which used the Towns method. Dr. Cabot was as distinguished as Lambert and is credited with having inaugurated social work in American hospitals and pioneering psychiatric social work training. His contributions to social work, his medical services, and teaching of physicians were of the highest quality. His adoption of the Towns method can hardly be attributed to mercenary motives or ignorance. See his entry in *Dictionary of American Biography,* vol. 22, Suppl. 2 (New York: Scribner's, 1958).

57 Alexander Lambert, "Obliteration of the Craving for Narcotics," *JAMA 53* : 989 (1909).

Chapter 5

1 *Laws of Pennsylvania of the Session of 1860,* Act no. 374, Title I, Section 70, "Selling Poisons," p. 401; *Ohio Laws: 1885–1887,* vol. 82, p. 49, passed 6 Feb. 1885. The Illinois law against cocaine was approved 11 June 1897 (*Laws of Illinois* [1897], p. 138). It allowed cocaine sale only on a physician's or dentist's prescription and refilling was prohibited.

2 Martin I. Wilbert and Murray Galt Motter, *Digest of Laws and Regulations in Force in the United States Relating to the Possession, Use, Sale,*

and Manufacture of Poisons and Habit-forming Drugs, Public Health
Bulletin no. 56, Nov. 1912 (GPO, 1912).

3 The belief in two classes of addicts, one bad and one either good or
   morally neutral, is a common conclusion of writers on narcotic use. Dr.
   George Wood (1868) describes the benevolent effects of opium on the
   healthy, but its baneful effects on the weak-willed. In this century in the
   U.S., the "underworld" user of narcotics was to be dealt with severely,
   but the "average" addicted person was to be pitied. Similarly in the
   Treasury Committee Report of 1919 the two classes of addicts were
   distinguished (*Special Committee of Investigation Appointed March 25
   1918, by the Secretary of the Treasury: Traffic in Narcotic Drugs,* GPO,
   1919).

4 When addiction maintenance became specifically legalized in New York
   State (July 1917) the *Medical Economist* began a series of articles
   enumerating reasons for a physician to use opiates, partly as an induce-
   ment to the mass of physicians to assume some of the supply to addicts
   which had previously been borne by peddlers and other sources. "Opium
   —The Obligation of the Physician to Use It" appeared monthly from
   July through December 1917. The journal's attitude is characterized by
   a statement appearing in the August installment (5 : 143): "the law has
   deliberately said that [the physician] alone can use it and thus this wonderful medicine is wholly in our hands for use in the healing and medi-
   ating art of medicine." Most physicians, to judge from the tone of the
   series, were not inclined to treat addicts, even if such care was legal.

5 J. H. Young, *The Toadstool Millionaires* (Princeton Univ. Press, 1961),
   pp. 211–14, 237.

6 L. F. Kebler, *Habit-forming Agents: Their Indiscriminate Sale and Use,
   a Menace to the Public Welfare,* Agriculture Dept., Farmer's Bulletin no.
   393, April 1910 (GPO, 1910), pp. 15–18.

7 This amendment declared a label or package misbranded if any "statement, design, or device regarding the curative or therapeutic effect of
   such article or any of the ingredients or substances contained therein
   . . . is false and fraudulent." The amendment was approved 23 Aug.
   1912 (ch. 352, 37 *Stat. L.,* 416). See J. H. Young, *Medical Messiahs*
   (Princeton Univ. Press, 1961), pp. 49–51.

8 "Report of the Commission on Proprietary Medicines, American Pharmaceutical Association," *JAPhA* 5 : 1376–81 (1916).

9 J. P. Street, "The Patent Medicine Situation," *Amer. J. Publ. Health* 7 :
   1037–42 (1917).

10 For the role of the Public Health Service in the federal government see
   A. H. Dupree, *Science in the Federal Government* (Cambridge: Harvard
   Univ. Press, 1957), pp. 262 ff.

11 My interview with Dr. Robert Fischelis, Washington, D.C., 28 July 1970.

12 J. K. Thum, "Martin I. Wilbert," *Amer. J. Pharmacy* 89 : 49–61 (1917).

13 Wilbert and Motter, *Digest of Laws.*

14 Thum, "Martin I. Wilbert," p. 51.

15 Charles E. Terry and Mildred Pellens, *The Opium Problem* (New York:
   Bureau of Social Hygiene, 1928; reprint ed., Montclair, N.J.: Patterson

Smith, 1970). Terry (1878–1945) received his M.D. degree from the University of Maryland in 1903 and later became the first full-time health officer of Jacksonville (1910–17). After serving as medical editor of *Delineator* magazine, he became executive secretary of the Committee on Drug Addictions formed in 1921, funded by the Bureau of Social Hygiene, a private research organization supported by such philanthropists as Paul M. Warburg and John D. Rockefeller, Jr. He prepared *The Opium Problem* with the aid of Mildred Pellens, whom he later married. When his position on the bureau terminated, he served at the Harlem Valley Hospital in New York until his death. Terry was closely associated with the American Public Health Association, and many of his articles appeared in the *Journal* of the APHA between 1912 and 1923. For further details see Edward R. Smith, "Seven Years of Pioneering in Preventive Medicine," *J. Florida Med. Assoc.* 53 : 725–28 (1966). I am indebted to Dr. Smith of the Florida State Department of Health and Welfare for providing information on Dr. Terry's life.

16 Charles E. Terry, "Drug Addictions, A Public Health Problem," *AJPH* 4 : 28–37 (1914), p. 28. Subsequent information and quotations are from the same source.

17 *Public Acts of Tennessee, 1913,* ch. 11, pp. 403–07, approved 25 Sept. 1913, effective 1 Jan. 1914.

18 Lucius P. Brown, "Enforcement of the Tennessee Anti-narcotic Law," *AJPH* 5 : 323–33 (1915). Subsequent information and quotations are from the same source.

19 Edward Marshall, "Drug Evil Now the Target of Fierce Attack," N.Y. *Times,* 9 Feb. 1913. See above, Chapter 4, for a full description of medical support for Towns.

20 His hospital acquired "medical consultants" like Alexander Lambert and Samuel W. Lambert who at the time was dean of the College of Physicians and Surgeons (Columbia); Smith Ely Jelliffe was founder of the *Psychoanalytic Review* and co-author (with William Alanson White) of the leading American text of psychiatry; the other consultants to the Towns hospital were Drs. George Montague Swift and James Watt Fleming.

21 Edward Marshall, "Drug Evil," N.Y. *Times,* 9 Feb. 1913.

22 Innumerable jibes and attacks directed at Towns appeared in the *Medical Economist,* e.g. "Townes [*sic*] on the Law and Medicine on Townes" (2 : 327–35 [1914]). Yet to medical specialists he seemed reputable as evidenced by his staff of consultants, and also respected by laymen such as Henry Ford, who chose to send addicted and alcoholic workers to the Towns Hospital for treatment (N.Y. *Times,* 8 July 1915).

23 *Laws of New York, 1913,* ch. 470, pp. 984–91; approved 9 May 1913.

24 Earlier restrictions in the public health laws forbidding refilling of prescriptions and sale of dangerous drugs without prescription were admitted to be commonly violated and rarely enforced (*Amer. Drug. Pharmaceut. Rec.* 52 : 255 [1908]).

25 See e.g. N.Y. *Times,* 1 Nov. 1915, which reports 700 violations after enactment of the Boylan law. Also see C. F. Collins, "The Drug Evil and

the Drug Law," *Monthly Bull. Dept. Health N.Y. City* 9 : 1–24 (1919), esp. p. 4.

26 N.Y. *Times,* 22 Jan., 31 Jan. 1914. Also see Collins, "Drug Evil," p. 4.

27 The Vanderbilt Committee was composed of numerous officials and authorities already active in the narcotic problem, e.g. Katherine Bement Davis, New York City Commissioner of Corrections, and later executive secretary of the Bureau of Social Hygiene; Justice Cornelius Collins, chief magistrate of New York City, and so on. In 1916 the various officials and committees concerned with narcotic control in New York City were consolidated into one group (Collins, "Drug Evil," pp. 4–6). The bill the Vanderbilt Committee favored was introduced by Senator J. J. Frawley in March 1914, and the Towns measure was again introduced by Senator Boylan. A modified form of the Boylan bill was later endorsed by the Vanderbilt Committee, and the Boylan Act was signed by the governor on 14 April 1914. A long article by Marshall on Towns's efforts was again carried in the N.Y. *Times* on 22 February 1914. The *Times* on 17 April erroneously ascribed the Boylan bill to the Vanderbilt Committee's efforts, which prompted Boylan's outburst. See Letters to the Editor, N.Y. *Times,* 20 April 1914.

28 *Laws of New York, 1914,* ch. 363, pp. 1120–24.

29 Ibid., sect. 249a, pp. 1123–24.

30 J. A. Cutter, in the *Medical Economist,* commented that the general press omitted mention of this feature of the Boylan law ("Medical Economics of the Boylan Law," 2 : 296 [1914]).

31 N.Y. *Times,* 21 June 1914; also see N.Y. *Times,* 1 July 1914.

32 N.Y. *Times,* 8 July 1914.

33 N.Y. *Times,* 15 July 1914; also 6 Jan. 1915. See also Collins, "Drug Evil," pp. 4–5.

34 Amendments to the Boylan Act, *Laws of New York, 1915,* ch. 327, pp. 1017–22; became law on 17 April 1915 to take effect immediately.

35 Collins, "Drug Evil," p. 5.

36 N.Y. *Times,* 15 April 1915.

37 Ibid.; similarly, Philadelphia provided hospital beds (C. B. Farr, "Narcotic Habitués and Their Treatment," *JAMA* 64 : 1270–71 [1915]); as did Chicago (C. E. Sceleth, "What We Believe to Be Facts Concerning Drug Addicts," *Ill. Med. J.* 46 : 70–72 [1924]).

38 F. A. McGuire and P. M. Lichtenstein, "The Drug Habit," *Med. Record* 80 : 185–91 (1916); the authors treated in The Tombs 12,000 addicts in 12 years and reported no deaths from withdrawal of opiates. They concluded that no physician should be allowed to treat a patient outside a sanitarium or hospital, that heroin addicts tended to be young, white Americans, and that opiate addicts tended to steal to maintain their habit and were not given to violence.

39 Leaders of the AMA and the New York medical groups shared society's disapproval of the medical profession for "creating addicts," and some were prepared to support very stringent steps to limit the freedom of addicts.

40 This editorial also criticized the Boylan and Harrison Acts for not making

provision for long-term addicts. The N.Y. *Times* picked up this idea in a sympathetic editorial on 18 May 1915.

41 O. Rotter, "Causes, History, and Achievements of the Medical Economic Movement in N.Y.," *Med. Economist 1* : 4–11 (1913); "New Police Regulations for Doctors' Autos," editorial, *ibid. 6* : 41 (1918); L. D. Volk, "The Existing Economic Evils of the Medical Profession," ibid. *2* : 276–82 (1914). By 1914, the League had changed its name to The Federation of Medical Economic Leagues.

42 A. Goldman, "An Appeal to the Few from the Many," ibid. *1* : 60–64 (1913); Goldman claimed that those on top "with their prestige and power . . . could exert tremendous influence for our economic progress. Through their connections with various institutions, they could bring about reforms in a gradual and orderly way. But right here is where they fear to be identified with our movement. They leave our ranks and align themselves with opposing forces."

43 Membership estimates for the Federation of Medical Economic Leagues are based on statements made in the *Medical Economist* (*1* : 11, *2* : 138, *4* : 221): in August 1913, 1,000; the following year, 350 in Kings County and a total of "several thousand in Manhattan, Bronx and Kings"; and in 1916, 3,000. The number of physicians in New York State rose from 14,117 to 15,877 from 1910 to 1920 (James G. Burrow, *AMA, Voice of American Medicine* [Baltimore: Johns Hopkins Press, 1963], p. 403), and the number in New York City was about 7,000 in 1911 (*Medical Directory of New York, New Jersey and Connecticut*, Medical Society of the State of New York, 1911, vol. 13, p. 15).

44 Lester David Volk (1884–1962). See obit., N.Y. *Times,* 1 May 1962; also *Biographical Directory of American Congressmen, 1774–1961*, p. 1756.

45 L. D. Volk, "Organization of the Medical Profession," *Med. Economist 3* : 202–04 (1915).

46 The New York City Health Department, however, opposed addiction maintenance, and the regular medical societies as well as the Federation of Medical Economic Leagues opposed such severe restrictions on the private physician. The various forces now committed to the narcotic fight—the Hearst papers, Towns, various medical groups including private practitioners and public health officials, the drug trades, and rising public concern—led in 1916 to an impasse in the legislature. Dr. John P. Davin led the fight against the Towns-Hearst bill for the Medical Economic League and became a familiar medicopolitical figure in New York State by opposing any encroachments by the state on the private practitioner. After the bill was defeated, Volk wrote a glowing report of the success of the league in fighting on behalf of the humble practitioner ("The Defeat of the Boylan Bill," *Med. Economist 4* : 100–03 [1916]).

47 Authorized by a concurrent resolution of the Senate and Assembly in April 1916, appointed in September. The preliminary report appeared in February 1917. Members of the committee were George H. Whitney, chairman, George R. Brennan, R. M. Prangen, John J. Boylan, and Maurice Bloch. The committee gave considerable prominence to Dr.

Bishop's theories in the preliminary report and could be said to have accepted his view of addiction disease, which included the need for maintenance in many instances ("Preliminary Report of Joint Legislative Committee Appointed to Investigate and Examine the Laws in Relation to the Distribution and Sale of So-called Habit-forming Narcotic Drugs," N.Y. State Legislature, Senate Doc. no. 31, 17 Feb. 1917, Albany).

48   N.Y. *Times,* 14 Dec. 1916.

49   Dr. Emerson (1874–1957) was one of the leading public health educators and administrators in the nation. He was Health Commissioner of New York City from 1915 to 1917 and later professor of public health administration at Columbia (1922–40). In 1922 he headed a committee of the Council on Public Health and Instruction of the AMA which sought to write a model state antinarcotic law with the support of the NDTC and other health professions. The model law prepared in March 1922 closely followed contemporary strict interpretations of the Harrison Act (see Terry and Pellens, *Opium Problem,* pp. 893–96, 904–05). For provisions prohibiting addiction maintenance and some of the drug trades' opposition to "excessive" legal restrictions on the health professions, see "An Unsatisfactory 'Model' Law," *Druggists Circular 66 :* 423–24 (1922).

50   Although authorized to maintain addicts "pending treatment" after 1 July 1917 (*Laws of New York, 1917,* ch. 431, sect. 249a), the N.Y. City Health Department did not do so and preferred to send the addict directly to a hospital for detoxification. See "Drug addicts: A Public Health Problem," *Weekly Bull. Dept. Health City of N.Y. 6 :* 305–07 (29 Sept. 1917). Later regulations emphasizing "temporary" maintenance before treatment were issued by State Health Commissioner Herman Biggs (see ibid., pp. 394–95).

51   N.Y. *Times,* 5 Dec. 1916.

52   Bishop's views were fairly closely followed in the preliminary report (see above, ch. 5, n. 47); also see N.Y. *Times* editorial of 11 Dec. 1916.

53   Quoted by Collins, "Drug Evil," pp. 12–13.

54   *Med. Economist 4 :* 109–10 (1916). The league took pride in its influence on the committee. See ibid. *5 :* 72–73 (1917), where excerpts from the two reports are compared in parallel columns.

55   Ibid. See also ibid. *6 :* 445 (1918), where approval seems dependent on Senator Whitney's becoming head of the proposed State Narcotic Control Commission.

56   *Laws of New York, 1917,* ch. 431, 9 May 1917 (effective 1 July 1917).

57   *Laws of New York, 1917,* ch. 431, sect. 248; "Report, Special Meeting of Medical Society of the County of New York, 23 June 1919," *N.Y. Med. J. 110 :* 130–31 (1919).

58   *Laws of New York, 1917,* ch. 431, sect. 249a.

59   Collins, "Drug Evil," pp. 8–9.

60   "Report of Committee on the Drug Evil," Jan. 1918, in Collins, "Drug Evil," p. 9.

61   "Final Report of the Joint Committee Appointed to Investigate the Laws

in Relation to the Distribution and Sale of Narcotic Drugs," New York State Legislature, Senate Doc. no. 35, 1 March 1918, p. 3.

62 Concern over addiction among returned servicemen was commonly expressed. Towns feared 500,000 addicts would return from the war. German spies and machinations to spread addiction appeared in several articles in the N.Y. *Times*: "Narcotic Inquiry in Camps" (28 May 1918); "Germans Sold Drugs to Debauch Soldiers" (20 Aug. 1918); and on 13 September 1918 the Preliminary Report of the Secretary of the Treasury Committee on Narcotics is quoted as evidence that thousands of draftees were being rejected in New York because of preexisting addiction, and that perhaps 200,000 addicts between ages 21 and 31 lived in New York. A stricter federal law was demanded. An unusual and now amusing account of German ingenuity was described in a *Times* editorial of 18 December 1918. The *Times* cautioned that the story was "probably a mere invention" but described how the Kaiser's scientists planned to addict the world by secretly inserting addictive drugs into tubes of exported toothpaste. The drugged toothpaste allegedly had been test-marketed among African natives.

  Actually, of 2,510,791 men examined at local draft boards, 1,488 addicts were discovered, of whom 54 were permitted to enter the service. Addicts were found to come predominantly from large urban centers, New York City in particular (1,022 urban, 466 rural). Of the urban group, 383 came from New York State (A. G. Love and C. B. Davenport, *Defects Found in Drafted Men*, War Dept. [GPO, 1920], pp. 359–60, esp. p. 766). One factor that might have alarmed the federal government was that more addicts than alcoholics were discovered among the examined men; only 853 cases of alcoholism were diagnosed among the men between the ages of 21 and 31 (pp. 359–60).

63 Collins, "Drug Evil," p. 7, quoting his "Report to the State Association of Magistrates" of Feb. 1915.

64 A separate commission was established rather than giving the task to the State's Health Department, which was weary and discouraged after its responsibility for narcotic control under the First Whitney Act; see N.Y. *Times* of 8 May 1919; also "Statement of Deputy Commissioner Matthias Nicoll, Jr." (*Proceedings of Conference of State and Provincial Health Authorities* 37 : 116 [1922]): "These are primarily police matters and I speak from experience of one year during which the State Health Department was given legislative control of narcotic drugs in warning you to make every effort to prevent such a prerogative being forced upon you by legislative action. You will accomplish little or nothing and what you do accomplish will be at the expense of strictly public health work." In 1923 Dr. Nicoll succeeded Dr. Herman M. Biggs as State Commissioner of Health.

65 "Final Report," New York State Legislature, Senate Doc. no. 35, 1 March 1918.

66 See above, ch. 5, n. 54.

67 New York State Narcotic Control Commission, hereafter cited as

NYSNCC, *First Annual Report,* 10 April 1919 (Albany, N.Y.: J. B. Lyon and Co., 1920), pp. 3–4; NYSNCC, *Second Annual Report,* 15 April 1920 (Albany, N.Y.: J. B. Lyon and Co., 1920), p. 4.

68 NYSNCC, *Second Annual Report,* p. 8.
69 NYSNCC, *Second Annual Report,* p. 21.
70 *Weekly Bull. Dept. Health N.Y. City 10* : 17–18 (15 Jan. 1921).
71 NYSNCC, *Second Annual Report,* pp. 39–40; N.Y. *Times,* 14 Nov. 1920.

Chapter 6

1 One of the best studies of the agency for this period is *The Bureau of Internal Revenue: Its History, Activities, and Organization,* by L. F. Schmeckebier and F. A. Eble, Service Monograph of the Government, Institute for Government Research (Baltimore: Johns Hopkins Press, 1923), esp. pp. 42–43. A history of that part of the Internal Revenue Bureau relating to alcohol and the subdivision established to enforce the 18th Amendment is L. F. Schmeckebier, *The Bureau of Prohibition: Its History, Activities, and Organization,* Monograph no. 57, Institute for Government Research (Washington, D.C.: The Brookings Institution [Lord Baltimore Press], 1929), esp. pp. 3–4, 136–45.

2 U.S. Treasury Dept., Bureau of Internal Revenue, "Report of the Commissioner for the Fiscal Year Ending June 30, 1915" (GPO, 1915), p. 147. (Hereafter cited as BIR annual report).

3 The *Medical World* of Philadelphia thought protection of dispensing rights of the physician lay in the Harrison Bill (see "Our Ancient Privilege in Danger," editorial, *31* : 439–42 [1913]). If the Harrison Bill was not passed, the journal feared retail druggists might succeed in the next session of Congress in prohibiting dispensing by physicians. It was, therefore, better to make some compromise (see "The National Antinarcotic Bill," editorial, ibid. *32* : 91–92 [1914]). See *JNARD 16* : 1404 (1913), for the pharmacists' view.

4 Internal Revenue Regulations no. 35, "Law and Regulations Relating to the Production, Importation, Manufacture, Compounding, Sale, Dispensing, or Giving Away of Opium or Coca Leaves, Their Salts, Derivatives, or Preparations," Commissioner of Internal Revenue, 15 Jan. 1915 (GPO, 1915).

5 Ibid., article 10, p. 13.

6 Eugene C. Brokmeyer to HW, 24 Oct. 1914 (WP, entry 36).

7 In articles of Internal Revenue Regulations no. 35 (1915), no provision is made for registration of consumers, and in Treasury Decision of 9 March 1915 (TD 2172) consumers, "as such," are forbidden to register under the Harrison Act.

8 U.S. Treasury Decision 2172, 9 March 1915.

9 C. McFarland to the Attorney General, 18 May 1915 (JDR); Wm. Wallace, Jr., Asst. Attorney General, to C McF, 27 May 1915 (JDR); WW Jr. to U.S. Attorney H. F. Fisher, Memphis, Tenn., 16 June 1915 (JDR): "The Act is undoubtedly a difficult one to construe and effectively enforce,

but it is one of great importance to the public." And see exchanges with other U.S. attorneys discussing cases in various district courts, below (JDR).

The Justice Department felt that cure was an easy matter particulary if the addict was held in custody for a substantial period. Their evidence for this optimistic belief came from Federal Penitentiary annual reports: "Our success in the treatment of the narcotic cases is very encouraging . . . all cured. This was accomplished without undue suffering on the part of the unfortunate individual" ("Annual Report," U.S. Penitentiary, Leavenworth, Kans., 1913, p. 42). "I am pleased to again report success in the treatment of our narcotic cases. My experience this year with these cases has strengthened my opinion, as expressed in the last annual report that this class of prisoners should have a sentence sufficiently long to enable them to become fully restored physically and mentally, particularly, to have restored their will power, which, in my opinion cannot be accomplished with less than a ten-year sentence." ("Annual Report," U.S. Penitentiary, Leavenworth, Kans., 1914, p. 50).

10 One medical journal called the decision a "cruel injustice" without ground or authority, *N.Y. Med. J.* 103 : 1036 (1916).

11 "Penalties Imposed by the Harrison Antinarcotic Law," editorial, 33 : 459 (1915). Also, "If any doctor is found guilty of using his professional rights and position to foster the continuance or increase of addiction to narcotic drugs, he should be stopped with a firm hand and punished. Such a man should be driven from the profession in disgrace" (*Med. World* 33 : 416 [1915]).

12 C. F. J. Laase, "The Practitioner of Medicine and the Narcotic Addict," *Med. Economist* 6 : 37–41 (1918), esp. p. 38.

13 "The Harrison Law and the Commissioner's Rulings," editorial, 33 : 203 (1915). Also see editorial, *Boston Med. Surg. J.* 174 : 434 (1916) which favored the Harrison Act and opposed physicians who prescribed narcotics for maintenance.

14 Montana: *U.S. v. Woods*, 224 Fed. Rep. 278 (3 July 1915); Pennsylvania: *U.S. v. Jin Fuey Moy*, 225 Fed. Rep. 1003 (13 May 1915); Tennessee: *U.S. v. Friedman*, 224 Fed. Rep. 276 (1 June 1915).

15 The conspiracy charge would be based on ch. 1, sect. 6, "Seditious Conspiracy," of *U.S. Statutes at Large*, vol. 35, part 1, ch. 321 (4 March 1909), Revision of the Criminal Code. Charges of aiding and abetting would be based on sect. 332 of ch. 321. For examples of advice to U.S. attorneys to take these two courses, see WW Jr. to U.S. Attorney R. E. Byrd, Roanoke, Va., 10 June 1915; to H. F. Fisher, Memphis, Tenn., 16 June 1916 (JDR). The philosophy Wallace advised U.S. attorneys to pursue was that "doctors and druggists should not be prosecuted where there is room to believe that they are acting in good faith, and that only those doctors and druggists should be prosecuted whose actions clearly show that they are merely pandering for gain to the desires of drug addicts." Lack of good faith would require evidence of "continuous acts upon the part of the doctor and druggist, showing utter disregard of the needs of the patient, the amount of the drug prescribed or dispensed, and

the frequency of its prescription and dispensing," WW Jr, to Perry B. Miller, U.S. Attorney, Louisville, Ky., 18 January 1916 (JDR).

16 See above, ch. 6, n. 14.

17 H. F. Fisher to Attorney General, 13 May 1915 (JDR).

18 For further discussion of prosecution problems, see H. S. Phillips, U.S. Attorney, Southern District of Florida, to L. L. Froneberger, Deputy Collector of Internal Revenue, Jacksonville, Fla., 15 July 1915 (JDR).

19 WW Jr. to H. B. Tedrow, U.S. Attorney, Denver, Colo., 15 Sept. 1915 (JDR); HBT to Attorney General, 9 Sept. 1915 (JDR).

20 See above, ch. 6, n. 14.

21 F. Robertson, U.S. Attorney, Kansas City, Kans., to Attorney General, 2 Oct. 1915 (JDR). WW Jr., to F. Robertson, 11 Oct. 1915 (JDR).; this letter contains a good summary of the government's reasoning in defense of the Harrison Act's antimaintenance powers. WW Jr. to S. K. Dennis, U.S. Attorney, Baltimore, 7 Oct. 1915 (JDR).

22 J. J. Scott, Collector of Internal Revenue, San Francisco, Calif., to W. B. Woodburn, U.S. Attorney, Carson City, Nev., 15 Nov. 1915 (JDR). WBW to JJS, 16 Dec. 1915 (JDR). JJS to WBW, 23 Dec. 1915 (JDR); the correspondence was sent to the Attorney General by Woodburn on 31 Dec. WW Jr. to WBW, 7 Jan. 1916 (JDR).

23 _U.S._ v. _Jin Fuey Moy_, 241 U.S. 394, decided 5 June 1916. Justice Holmes delivered the majority opinion; no dissenting opinion was filed by the minority. In one medical journal's opinion the decision was regrettable: "the Act now seems so leaky that it will hold nothing unless Congress does some recasting" (_N.Y. Med. J. 104_ : 905–06 [1916]). See also J. H. W. Rhein, "Some Phases of the Drug Habit Problem, Especially in Relation to the Harrison Act," _Penna. Med. J. 20_ : 97–101 (1916): Dr. Rhein condemned outpatient reduction of drugs as a mere device to evade the law and recommended stricter laws since after the Jin Fuey Moy decision the federal laws were inadequate.

24 The Court's doubts on opium production were well founded, since opium has been produced in the United States, although not with great commercial success. The majority opinion did not claim that none of the Harrison Act was in fulfillment of international obligations, only that the particular revenue specified in Section 8 was not required by the Opium Convention, and that, in addition, nowhere in the Act was there any reference to the Convention (241 U.S. 401–402). For an example of the various documents leading up to the Harrison Act which specified that the Act would be in fulfillment of treaty obligations, see "Registration of Producers and Importers of Opium, etc.," House Rept. 23, 24 June 1913, 63rd Cong., 1st Sess. (GPO, 1913).

25 BIR annual report, for year ending June 30, 1916, pp. 24–25. Even before the Jin Fuey Moy decision in 1916, the Commissioner recommended changes in the Harrison Act to facilitate "restricting or entirely eradicating the use of narcotics for other than medicinal purposes, which prior to [the Harrison Act] had become an evil of the gravest menace." He recommended inclusion of chloral hydrate and cannabis, tax on drugs by weight, repeal of the Act's Section 6 regarding exemptions for proprie-

taries, record-keeping requirements for all narcotic drugs handled, and provision of treatment by the Public Health Service, or another appropriate agency, for indigent addicts deprived of their drugs by effect of the Harrison Act (BIR annual report for year ending June 30, 1915, pp. 29–31).

26 After the Jin Fuey Moy decision in mid-1916, the request for amendment became even more insistent, for the decision was said to have severely crippled the federal government's campaign against illicit narcotic use by unregistered persons (which would include addicts and peddlers). See BIR annual report for year ending June 30, 1916, pp. 24–25. This plea is repeated in the BIR annual reports for 1917 and 1918 and set the basis for appointment of the Treasury Special Committee. See BIR annual report 1916, p. 24. The Justice Department doubted that the Harrison Act could be given strengthened police powers by congressional amendment because the Act seemed at the borderline of constitutionality in its present weakened interpretation. See W. C. Fitts, Asst. Attorney General to Senator William Calder, 2 Nov. 1917 (JDR).

27 Reorganization, vast new tax-collecting responsibilities brought on by the threat and then the reality of war, gave the Internal Revenue Bureau inadequate personnel and little time for enforcing the Act. See Schmeckebier and Eble, *Bureau of Internal Revenue*, pp. 44, 47, 52. This inevitable neglect of the Harrison Act was seen as one reason to give the whole task to the Public Health Service in *JAPhA* 7 : 572 (1918). BIR annual report for year ending 30 June 1916, p. 45. The standard study of the period is Robert K. Murray's *Red Scare: A Study of National Hysteria, 1919–1920* (Minneapolis: Univ. of Minnesota Press, 1955). My account is also dependent on the chapter "Red Scare" in William E. Leuchtenburg, *The Perils of Prosperity, 1914–1932* (Univ. of Chicago Press, 1958), pp. 66–83.

28 A direct connection between the efficiency needed for the war effort and the inefficiency caused by narcotic use was made by the Treasury Department. Warning of narcotic use as a threat to the war effort appeared in the Commissioner of Internal Revenue's annual report for 1917 (BIR annual report for year ending 30 June 1917, p. 16; see also Daniel Roper, *Fifty Years of Public Life* [Durham, N.C.: Duke Univ. Press, 1941], pp. 185–90). Rep. Rainey's fear of addiction's toll on draftees and youth in general has been mentioned. A popular expression of this fear is found in "Narcotics and the War," by Janette Marks (*North American* 206 : 879–84 (Dec. 1917). It was associated with the effect of opiate treatment of war injuries on the rate of addiction in the postwar period. Recognition that narcotics caused inefficiency could not be overlooked in light of the vigorous action of Congress in prohibiting the sale of liquor to members of the armed forces in May 1917, a month after the declaration of war. Also see Andrew Sinclair, *Prohibition: The Era of Excess* (Boston: Little, Brown, 1962), pp. 117–18; National Commission on Law Observance and Enforcement, "Report on the Enforcement of the Prohibition Laws of the United States," 7 Jan. 1931 (GPO, 1931), pp. 4–7. The manufacture of distilled spirits was forbidden by the Food Control Act in 1917 and

the withholding of supplies from brewers was made an option of the President. The Agricultural Appropriation Act of 1918 prohibited the manufacture of liquor in the United States after 30 June 1919 if a state of war still existed, and it banned the use of foods stuffs for making liquor. On 16 Sept. 1918 the President ordered that food no longer be used in the making of beer.

29 *Debs* v. *U.S.*, 249 U.S. 211 (decided 10 March 1919); a week earlier the Court had similarly upheld the conviction of an antidraft pamphleteer (*Schenck* v. *U.S.*, 249 U.S. 47 [3 March 1919]).

30 Leuchtenburg, *Perils*, pp. 120–39.

31 Murray, *Red Scare*, pp. 196 ff.

32 For another example of a mental health authority who before the war had described heroin and addiction without alarm see Pearce Bailey, "Applicability of the Findings of the Neuropsychiatric Examinations in the Army to Civil Problems," *Mental Hygiene* 4 : 301–11 (April 1920), p. 303. In describing addicts and diseased personalities Bailey warns, "It is in them that mental contagion which leads up to hysterical mass movements, spreads with the greatest rapidity, and in their minds sedition finds an easier route than realism. . . . Suggestible, they easily become the tools of designing propagandists in spreading seditious doctrines, or in the commission of acts in defiance of law and order" (p. 308). Bailey had been the army's chief neuropsychiatrist.

33 In 1916 (*U.S.* v. *Jin Fuey Moy*), Justice Holmes doubted that Congress wanted to make criminals out of citizens who had opium in their posession. But by 1919 Holmes subscribed to the opinion of Justice Day which held for the majority in *Webb* v. *U.S.* that to maintain an addict by medical prescription "would be so clear a perversion of meaning [of the word prescription] that no discussion of the subject is required" (249 U.S. 99–100). The mood of the Court shifts from a concern for citizens' rights against the government's encroachment to a belief that prescription of drugs to an addict could be prevented by federal law.

34 Mayor John F. Hylan to Health Commissioner Royal S. Copeland, 3 May 1919 (papers of Mayor Hylan, box 442, file "Health Department, 1919-I," N.Y. Municipal Archives). An exconvict had been arrested with narcotics and explosives in his possession. Coming during the tumult aroused nationally by the discovery of the May 1st bomb packages mailed to prominent antiradical Americans, the arrest made possible the combination of two current fears affecting New Yorkers. Also see N.Y. *Times*, 27 May and 30 May 1919. No other evidence linking bombs and narcotics appears to have been uncovered.

35 Daniel C. Roper to William G. McAdoo, 5 March 1918 (PHSR). Roper emphasized the need for action in the war emergency. Later that year another internal government memorandum within the Public Health Service gave the same reason for action, since "any work aiming at the reduction of the large number of drug addicts in this country is intimately connected with the official prosecution of the war" (Carl Voegtlin, Professor of Pharmacology, Hygienic Laboratory, to the Surgeon General PHS, 1 Aug. 1918, PHSR).

36 Rep. Henry T. Rainey (1860–1934) served in Congress from 1903 to 1921 and from 1923 to his death. He succeeded John Garner as Speaker of the House in March 1933. Rainey interested himself in narcotics issues and, until his absence of one term, was a leader in most antinarcotic legislation. When he returned, he continued to serve on committees reviewing narcotic issues but the leadership had passed to Republican Stephen Porter of Pennsylvania.

37 Dr. Rhees later served with the Narcotic Division of the Prohibition Unit as an agent. Charles F. Stokes (1863–1931) received his M.D. from Columbia in 1884 and was Surgeon General of the Navy from 1910 to 1914. He retired in 1917 with the rank of rear admiral. Stokes found his own cure for narcotics addiction, which differed from the Towns-Lambert treatment and the antitoxin theories of Bishop and Pettey, basing his regimen on attempting to reestablish a balance between the sympathetic and parasympathetic nervous systems. See C. P. Stokes, "Pathology and Treatment of Drug Addiction" *Med. Rec.* 91 : 969 (1917). He sought appointment to various other government committees. His was an influential voice warning of impending catastrophe in the growing fear of addicts in New York State in 1919 (N.Y. *Times,* 17 Feb. 1919).

38 Rainey introduced *HR 12,787* on 20 August 1918 with the goal of repairing damage done to the act by the Jin Fuey Moy decision of 1916 and also repealing Section 6 (Rainey to Surgeon General, PHS, 23 Aug. 1918, PHSR). Rainey's amendments were contained in sections 1006–09 of the Revenue Act of 1918, approved 24 Feb. 1919 (*Public Law no. 254,* 65th Cong.).

39 *Exportation of Opium,* hearings before a Subcommittee of the Committee on Ways and Means on *HR 14,500,* House, 66th Cong., 3rd Sess., 8, 11 Dec. 1920 and 3, 4 January 1921 (GPO, 1921). See pp. 47–48 for exchange between W. L. Crounse, general representative of the National Wholesale Druggists Association, and Rep. Rainey on this question.

40 *Amendments to the Harrison Narcotic Act,* hearings before a Subcommittee of the Committee on Ways and Means, House, 69th Cong., 1st Sess. 21, 22, 26 May 1926 (GPO, 1926), see pp. 23–24. See also *Exportation of Opium,* Hearings (1921), pp. 16, 43–44.

41 U.S. Treasury, *Preliminary Report* of the Special Committee of Investigation, August 1918 (GPO, 1918).

42 *Special Committee of Investigation, Appointed March 25, 1918, by the Secretary of the Treasury: Traffic in Narcotic Drugs* (GPO, 1919), pp. 3, 23–26, 29.

43 *Ibid.,* pp. 9–19.

44 Chiefs of Police of every American city of over 5,000 population were circularized, but only 32% returned any information. Leading causes of addiction were listed as prescriptions, association with other addicts, and liquor prohibition. Penal institutions—county, state, and federal—returned 3.9% of the questionnaires with information. From superintendents of state, county, and municipal almshouses, state hospitals, insane asylums, and county municipal hospitals (a total of 5,101), only about 6% reported "any information of value" (*Traffic in Narcotic Drugs,* pp. 14–19).

45 *Traffic in Narcotic Drugs,* pp. 19–22. Apparently one million was a compromise between the PHS's estimate of 750,000 and the Revenue Service's estimate of 1.5 million. See A. G. DuMez, "Some Facts Concerning Drug Addiction," memorandum prepared for the PHS and marked "Not for Publication in Present Form," 9 Dec. 1918 (PHSR).

46 *Traffic in Narcotic Drugs,* p. 22. That Prohibition would create more narcotic users was an old and enduring belief. Prohibitionists looked for contrary evidence, wets warned of a dire avalanche of addicts, and the federal and local governments took the possibility seriously. The New York City Health Department declared that the vigorous drive on addicts in that city in 1919 was prompted by just this fear of the effects of Prohibition (Department of Health of the City of New York, *Annual Report,* 1919, p. 193).

47 N.Y. *Times,* 10 April 1919. In September 1919 Porter was described in Justice Department documents as Supervising Internal Revenue Agent.

48 N.Y. *Times,* 17 Feb. 1919.

49 Copeland is quoted in the *Times* of 23 March 1919, where the figures for drugstore sales are also given. An estimate of how many addicts the heroin or morphine would supply can be computed by multiplying the number of grains in an ounce (437.5) by the approximate number of ounces of heroin and morphine (roughly 2,500) and then dividing by the average number of grains used by an addict monthly. The daily average in 1919 is often given as 10 grains, in which case the number of addicts supplied for a month by drugstore sales, if all went to addicts for simple maintenance, would be about 3,300. If one assumes a conservative daily average intake of 5 grains, the figure would be doubled.

50 As early as January 1919, Justice Collins had written that the City Health Department was ready to open clinics in New York if necessary (C. F. Collins, "The Drug Evil and the Drug Laws," *Monthly Bull. Dept. Health N.Y. City* 9 : 1–24 [1919], p. 13). In a *Times* interview of 31 March 1919, mention was made by Copeland that clinics were planned. The clinics' development is closely followed in the *Times* after 10 April 1919. Copeland's original optimism was recalled by the president of Chicago's Board of Education, J. D. Robertson, who also had predicted failure (*Limiting Production of Habit-forming Drugs and Raw Materials from Which They are Made,* House Committee on Foreign Affairs, Hearings on *HJR 430* and *HJR 453,* 67th Cong., 4th Sess., 13–16 Feb. 1923, rev. print., p. 107). For a more detailed account of the opening see *Weekly Bull. Dept. Health N.Y. City,* 19 April 1919, pp. 121–22.

51 New York State Narcotic Control Commission (NYSNCC), *First Annual Report,* 10 April 1919, Legislative Doc. no. 83 (Albany: J. B. Lyon, 1919), pp. 3–4.

52 Seven physicians worked all day to handle the addicts who came through at a rate of 100 an hour. Dr. Copeland warned the city that violence might break out if a supply were not kept flowing to the addicts. N.Y. *Times,* 11–13 April 1919. The determination to provide hospital and curative treatment for addicts is well documented in the many defeats suffered by the Health Department before it finally secured adequate

bed space. A large portable hospital offered by the Rockefeller Foundation was first briefly accepted and then rejected by the city, apparently on suspicion that strings were attached. It was feared that the Foundation, in the words of Corrections Commissioner Bird Coler, sought a "grip on the habits of men" and that it was pro-Prohibition (N.Y. *Times,* 19 July 1919). Secretary of the Navy Josephus Daniels gave the city permission to use the large Pelham Bay Naval Training Station for institutional treatment, but the community objected (ibid., 29 July 1919). Then the city turned to the tuberculosis center on Staten Island, Sea View Hospital, but the community again objected and threatened to picket the ferry and demonstrate if addicts were sent to the Island. Finally, Riverside Hospital on North Brother Island was selected and, since the city owned the island, the hospital, and access, agreement was obtained. In late August, Riverside Hospital became the major treatment facility for addicts transferred from the clinic for institutional care (ibid., 6–26 Aug. 1919).

53 Perhaps prompted by A. G. DuMez's work on the Treasury's Special Committee, the PHS began to consider in late 1918 and early 1919 how to become involved in the fight against addiction while preserving its traditional role as a catalyst only. In a memorandum prepared by the Hygienic Laboratory on 9 May 1919, it was considered proper for the service to warn against "ambulatory treatment" since an addict would not voluntarily withdraw himself, but "any statement as to the treatment of drug addiction, especially morphinism, must be made with caution at the present time as our knowledge of this phase of this subject is very indefinite." While gingerly approaching the proper boundaries of activity, the PHS was about to be solidly pushed toward direct patient care by the Commissioner of Internal Revenue. Commissioner Roper, in a memorandum of 15 July to the Secretary, with a copy to the Surgeon General, suggested that the PHS temporarily take care of all indigent addicts, apparently on a maintenance program, until expansion of the service's hospital facilities enabled admission for institutional treatment and "permanent cure" (PHSR). Mention of such possible activity by the PHS was written into the July 31st letter to revenue officials which was made public (U.S. Treasury Dept., Bureau of Internal Revenue, *Enforcement of the Harrison Narcotic Law,* "M-Mim 2212 to Collectors of Internal Revenue, Revenue Agents, and Others Concerned," 31 July 1919 [GPO, 1919]). The revenue officials were advised to confer with local authorities and U.S. attorneys in order to establish at the earliest date "public clinics" where relief in conformity with the law might be given. Roper did not believe addiction treatment was a proper matter for the government's tax-collecting agency to oversee (Roper to Surgeon General, 19 June 1919, PHSR). See also L. F. Schmeckebier, *The Public Health Service: Its History, Activities, and Organization,* Institute for Government Research (Baltimore: Johns Hopkins Press, 1923), pp. 47–52.

54 Surgeon General Blue found in the VD clinics a model for PHS response to demands for action. The clinics would reduce patients to a minimum comfortable dose and then "act as feeders to the institutions where real cure can be carried out." Blue's apparent optimism for a real cure was

actually only a belief that detoxification could be carried out in an institution because even before the New York City clinic had completed four months' operation, Blue believed that such cures would not secure permanent results until complete national and international control of drug output was secured (Blue to Roper, 28 July 1919, PHSR). The clinics in New York, New Orleans, and Memphis were given as examples of the kind of clinic desired.

55 Roper, *Fifty Years of Public Service,* p. 185. For actual figures of draft rejects in New York see above (ch. 5, n. 63). For a contemporary criticism of Roper's figures, see Pearce Bailey, "The Drug Habit in the United States," *New Republic,* 16 March 1921, pp. 67–69.

56 Roper, *Fifty Years,* pp. 186, 189–93.

57 Roper to Blue, 19 June 1919 (PHSR).

58 Senator Joseph I. France, Maryland, a physician, introduced S 2785 on 15 Aug. 1919 (66th Cong., 1st Sess.). In the House, Rep. Rainey introduced an identical bill, *HR 11, 778.*

59 Roper to Secretary of Treasury, 15 July 1919 (PHSR).

60 U.S. Treasury Dept., Internal Revenue Regulation no. 35 (GPO, 1919).

61 Blue to Roper, 28 July 1919 (PHSR).

62 One more example of the PHS reacting to the Revenue Bureau's attempt to deeply involve the medical branch of the Treasury in the narcotic problem was Roper's suggestion that the PHS agree to add provisions for more laboratory facilities in order to search for an effective treatment of addiction. The commissioner had become convinced that some treatment which counteracted or neutralized habit-forming drugs was necessary for an ultimate solution (Roper to Blue, 5 Sept. 1919, PHSR). The Surgeon General agreed (Blue to Roper, 16 Sept. 1919, PHSR).

63 "Report of the Committee on the Narcotic Drug Situation in the United States," approved by the House of Delegates, April 1920, New Orleans Convention, in *Digest of Official Actions, 1846–1958* (Chicago: American Medical Association, 1959), p. 502. The full report is reprinted in *JAMA 74* : 1324–28 (1920). The members of the committee were identified in Charles E. Terry and Mildred Pellens, *The Opium Problem* (New York Bureau of Social Hygiene, 1928; reprint ed., Montclair, N.J.: Patterson Smith, 1970, p. 887), as E. Eliot Harris, New York, chairman; Arthur T. McCormack, Kentucky; Paul Waterman, Connecticut; and Alexander Lambert, ex officio (as president of the AMA 1918–19). Among other recommendations were condemnation of ambulatory treatment of drug addiction, and endorsement of total prohibition of heroin.

64 *Care and Treatment of Drug Addicts,* Committee on Public Health and Quarantine, Senate Report no. 232, 66th Cong., 1st Sess., 10 Oct. 1919 (GPO, 1919). Printed in the report was a letter from Secretary of the Treasury Carter Glass describing the need for the France bill because of "a critically serious situation growing out of the enforcement of amendments to the Harrison Narcotic Act" (Glass to France, 3 Sept. 1919). Among others involved in trying to develop the most effective and palatable bill was Arthur D. Greenfield, the New York attorney who had gained the respect of the PHS by his attitude toward law enforcement and inter-

pretation of the Harrison Act, opposition to addict maintenance, and lack of any ax to grind or cure to promote. The France bill was not the first federal attempt to care for indigent addicts. Senator Jacob Gallinger had introduced a bill to provide treatment in the District of Columbia for habitués as early as April 1908 ("President's Home Commission," Senate Doc. no. 644, 60th Cong., 2nd Sess., 8 Jan 1909, p. 258). The France bill allotted $13 million in matching funds for the first year and $2 million for the second year of a national antinarcotic program. Each state would match the federal contribution to establish programs of care, prevention, and treatment of drug addicts. The Secretary of the Treasury would approve all state programs. The states would be permitted to use PHS facilities, and navy and army facilities not then needed could be borrowed by the PHS in furtherance of addiction control. Ten percent of the federal funds might be spent to "collect and spread information in regard to the care and treatment of drug addicts and for administration." The Treasury Department, containing both the PHS and the Bureau of Internal Revenue, considered these legislative recommendations the necessary sequel to providing temporary narcotic supply clinics. Definitive treatment was needed in institutions and the clinics would act as feeders to the institutions. (Quotations from S 2785 as amended by the Committee on Public Health and Quarantine, 1 Oct. 1919 are from a copy in the files of the PHS.)

65   A. G. DuMez, "Some Facts Concerning Drug Addiction," memorandum dated 9 Dec. 1918, sent to the Surgeon General from the Hygienic Laboratory, 16 Dec. 1918 (PHSR). DuMez's description is very similar to Dr. Bishop's concept of addiction disease and illustrates that what would in a year or so be taken as evidence of duplicity or dangerous ignorance was then respectable and seemingly scientific. DuMez also demonstrated his beliefs in a review article (*JAMA* 72 : 1069 [1919]) in which he credited Valenti's experiments. Bishop and DuMez were in error as to the indisputable evidence for a detectable antitoxin or antibody. Soon the error became medical heresy which endangered the careers of physicians who did not recant; Bishop is an example. By 1921, even the Surgeon General thought the phrase "physiological balance" was so "controversial" that he did not wish it to be mentioned publically. Cummings to Dowling, 12 Feb. 1921 (PHSR).

66   DuMez, "Some Facts."

67   A. G. DuMez, "Treatment of Drug Addiction," memorandum to the Surgeon General, 28 Feb. 1919 (PHSR).

68   A. G. DuMez to the Surgeon General, 14 June 1921, where it is claimed that the greatest hope for keeping addicts off drugs "lies in a more rigid and thorough enforcement of the present anti-narcotic law." Similarly, Dr. Pearce Bailey, former chief neuropsychiatrist for the army during World War I, complained that "one of the difficulties in the way of meeting the situation has been that drug addiction has too long been considered a medical problem. . . . The problem is not one to be handled by the Boards of Health or by special commissions, but by the Internal Revenue Department, which should check up all sales, by the municipal police,

and by the local and federal courts" ("The Drug Habit in the United States," *New Republic*, 16 March 1921, pp. 67–69). Early in 1919, the PHS and the Bureau of Internal Revenue agreed that the government had a moral obligation to provide cure if cure were made compulsory (e.g. Greenfield to Blue, 31 May 1919, PHSR, and Roper to Secretary of the Treasury, 15 July 1919, PHSR), but as the impossibility of providing any reasonable chance of cure with current regimens became apparent, the PHS backed away from claiming a major role for medical treatment in the curbing of addiction in the United States.

69   An attempt at this time by the PHS to contribute to the federal effort against narcotics was the near-establishment of a national advisory committee "to formulate such suggestions as will tend to make clear to physicians the exact nature and extent of their right to prescribe narcotic drugs, and to advise with respect to such legislation and such administrative procedure as may be called for by existing conditions" (Blue to Dr. Thomas Blair, Director of the Bureau of Drug Control, Pennsylvania Department of Health, 5 Nov. 1919, PHSR). The committee was first suggested by Arthur Greenfield to Blue as a response to physicians' confusion over what they could prescribe for and what not. Greenfield believed that an inquiry started under the aegis of the PHS would focus unsettled thinking and speed a "consensus of the best medical opinion" (Greenfield to Blue, 14 Aug. 1919, PHSR). The proposal received Blue's support and the enthusiastic support of the Bureau of Internal Revenue. Roper hoped that the committee would clarify standards of practice (Roper to Blue, 3 Sept. 1919, PHSR).

Among those appointed were Dr. Pellini, Dr. Thomas Blair of Pennsylvania, A. C. Webber of Boston, Mrs. Hamilton Wright, and Greenfield himself as chairman; all had taken strong stands against a concept of addiction disease which would lead to maintenance in many instances. The committee was disapproved by Secretary of the Treasury David Houston, who felt it would violate a statute agains expenditures incurred by a committee or commission of inquiry except for expenses specifically authorized. The Secretary's veto came even after invitations had been extended by the Surgeon General (Dr. Homer Cumming) and after approval by the assistant secretary in charge of the PHS and the Bureau of Internal Revenue. These subordinates to the Secretary even approved the committee, with the understanding that no expenditures would be incurred after the members had agreed to serve at their own expense (Asst. Surgeon General Schereschewsky to Greenfield, 23 July 1920, PHSR). Perhaps the powerful influence of Rep. Rainey had intervened to stop this new committee, which Secretary Houston claimed violated the spirit of the statute, for Rainey, in an exchange with Dr. Terry in January 1921, denied any need for an investigation beyond what the Treasury Committee had established in June 1919 (*Exportation of Opium*, Hearings before a Subcommittee of the Committee on Ways and Means on *HR 14,500*, House, 66th Cong., 3rd Sess., 8–11 Dec. 1920, and 3–4 Jan. 1921 [GPO, 1921], pp. 106–07). Secretary Houston reasoned that the answers sought by the investigation could be supplied by federal agencies responsible.

70 Nutt (1866–1938) was a practicing pharmacist in Ohio when he entered the Bureau of Internal Revenue in 1901. See below, ch. 8 for further details.

71 Schmeckebier, *Bureau of Prohibition,* pp. 309–10.

72 U.S. Treasury Dept., Bureau of Internal Revenue, "Digest of Responses to Questionnaire Submitted by the Bureau of Internal Revenue to Hospitals and Prominent Physicians Relative to the Methods of Treatment for Narcotic Drug Addicts," with a handwritten note on the cover "completed to December 5–19," (RPU). The opinions favored rapid or gradual withdrawal, hyoscine during withdrawal, institutional restraint, and custodial care for 90 to 180 days or longer. Selected responses from the collectors, dated between 30 July and 15 September 1919, seem in large part replies to M-Mim 2212 of 31 July 1919 (see ch. 6, n. 53 above), and are collected in a typewritten document "Digest of Correspondence from Collectors, Revenue Agents and District Attorneys Relative to the Narcotic Situation in the Various States" (U.S. Treasury, Bureau of Internal Revenue, n.d., RPU). Cooper's trip to points between Washington and Boston in October 1919 might similarly be considered a gathering of information about the effectiveness of the various clinics stimulated by Commissioner Roper's letter of 31 July. Cooper's memorandum was submitted to the Bureau 22 Oct. 1919 (RPU).

73 See above, ch. 6, n. 72.

74 Dr. J. C. Perry, Acting Surgeon General to Dr. Oscar Dowling, President, Louisiana State Board of Health, 29 Nov. 1920 (PHSR). The resolution was apparently submitted by Dr. George McCoy, Director of the Hygienic Laboratory. The full resolution, including condemnation of the use of heroin, had also been approved by the New York State Medical Society on 22 March and was based, according to Dr. Eliot Harris, its sponsor, on the evidence gained from the New York City clinic that addicts must be under "absolute control" when being taken off drugs.

75 For reference see above, ch. 6, n. 62; E. Eliot Harris to Commissioner of Internal Revenue, 1 May 1920 (RPU). A note to Prohibition Commissioner John F. Kramer from Narcotic Division Head Levi G. Nutt (5 May 1920, RPU) called his attention to the Harris letter and commented, "Time has arrived when action should be taken leading to the closing of these places." Nutt, however, was already taking steps to close the clinics.

76 U.S. Treasury Dept., Bureau of Internal Revenue, "Amending M-Mim 2212 dated 31 July 1919, and Outlining Treatment of Narcotic Drug Addiction Permissible under the Harrison Narcotic Law," Pro-Mimeograph, pro., no. 217, 19 Oct. 1921 (GPO, 1921). The 30-day limit prompted Rep. Volk to call for a congressional investigation of the narcotic situation and to describe the new rulings as the efforts of an "organized conspiracy" to drive the narcotic addict into established sanitaria (*Med. Record 101 :* 109 [1922]). As medical support for the 30-day limit, the ruling cited a

resolution passed by the Council on Health and Public Instruction of the AMA on 11 Nov. 1920. Since several members of this committee were New York City enemies of Volk's views, he found the connection further proof of the conspiracy.

77   Specified exceptions to withdrawal: "Those suffering from senility, or the infirmities attendant upon old age, who are confirmed addicts of years standing, and who, in the opinion of a reputable physician in charge, require a minimum amount of narcotics to sustain life" ("Amending M-Mim 2212" Section 3a). Doubtful cases could be investigated by the bureau on request and special instructions issued (p. 4). It is unlikely that any young heroin addict would be granted an exception, but the rule was not without some flexibility.

Chapter 7

1   Between the Jin Fuey Moy decision of June 1916 and the antimaintenance decisions of the Supreme Court in March 1919, there was little the federal government could do to prevent maintenance of simple addiction by physicians if all the tax regulations were followed. Pressure could be applied verbally, what Rep. Rainey admiringly called "simply bluffing the thing through" (*Exportation of Opium,* Hearings before a Subcommittee of the Committee on Ways and Means on *HR 14,500,* House, 67th Cong., 3rd. Sess., 8 and 11 Dec. 1920 and 3 and 4 Jan. 1921 [GPO, 1921], p. 47), but unless state laws opposed simple maintenance, as in Massachusetts, physicians were left to their own judgment. The Massachusetts law forbidding indefinite maintenance came into effect 1 January 1915 and was approved on 22 June 1914, before passage of the Harrison Act. The Massachusetts law (ch. 694, sect. 2, of Acts of 1914) made it unlawful for any physician or dentist to provide opiates or cannabis to any habitual user. In a test of a physician's intent or judgment, the Massachusetts Supreme Court upheld a lower court's decision against a physician for providing drugs to fifteen persons known to him to be habitual users (*Commonwealth* v. *Noble,* 230 Mass. 83). This is an antimaintenance statute in a state which had a problem of narcotic addiction and sought to curb addiction by means very similar to the Supreme Court's decisions in *U.S.* v. *Behrman,* 258 U.S. 280 (27 March 1922). Three years after Massachusetts, Pennsylvania outlawed addiction maintenance (*Laws of Pennsylvania,* Act no. 282, sect. 8, approved 11 July 1917). In contrast, New York permitted maintenance under state law.

2   Between 1910 and 1920 there was rapid development in the U.S. of the concept of a health district with a health center providing care and education. For a discussion, see George Rosen, *A History of Public Health* (New York: M.D. Publications, 1958), pp. 470–78.

3   Correspondence and records of the various narcotic clinics were collected by the Narcotic Division of the Prohibition Unit and are now in possession of the Bureau of Narcotics and Dangerous Drugs. Each file contains investigations of the clinics or descriptions of its activity and closure. With the permission of the bureau I examined these records in 1971. Unless

noted otherwise, records quoted in this chapter are from this collection.

4   A clinic was under consideration in San Francisco in 1919 and the suggestion received the approval of the PHS (Surgeon General Rupert Blue to W. C. Hassler, 3 Sept. 1919, PHSR). In St. Louis a "free narcotic clinic" was planned under the Board of Health (Revenue Agent in Charge, St. Louis, to Commissioner of Internal Revenue, 8 Sept. 1919, in U.S. Treasury Dept., Bureau of Internal Revenue, "Digest of Correspondence from Collectors, Revenue Agents and District Attorneys Relative to the Narcotic Situation in the Various States," n.d., RPU). The revenue agents registered addicts in Kansas City, Mo., and physicians were allowed to prescribe for them. The mayor of Kansas City disapproved a public clinic, so physicians were permitted under approval of the Board of Health to prescribe for addicts (E. C. Ruth, Internal Revenue Agent in Charge, St. Louis, to Commissioner of Internal Revenue, 4 Dec. 1919).

5   The number of clinics known to the Narcotic Division was about 40. Registrants at the clinics totaled 2,485 according to a compilation of 44 clinics dated 30 April 1921. In the 26 clinics of which detailed investigations had been made, only 10.5% of the registrants were considered to have a disease other than addiction (O. G. Forrer, Assistant Director, Narcotic Field Force, to L. G. Nutt, Director, 30 April 1921). This compilation does not include the experimental New York City clinic. Forty-four is the usual number of clinics estimated, although it is likely that a close study of local methods of dealing with addicts in 1910–25 would reveal more.

6   Atlanta had an older clinic population in comparison to Albany and New Haven. Atlanta's age range was from 20 to 87; males averaged 43 and females 46. In New Haven the average ages were 33 and 32 respectively; in San Diego the average age of both sexes was 27. The Albany clinic was evenly divided between males and females; Providence had three times as many females as males (74 and 27), while New Haven's ratio was almost reversed (66 males and 26 females). Generally more males than females attended the clinics; in the 26 clinics closely examined in 1921, there were 966 males and 591 females.

7   The medical profession was evincing a sharpened interest in regard to state controls. Dr. James F. Rooney, chairman of the State Medical Society's Legislative Committee, declared in May 1921: "Regulations as to the use of narcotic drugs and alcohol are merely the beginning of an attempt to completely control therapeutic methods." Dr. Rooney was elected president of the State Medical Society the following month. ("Report of the Committee on Legislation," *N.Y. State Med. J. 21* : 209–13 [1921]). Pharmacists' opposition to regulation of narcotic dispensing within New York State is described in "No Time to Adopt a 'Model' Law" (*Amer. Druggist Pharmaceut. Rec. 66* : 391–94 (1922).

8   Alexander Lambert is representative of AMA reformers. As chairman of the Judicial Council of the AMA in 1916 which had submitted to the House of Delegates a favorable report on health insurance, Lambert favored some kind of health reform similar to that adopted in Germany and Great Britain. He was also active in the American Association for

Labor Legislation, which promoted health insurance in various states, and the improvement of workmen's compensation laws which had slowly gained acceptance during the years before World War I. In New York Lambert favored a fixed-fee schedule for physicians as a corollary to workmen's compensation. Lambert proposed to bring delivery of medical services in the U.S. into alignment with other Western industrial nations as the proper solution to the great need of the poor and the middle class. He was elected president of the New York State Medical Society in 1918 and of the American Medical Association in 1919.

9   Rosen, *History of Public Health*, p. 455.

10 An editorial in the *Medical Record* of New York associated Prohibition, compulsory reporting of venereal disease, antivivisectionism, and the Harrison Act in a complaint about "The Growing Enslavement of the Profession of Medicine" (99 : 18 [1921]).

11 See Pearce Bailey, "The Drug Habit in the United States," *New Republic*, 16 March 1921, pp. 67–69; see also "Report of the Committee on the Narcotic Drug Situation in the United States," *JAMA* 74 : 1324–28 (1920).

12 Francis O. Caffey, U.S. Attorney, New York City, to Commissioner of Internal Revenue, 27 Sept. 1919. The letter describes meetings held 6 and 17 Sept. 1919 (JDR). This confidential communication estimated the number of addicts in New York City as "at least four or five thousand."

13 N.Y. *Times*, 10 April 1919. The fear that perhaps half a million addicts would be created by the war is found in *Medico-Legal Journal* 35 : 17–20 (1918), p. 20. Charles Towns had predicted that gassing of soldiers would lead to opiate use and then addiction on a wide scale ("The War and the Dope Habit," *Literary Digest*, 9 June 1917, pp. 1776–77). The later belief that many of New York City's addicts were returned veterans, for which no evidence has so far been located, was only to confirm a fear of several years' standing.

14 Porter quoted in N.Y. *Times*, 11 April 1919; he gave as an illustration one physician providing "treatment" to 271 addicts in two hours.

15 John P. Davin, who had ably represented the Medical Economic League in Albany in defending the prescribing rights of the private practitioner now, on behalf of the Physicians' Protective Association, attacked the arrests of physicians by the federal government and establishment of a public clinic by Dr. Copeland (N.Y. *Times*, 13 April 1919). Dr. Davin was an active member of the Federation of Medical Economic Leagues and was an associate editor of the *Medical Economist*. His attacks were balanced by the early release of parts of the Treasury's Special Committee Report, *Traffic in Narcotic Drugs*, which, as reported that day in the N.Y. *Times*, claimed that 1.5 million addicts were abroad, that the addictive drugs, particularly heroin, were "German products," and that a strict campaign against addiction was now to begin.

16 See N.Y. *Times*, 14 June 1919. At the special meeting called to consider the narcotic situation in New York City, the physician protestors, led by Davin, were defeated, as we see from the minutes of the County Medical Society. Davin's nemesis, Dr. E. Eliot Harris, as Chairman of the Public Health Committee, offered the following resolution.

Resolved that the Medical Society of the County of New York expresses the wish to co-operate with the State Narcotic Drug Commissioner, Hon. Walter R. Herrick, in every legitimate and constructive way to eliminate narcotic drug addiction and to help cure the addict.

Dr. John P. Davin offered a substitute resolution, which was declared to be out of order.

On appeal from this decision from the Chair was sustained (54-41).

On motion the resolution of the Public Health Committee was adopted (Archives of the Medical Society of the County of New York, New York City).

At about the same time, the president of the AMA condemned the position advocated by Dr. Davin:

There is a condition in the United States which involves seriously the interests, and even the reputation, of the medical profession: that is, the complicated situation arising out of the narcotic drug laws . . . .

The situation has become such that several states have passed their own narcotic laws to supplement the federal law endeavoring to control a problem which was fast becoming desperate. These laws are making it more and more burdensome for physicians using the narcotics legitimately, but that is a mere annoyance. The responsibility on the medical profession is becoming greater and greater to see to it that some action should be taken against a few renegade and depraved members of the profession who, joining with the criminal class, make it possible to continue the evil and illicit drug trade.

[That portion of addicts who are] real degenerates and criminals are extremely difficult to deal with, and practically cannot be kept from their drug as long as it is possible, through inadequate legal control, to continue the illicit drug trade (Alexander Lambert, "Address of the President Elect," *JAMA 72* : 1767–68, 1919).

Dr. Davin quickly offered a rebuttal to Lambert and other leaders of the profession and at the same time announced the formation of the American Federation of Physicians, whose goal was the abolition of the New York State Narcotic Control Commission (J. P. Davin, "For repeal of the Narcotic Drug Law" [letter to the editor], *Med. Rec. 96* : 161–62, 1919).

As another example of influential physicians applauding the government's actions, see editorial with resolutions of commendation in the *New York Medical Journal*, 14 Feb. 1920, pp. 292–93.

17 Bird S. Coler, quoted in the N.Y. *Times*, 13 April 1919. Prohibitionists were unable to locate evidence for this prediction after the start of national Prohibition; see *Literary Digest*, 16 April 1921, pp. 19–20.

18 Pleas were made because the arrest of "mere dope doctors" scared other doctors who were maintaining some addicts. The line between the two types of practice was somewhat subjective. Dr. Copeland reassured "reputable" doctors that they could continue to treat addicts (N.Y. *Times*, 17 and 21 April 1919), and the *New York Medical Journal* editorially

assured physicians that only the most blatant examples of profiteering and selling of drugs by physicians were receiving police attention (22 Feb. 1920).

19   Regulations reprinted in the *Weekly Bull. Dept. of Health N.Y. City,* 12 April 1919, pp. 115–17. According to Dr. Copeland (N.Y. *Times,* 16 July 1919), within a few months an estimated 10,000 addicts were using the triplicate system. This figure appears to have included 5,000 treated at the city's clinic and 1,200 registered with the State Commission of Narcotic Drug Control's office on Prince Street.

20   N.Y. *Times,* 12 and 13 April 1919. R. S. Copeland to Thomas Cooper, Treasury Department, Bureau of Internal Revenue, 16 Oct. 1919, gives details of treatment and hospital operation at that time. Copeland was at this time faulting the availability of drugs on the outside as the reason for lack of substantial success.

21   These statistics are from the summary of clinic operations up to 1 Jan. 1920; see S. D. Hubbard, "New York City Narcotic Clinic and Differing Points of View on Narcotic Addiction," *Monthly Bull. Dept. of Health N.Y. City 10* : 33–47 (1920), pp. 45–47. Information on the number of clinic applicants between 10 April and 1 July 1919 is reprinted in Alexander Lambert, "The Underlying Causes of the Narcotic Habit," *Modern Med. 2* : 5–9 (1920). Early statistics reveal 725 registrants between ages 15 and 19 out of 2,723 total "narcotic applicants." Further information can be found in the department's *Annual Report* for 1919, p. 194. The several compilations are not totally consistent but in the main agree. The Department of Health was searched without success in the summer of 1971 for the original of these statistics and any other clinic information that might have been retained in its files and archives.

22   Hubbard, "Narcotic Clinic," pp. 46–47, 40.

23   The clinic closed 6 March 1920 (N.Y. *Times,* 7 March 1920) but the Riverside Hospital continued to receive addicts for institutional treatment under the auspices of the Health Department. (See *Weekly Bull. Dept. Health N.Y. City,* 16 Oct. 1920, p. 332.)

24   Registrations were approximately 13,000 in the entire state by April 1920; this was thought to be one-third of the total.

25   Lambert, "Underlying Causes," p. 8.

26   Hubbard, "Narcotic Clinic," p. 34. Some of the credence given Hubbard's conclusions can be measured from the fact that versions of his article were reprinted within a few months by the American Medical Association ("Some Fallacies Regarding Narcotic Drug Addiction," *JAMA 74* : 1439–41 [1920]) and the Public Health Service ("Municipal Narcotic Dispensaries," *Public Health Reports 35* : 771–73, 26 March 1920).

27   The regimen followed in the hospital and its results are described in *Weekly Bull. Dept. Health N.Y. City,* 27 Sept. 1919, pp. 305–06; A. R. Braunlich, "Treatment of Drug Addiction at Riverside Hospital," *Monthly Bull. Dept. Health N.Y. City,* Feb. 1920, pp. 47–49; T. F. Joyce, "The Treatment of Drug Addictions," *Weekly Bull. Dept. Health N.Y. City,* 9 Oct. 1920, pp. 322–24.

28   Department of Health, City of New York, *Annual Report,* 1920, p. 257.

For another hostile reaction to addicts who failed to be cured, see T. F. Joyce ("Denarcotizing the Addict," *Monthly Bull. Dept. Health N.Y. City,* June 1921, pp. 132–36), "I still insist that if there is any more destructive, more troublesome, more nerve wracking, more ungrateful class of patients . . . we have not as yet met them" (p. 136).

29 Braunlich, "Treatment of Drug Addictions," p. 49.

30 For the Narcotic Division of the Revenue Service, the failure of the New York clinic was due to the availability of illicit supplies on the streets. The clinic experience made apparent the prior necessity to secure the control of illicit narcotics. This was also Copeland's conclusion (Copeland to Cooper, 16 Oct. 1919), and the deduction drawn by the Revenue Service's inspector Thomas Cooper: "If it were not possible for the addict to secure the drug clandestinely, the New York plan ought to be absolutely and completely successful" (Memorandum for the Bureau of Internal Revenue, 21 Oct. 1919). The New York clinic became the proof that clinics could not work. Simple maintenance clinics were not even considered legitimate because they did not attempt to cure.

31 Hubbard, "New York City Narcotic Clinic," pp. 42–44. Similarly, the experience at The Tombs had suggested that withdrawal was quite safe, if painful (see above, ch. 5).

32 Braunlich, "Treatment of Drug Addictions," p. 49.

33 Hubbard, "Some Fallacies," pp. 1440–41. Joyce stated ("Denarcotizing the Addict"), "If our legal brothers would cooperate with us, by enacting drastic laws, they would deter the habitual repeater as well as the distributor, and we might get better results" (p. 135).

34 Hubbard, "New York City Narcotic Clinic," pp. 42, 43; also "Some Fallacies," pp. 1440–41.

35 Lambert, "Underlying Causes," p. 5.

36 One comment on the Shreveport clinic by the (later) Federal Bureau of Narcotics captures its attitude toward that clinic and clinics in general: "It was estimated that 75 per cent of the drug addicts in Texas made their headquarters at Shreveport following the operation of that clinic" (Federal Bureau of Narcotics, *Narcotic Clinics in the United States* [GPO, 1955], p. 12). Prof. Lindesmith, on the other hand, wrote in 1965: "It is the general impression today that the [clinic] in Shreveport, Louisiana, was one of the most efficiently operated" (*The Addict and the Law* [New York: Vintage Books, 1965], p. 149).

37 Oscar Dowling (1866–1931) was born in Alabama and received his M.D. from Vanderbilt in 1888. He specialized in eye, ear, nose and throat diseases. In 1906 he was appointed to the Louisiana State Board of Health and served as its president for many years. In the teens of this century he took an active role in fighting patent medicines, alcohol, and narcotics. As late as 1 May 1920 Dr. Dowling was trying to get approval from Levi Nutt for a clinic operation that maintained addicts but permitted administration of the drug only in the clinic. Nutt, in a memo to the Legal Division of the Prohibition Unit, opposed any concessions on clinic operations. "In view of the proposed plan to abolish clinics throughout the country," he wrote, "I doubt the advisability of committing

ourselves . . . at this time." In spite of the New York City experience, Dr. Dowling thought dispensing was not without merit until states could provide institutional curative treatment (Oscar Dowling, President, Louisiana State Board of Health, to L. G. Nutt, Director, Narcotic Division, Prohibition Unit, 1 and 5 May 1920; L. G. Nutt to Legal Division, Prohibition Unit, 6 May 1920).

38 Evidence for Dr. Dowling's fear of indictment is found in a memorandum of his visit to the Narcotics Division in December 1920 prepared by R. C. Valentine of the General Counsel's office. Valentine described Dowling as "afraid that he himself may be arrested under the Federal law . . . and states he is anxious to follow instructions of the Federal Government. He evidently wants us to stand by our guns. We have no choice in the matter in view of the action taken in the New York State Clinics, but I explained the reason for our allowing an extension of the New Orleans' clinic closing date was based upon a necessity of securing, as far as practicable, the cooperation of State governments in enforcement of narcotic laws" ("Note for Case New Orleans File," 11 December 1920, signed "RCV," [RPU]).

39 *State of Louisiana Public Act no. 252,* approved 11 July 1918, promulgated 3 Aug. 1918.

40 "News Report," *JAPhA* 7 : 572 (1918). The survey was also noted in a memo summarizing the New Orleans clinic's history, "Report of Dr. M. W. Swords, in Charge of Narcotic Clinic, Louisiana State Board of Health, to the Honorable Mr. J. O. Bender, Internal Revenue Agent, United States Government, New Orleans, Louisiana, District" (11 June 1919). Dr. Rosewater is apparently the same Dr. Charles Rosenwasser who practiced in New Jersey and testified before the New York State Whitney Committee in 1917.

41 The clinic in New Orleans opened on 6 Feb. 1919 and is discussed in the memo to Agent Bender, and in an article by Swords, "Drug Addiction and Its Relation to Public Health," *New Orleans Med. Surg. J.* (1921), p. 272.

42 The exchange with the state's attorney general and his opinion (see minutes of the Louisiana State Board of Health, meeting of 20–21 Feb. 1919), are quoted in the memo by Swords.

43 "Memorandum on the Narcotic Situation in New Orleans and the Status of Clinics Nationally" was prepared by Dr. Oscar Dowling and sent to Nutt under cover of a letter dated 12 Feb. 1921; Nutt to Arthur D. Greenfield, New York, 23 Nov. 1920.

44 New Orleans *Times-Picayune,* 27 Nov. 1920.

45 Dowling to members of the Louisiana State Board of Health, 26 Oct. 1920; John F. Kramer, Prohibition Commissioner, to Dowling, 8 Nov. 1920; W. T. Truxtun, Internal Revenue Agent, to David A. Gates, Supervising Federal Prohibition Agent, Little Rock, Ark., 12 Oct. 1920.

46 Truxtun's second report was sent to Governor J. M. Parker on 6 February 1921. Truxtun spent considerable time locating any registrants with a criminal record or using a false name since he felt these discoveries would discredit the clinic. The government's attitude toward the clinic

was affected by a confidential letter to Nutt from Dr. William Edler, a physician who had been assigned to the anti-VD program of the state by the federal government. After 18 months in New Orleans, Dr. Edler described the clinic as "a social menace exceeded by nothing—and that is saying a great deal for a city like New Orleans." Dr. Edler admitted he had never been in the clinic, but he observed that it attracted undesirables and "merely dispensed morphine at a profit" (Edler to Nutt, 1 Dec. 1920).

47 Evidence that Truxtun was indeed slanting information to make Dr. Swords and the dispensary appear irresponsible and venal comes from another agent's report (dated 21 Jan. 1921). It was not to a state official but to the Narcotic Division on the matter of Swords's heroin, cocaine, and laudanum purchases. The agent looked into the sales of drugs to the clinic by two wholesalers in New Orleans and discovered that purchases had indeed been made; the heroin and cocaine were purchased on 5 February 1919, at the very beginning of the clinic's operation. Dr. Swords explained that he had at first believed that these two drugs were required by addicts, the same early belief held by the New York City clinic in April 1919. He decided later that heroin and cocaine use was a vice but that morphine was satisfactory for maintenance. He then sent the two drugs to the state chemist for safekeeping, with whom they remained. The dispensing of laudanum to a woman was found to be approved in writing, both by Dr. Dowling and another New Orleans physician, Dr. J. Barth, although the report to the governor in the following month made the dispensing seem an irresponsible and personal violation by Dr. Swords (John M. Tully, Agent, to Truxtun, 21 Jan. 1921).

48 Swords to Truxtun, 4 Dec. 1920; Dowling to Nutt, 17 Jan. 1921.

49 Dowling to USPHS Surgeon General, 15 and 17 Feb. 1921 (PHSR). Henry Mooney, U.S. Attorney, New Orleans, to Nutt, 17 Feb. 1921.

50 At the time of the February meeting the clinic was also investigated by a designee of the Surgeon General—R. M. Grimm, an officer in the Hygienic Laboratory. Grimm did not report to the Public Health Service the black situation that the narcotic agent described; nevertheless he indicated the concurrent opinion of the PHS that a clinic was not a sufficient solution, "a feeble attempt to treat a social condition which is generally recognized to be far-reaching in its effects" (R. M. Grimm to Surgeon General, USPHS, 25 March 1921 (PHSR).

51 W. S. Drautzburg and Ralph H. Oyler to Nutt, 27 March 1920.

52 B. R. Rhees and O. A. H. de la Gardie to Nutt, 23 Oct. 1921.

53 Dr. Terry began to request information from Dr. Butler at least as early as December 1922 and considered Butler's reports of great significance (Terry to Butler, 27 Dec. 1922, BuP).

54 W. P. Butler, "How One American City Is Meeting the Public Health Problems of Narcotic Drug Addiction," *Amer. Med.* 28 : 154–62 (1922).

55 J. B. Greeson, Kansas City, Mo., to Federal Prohibition Commissioner, 6 Oct. 1922.

56 H. H. Wouters, Special Narcotic Agent, to Nutt, 6 Oct. 1922; Wouters to W. S. Blanchard, Acting Prohibition Commissioner, 29 Sept. 1922.

57 Butler to Edward Wilson, Atlanta *Georgian,* 2 Feb. 1923 (BuP).

58 Anonymous to Colonel Lee (*sic*) G. Nutt, 10 Sept. 1922; Nutt to William Blanchard, 19 Sept. 1922. Wouters also saw Nutt in Chicago and discussed the Shreveport clinic and was ordered to investigate it (Wouters to Blanchard, 28 Sept. 1922).

59 Wouters's Report to Nutt, 6 Oct. 1922.

60 Handwritten note dated "11/2" attached to Wouter's report to Valentine, Legal Division, initialed "AYS" [?].

61 Dowling to Nutt, 15 Dec. 1922.

62 2 Feb. 1923 (BuP).

63 Butler to Terry, 15 Feb. 1923 (BuP).

64 Shreveport *Journal,* 7 and 9 June 1923.

65 As early as 1915 a U.S. Senator from Louisiana and the local representative requested a hospital for the treatment of addicts in Shreveport (Acting Surgeon General Glennan to Senator Joseph E. Ramsdell, 19 May 1915; Rep. J. T. Watkins, 4th Louisiana District, to Surgeon General, USPHS, 11 May 1915, PHSR). When the Harrison Act began to cut off sources of drug supply for addicts, Dr. Dowling suggested that a clinic be established in the Shreveport area "to protect them from the peddler and to control illegal traffic" (Dowling to Dr. Frank H. Walke, Parish Health Officer, Shreveport, 12 March 1919 [Copy in BuP]).

66 Charles E. Terry, Executive, Committee on Drug Addictions, Bureau of Social Hygiene, to Butler, 7 Nov. 1928 (BuP).

67 Lindesmith, *Addict and the Law,* p. 160.

68 Senator Duncan U. Fletcher asked for an explanation of the closing of the Jacksonville clinic in a letter to Nutt of 2 May 1921. He was assured that this was not directed at Florida—that all clinics were being closed.

69 Erwin C. Ruth, Special Narcotic Agent, to L. G. Nutt, 19 April 1921 (the copied report in the file is dated March, but from the covering letter and the report itself, April must have been the month in which it was prepared). Ruth was later arrested and dropped from the service, charged with blackmailing addicts and shaking down druggists and doctors. Sidney Howard, "The Inside Story of Dope in this Country," *Hearst's International,* Feb. 1923, p. 142.

70 T. E. Middlebrooks, Narcotic Agent in Charge, Atlanta, to L. G. Nutt, 17 Feb. 1922.

71 T. E. Middlebrooks to W. S. Blanchard, Acting Head, Narcotic Division, 30 Nov. 1923.

72 New Haven *Register,* 17 Aug. 1918. A similar arrangement whereby one physician was authorized to provide prescriptions for the city's addicts was followed in Memphis; the number totaled about 350 daily ("Drug Addicts in the South," *Survey,* 26 April 1919, pp. 147–48).

73 New Haven *Register,* 17 Aug. 1918.

74 Memorandum on the New Haven Clinic by Agents H. S. Forrer and O. W. Lewis to Prohibition Commissioner, 17 June 1920.

75 *Register,* 17 Aug. 1918.

76 Forrer and Lewis report, 17 June 1920.

77 E. C. Ruth, Special Narcotic Agent to L. G. Nutt, 6 Oct. 1920.

78 Report on the Albany Clinic by H. S. Forrer and O. W. Lewis to Nutt, marked confidential, dated 25 June 1920.

79 V. Simonton, Head, Narcotic Unit, Federal Prohibition Office, New York, to L. G. Nutt, 1 Sept. 1920.

80 See Charles E. Terry and Mildred Pellens, *The Opium Problem* (New York: Bureau of Social Hygiene, 1928; reprint ed., Montclair, N.J.: Patterson Smith, 1970), p. 843. The legislature passed several narcotic bills as well as one abolishing the Department of Narcotic Drug Control and presented the contradictory bills to Governor Nathan L. Miller. The governor vetoed all but the bill of abolishment. He explained that physicians could not agree on how to treat addiction and until this question was resolved, it was best to defer state laws designed to complement federal statutes. See *Public Papers of Governor Miller*, "Memoranda on Legislative Bills Approved," section entitled "To Repeal Article 22 of the Public Health Law and Abolishing [the] Department of Narcotic Drug Control," 13 March 1921 (Albany: J. B. Lyon, 1924), p. 178. New York City responded by passage of an antinarcotic section to the Sanitary Code on 25 July 1921 which reinstated some state controls.

81 Some clinics were brought into being by Commissioner Roper's letter to agents, 31 July 1919 (U.S. Treasury Dept., Bureau of Internal Revenue, *Enforcement of the Harrison Narcotic Law*, "M-Mim 2212 to Collectors of Internal Revenue, Revenue Agents, and Others Concerned," 31 July 1919, GPO, 1919), as a temporary method of handling the anticipated influx of addicts deprived of their drugs. Less than a year later the Prohibition Unit's legal division prepared a memorandum for Nutt: "The Proposed Plan to Abolish Clinics Throughout the Country" (6 May 1920). Between these two dates the decision to close the clinics was made. Probably the decision was made some time after Cooper's glowing reports of the clinics were submitted to the bureau (22 October 1919) and before Nutt's trip across the nation (March 1920) to evaluate for himself, always negatively, any clinic practicing maintenance.

82 J. E. Conway to R. C. Valentine, Head, Legal Division, Narcotic Field Force, Prohibition Unit, 5 May 1920: "The mere bringing of an indictment might have beneficial results, even if it is later decided, upon an understanding being reached with the offending officials, that prosecution could not be maintained."

83 Terry and Pellens, *Opium Problem*, p. 843.

Chapter 8

1 L. F. Schmeckebier, *The Bureau of Prohibition: Its History, Activities, and Organization*, Monograph no. 57, Institute for Government Research (Washington, D.C.: The Brookings Institution [Lord Baltimore Press], 1929), pp. 7–35, 136–45, 150–51, 170–72, 225–28, 309–12, for descriptions of the responsibilities, bureaucratic structure, salaries, and appropriations for narcotic enforcement.

2 "Presidential Message," *Cong. Rec. 64, pt. 1* : 215, 67th Cong., 4th Sess., 8 Dec. 1922.

3   "Report of Committee on Narcotic Drugs of the Council on Health and Public Instruction," *JAMA* 76 : 1669–71 (1921). Malachi Harney, a long-time enforcement officer in the Treasury Department, both in liquor and narcotics, recalls that the narcotic agents were sorely embarrassed by their close association with Prohibition agents who had lost public respect. Narcotic agents also performed a task which was much less controversial than dry agents (my interview with Harney; 4 June 1970, Washington, D.C.).

4   L. F. Schmeckebier and F. A. Eble, *The Bureau of Internal Revenue: Its History, Activities, and Organization,* Service Monograph of the U.S. Government, Institute for Government Research (Baltimore: Johns Hopkins Press, 1923), pp. 61–62.

5   Schmeckebier, *Bureau of Prohibition,* pp. 309–12. The number of agents and the appropriations and expenditures can be followed in the annual appearance of narcotic officials before the House Appropriation Committee.

6   The average number of federal liquor convictions with prison sentences during the years 1922–24 was about 31,000 annually, the average sentence between 20 and 30 days. For the same period the annual average number of federal narcotic convictions with prison sentences was about 4,000 with an average sentence that grew from 10 months in 1922 to 14 months in 1924 ("Hearings before the House Appropriation Committee," Treasury Dept. Appropriation Bill 1926; 4 Dec. 1924, 68th Cong., 2nd Sess., p. 472). Sentences for Harrison Act violations continued to rise until the average in 1928 was 1 year 10 months ("Hearings before the House Appropriation Committee," Treasury Dept. Appropriation Bill 1930, 23 Nov. 1928, 70th Cong., 1st Sess., p. 473). The number of violations of the Harrison Act from fiscal year 1916 to the nearest hundred (p. 475):

1916: 1,900	1921: 4,300	1925: 10,300
1917: 1,100	1922: 6,700	1926: 10,300
1918: 1,300	1923: 7,200	1927: 8,900
1919: 2,400	1924: 10,300	1928: 8,700
1920: 3,900		

The decline in violations after the first Jin Fuey Moy decision (1916) is of interest, as is the rapid rise in violations when a separate narcotic division was created in 1920 and after the Supreme Court decision against maintenance in 1919.

7   At the close of fiscal year 1928, just before the two narcotic farms were authorized by Congress, the number of prisoners in federal penitentiaries for violation of the Volstead Act was 1,156 (Schmeckebier, *Bureau of Prohibition,* p. 79). Those imprisoned for drug law violations were 2,529 and those for auto theft 1,148. The total number of prisoners was 7,738 so that the Harrison Act engendered the largest class of violations and represented about a third of all prisoners (p. 143).

8   Editorial, *JAMA* 60 : 1364 (1913).

9   In one rare instance a high FBN official admitted that enforcement in

the 1920s was perhaps as bad as the physicans and druggists claimed. Speaking at the Fourth Annual Conference of Pharmaceutical Law Enforcement Officials in Toronto on 25 August 1932, H. T. Nugent, Field Supervisor of the FBN, told how the new Narcotics Commissioner, Harry Anslinger, hoped that new rules for the agents would cut down on harassment of health professionals. According to Nugent, Anslinger thought that cooperation with the professionals would work "better than if we undertook to go out and, as the field man sometimes term it, black-jack them into line." Two months after assuming office, Anslinger issued orders that no agent should begin criminal investigation of professionals without written orders from the agent in charge, a copy of which was also sent to the commissioner's office. Nugent explained: "In that way he hoped to eliminate the complaint, and probably the justifiable complaint on the part of some of the professional men against the desire of some of our field men to build up a good record at the expense of the professional classes, and made up probably a lot of petty cases which we didn't feel should be called to the attention of the United States Attorney, or even reported to the Bureau." As a result of these measures, "we find now that the number of cases reported in professional classes has improved materially . . . that instead of getting a lot of petty cases, we are getting cases that have merit" (Stenographic typescript of Proceedings, located in box 31, American Pharmaceutical Association Archives, Washington D.C., pp. 86–87).

10　"Hearings before the House Appropriation Committee," Treasury Dept. Appropriation Bill 1933, 14 Jan. 1932, 72nd. Cong., 1st Sess., p. 376.

11　*U.S. v. Behrman,* 258 U.S. 280, decided 27 March 1922; also ibid., p. 289; that good faith was not a defense was suggested by the New York attorney Arthur D. Greenfield in "Some Legal Aspects of the Narcotic Drug Problem," *N.Y. Med. J. 110* : 100–03 (1919).

12　"House Investigation of Narcotics," *House Res. no. 258,* 67th Cong., 2nd Sess., 4 Jan. 1922, *Cong. Rec., vol. 62, pt. 1,* p. 808. Earlier, in November 1921, an investigation was approved by the American Public Health Association, perhaps following up Dr. Terry's suggestion to the House Committee in January 1921. It was endorsed by the House of Delegates of the AMA on 23 May 1922. Volk's onslaught against the Narcotic Division is found in Appendix to the *Cong. Rec., House, 62, pt. 13* : 13, 340–45, 67th Cong., 2nd Sess. (1922), and a second attack against the coterie of his enemies and a defense of Dr. Bishop and addiction maintenance is found in *Cong. Rec., House, 62, pt. 10* : 9, 789–96, 67th Cong., 2nd Sess., 30 June, 1922. Rebuttal to Volk's attack on prominent New York physicians such as Alexander Lambert was given by Rep. Ogden Mills, who demanded some proof from Volk that, among other allegations, these physicians and Greenfield profited from sanitaria; see *Cong. Rec., House, 62, pt. 2* : 1665, 67 Cong., 2nd Sess., 24 Jan. 1922. For a picture of the combat over maintenance which is as conspiratorial as Volk's but on the opposite side, see A. C. Prentice, "The Problem of the Narcotic Drug Addict" *JAMA 76* : 1551–54 (1921).

13　The resolution adopted had been prepared and submitted by Dr. Rooney,

House of Delegates, "Proceedings of the St. Louis Session, 23 May 1922," *JAMA 78* : 1715 (1922). State medicine was defined as "any form of medical treatment provided, conducted, controlled, or subsidized by the federal or any state government," with a few exceptions, such as to the uniformed services and in cases of communicable disease, mental health, and the indigent sick.

14   *Amendments to the Harrison Narcotic Act,* Hearing before a Subcommittee of the Committee on Ways and Means, House, 69th Cong., 1st Sess., 21–22, 26 May 1926 (GPO, 1926), pp. 5–6. The government's practice was declared unconstitutional in *Starnes v. U.S.,* 282 Fed. 236, decided 21 July 1922, and the decision was applauded by the AMA in "Lawless Law Enforcement," *JAMA 85* : 680–81 (1925); also see "Strengthening the Harrison Narcotic Act," editorial, *JAMA 86* : 1473–74 (1926).

15   *Eckert* v. *U.S.,* 8th Circuit Court of Appeals (8 Fed. Rept. [2] 257), 6 Aug. 1925.

16   *U.S.* v. *Daugherty,* 269 U.S. 360, decided 4 Jan. 1926, pp. 362–63.

17   *HR 11, 612* printed in *Amendments to the Harrison Narcotic Act,* hearings pp. 1–2.

18   *Linder* v. *U.S.,* 268 U.S. 5, decided 13 April 1925, at p. 22.

19   252 U.S. 416, decided 19 April 1920.

20   L. C. Andrews, Secretary of the Treasury to Rep. William R. Green, chairman, House Committee on Ways and Means, 29 March 1926; letter reprinted in *Amendments to the Harrison Narcotic Act,* hearings, p. 2.

21   Testimony of L. C. Nutt, *Amendments to the Harrison Narcotic Act,* hearings, 26 May 1926, pp. 46–49.

22   276 U.S. 332, decided 9 April 1928. The majority opinion was written by Chief Justice Taft, who was joined by Justices Stone, Sanford, Van Devanter, Holmes, and Brandeis.

23   "United States Supreme Court Distrusts the Harrison Narcotic Act," editorial, *JAMA 86* : 627–28 (1926).

24   Oscar Dowling, "Three Great National Health Problems," *JAMA 85* : 484–88 (1925). Dowling chose for discussion drug addiction, rabies, and venereal diseases. He was discouraged by the battle against addiction; he believed the Harrison Act had made little progress and represented "an attempt to cure a deep rooted evil with one stroke of the pen." He criticized the lack of planning to care for addicts, and so on. Dowling's views were somewhat confused and did not add anything new to the debate, but his comments do reflect anger at government interference, which arose undoubtedly as much from his personal experience with Nutt's agency as from the growing resistance of the AMA, of which he was a high official, to federal encroachment on the states' powers to control the practice of medicine.

25   *The National Prohibition Law,* Hearings of a Subcommittee of the Senate Committee on the Judiciary, April 1926, 69th Cong., 1st Sess.

26   Charles Merz, *The Dry Decade* (Seattle: Univ. of Washington Press, reprinted 1970), pp. 186–87.

27   Schmeckebier, *Bureau of Prohibition,* p. 57. The Wickersham Report

stated that 59% had failed (*Report on the Enforcement of the Prohibition Laws of the United States*, National Commission of Law Observance and Enforcement, House Doc. no. 722, 71st Cong., 3rd sess., 7 Jan. 1931, p. 15).

28　Nutt estimated 110,000 addicts in the United States in 1925 ("Hearings before the House Appropriation Committee," Treasury Dept. Appropriation Bill 1927, 2 Dec. 1925, 69th. Cong., 1st Sess., pp. 438–39). The following year he reported on a survey conducted by the 300 narcotic agents in May 1926 which revealed only 95,000 addicts. Details of the survey were not revealed ("Hearings before the House Appropriation Committee," Treasury Dept. Appropriation Bill 1928, 18 Nov. 1926, 69th Cong., 2nd Sess., p. 345). In May 1924, Drs. Kolb and DuMez had estimated about 110,000 addicts in the U.S.

29　"Hearings before House Appropriation Committee," Treasury Dept. Appropriation Bill 1931, 29 Nov. 1929, 71 Cong., 2nd Sess., p. 345. The appropriation for 1930 was $1.4 million, and a deficiency appropriation raised the total to $1.6 million. At these hearings Nutt estimated that there were fewer than 100,000 addicts in the U.S. and strongly disagreed that the addiction problem was increasing (p. 350).

30　Arnold H. Taylor, *American Diplomacy and the Narcotics Traffic, 1900–1939* (Durham, N.C.: Duke Univ. Press, 1969), pp. 141–45.

31　The International Narcotic Education Association "undertakes to organize, develop, and standardize narcotic education in the schools . . . of this country and ultimately of other countries" (*Narcotic Education* 1 : 6 [1927]). Other organizations with somewhat similar goals include Charles B. Towns's International Narcotic Association, which began apparently in late 1918 and of which little is known (Memorandum from Hygienic Laboratory to the Surgeon General, USPHS, 22 April 1919, PHSR). In the hearings on *Establishment of Two Federal Narcotic Farms* (House Judiciary Committee on *HR 12,781* and *HR 13,645*, 26–28 April 1928, 70th Cong., 1st Sess., rev. print. 1928), Mrs. Sarah Graham-Mulhall submitted a statement on behalf of the World Anti-narcotic Union, which she described as "containing millions of the greatest mothers, wives and sisters in the Union," and which apparently was closely associated with women's clubs. Mrs. Graham-Mulhall was president of the New York City Federation of Women's Clubs (pp. 87–90). She had served as a deputy commissioner of the short-lived New York State Narcotic Control Commission. Another group, the Narcotic Drug League, brought together in 1922 the leaders in the American antinarcotic campaign, including Bishop Brent, Dr. Alexander Lambert, Mrs. Graham-Mulhall, and Prof. Joseph Chamberlain, all of whom strongly supported the most stringent interpretation of the Harrison Act. For a description of this meeting see Survey 4 Feb. 1922, p. 218.

32　The longest and most direct rebuttal of the Kolb–Du Mez study came from New York's warden of the City Prison, S. W. Brewster, whose essay, "Survey of the Prevalence and Trend of Drug Addiction," appeared in a Hobson-inspired hearing before the Committee on Education of the House of Representatives (*Conference on Narcotic Education,* Hearings

on *HJR 65*, 69th Cong., 1st Sess., 16 Dec. 1925, pp. 177–90). The resolution for which the hearing was held had been introduced by a strong
supporter of Hobson, Rep. Walter F. Lineberger of California. It called
on the federal government to participate in Hobson's Conference on
Narcotic Education to be held in Philadelphia in the summer of 1926.
The record of the hearings illustrates Hobson's ability to publicize his
views and his own role. Hundreds of replies from prominent Americans
and requests for support of the conference were printed. Rep. Lineberger
wrote, on Captain Hobson's request, to 5,000 county and city superintendents of education; presidents of colleges, universities, and junior
colleges; state presidents and secretaries of Parent–Teachers' associations;
and "distinguished citizens from *Who's Who in America*." These letters
stressed the dangers of heroin addiction, claimed that there were more
than a million addicts in the United States, and enclosed copies of Hobson's "The Peril of Narcotic Drugs," which Lineberger had introduced
into the *Congressional Record* when Hobson's earlier campaign to print at
government expense 50,000,000 copies was not authorized by Congress.
The description of heroin was particularly misleading. The letter to the
names taken from *Who's Who*, for example, states that "heroin changes
a misdemeanant into a desperado of the most vicious type," while the
Hobson pamphlet became almost lyrical on the hazards of heroin to
evolutionary progress. The conference, according to Rep. Lineberger, was
primarily to meet the menace of heroin, which had caused "organized
banditry" in all parts of the nation (hearings, p. 10). Gerhard Kuhne, of
the Department of Correction of New York City, claimed that 75% of
crime would be eliminated if drug addiction could be stopped, for he
claimed that drugs were "a false stimulant" to crime. Alcohol, on the
other hand, he considered a minor cause of crime (hearings, p. 175).
For the AMA's rebuttal of the Hobson statistics, see "Drug Addiction in
the United States," *JAMA 82* : 1974–75 (1924).

33 Hobson's success with the media illustrates his efficiency and the existence
of a prepared audience. In 1924 Hobson tried to get a congressional
appropriation for the printing of "The Peril of Narcotics—A Warning to
the People of America," so that every home could have a copy. But, aside
from the cost, the Federal Narcotics Control Board denied Hobson's
claim that one ounce of heroin would cause 2,000 addicts and found
fantastic Hobson's warning that, "In using any brand of face powder
regularly, it is a wise precaution to have a sample analysed for heroin"
(Federal Narcotic Control Board, the Secretaries of State, Treasury and
Commerce, to Senator George H. Moses, chairman, Committee on
Printing, U.S. Senate, 27 May 1924, in *Conference on Narcotic Education*,
hearings, pp. 2–3). Hobson brushed aside such carping for he fought a
"biological struggle for the life of our people and the species" (hearings,
p. 5). One witness supporting Hobson assumed that the large number of
addicts in federal prisons reflected addiction as a cause of crime, instead
of their being in jail as the result of Harrison Act violations. The most
concise and forceful opponent of Hobson was Dr. Kolb who refuted in
detail Hobson's exaggerations. Yet Dr. Kolb did not favor maintenance of

addiction merely to satisfy addiction, and he wished continued enforcement of the Harrison Act. He simply did not think that addiction was the major threat that Hobson described; in fact, he said, "addiction is really a very rare thing throughout the United States." Dr. Kolb also denied any difference between morphine and heroin (hearings, pp. 33, 28). A somewhat revised version of "The Peril of Narcotic Drugs," along with some other propaganda of the Narcotic Education Association, was later printed in the *Congressional Record* at Rep. Lineberger's insistance (*Cong. Rec. House, 66, pt. 4* : 4088–91, 18 Feb. 1925, 68th Cong., 2nd Sess.). This extract from the *Record* was distributed via franked mail to leaders of American institutions, as he described in *Conference on Narcotic Education* (see above, ch. 8, n. 32). A general outline of Hobson's approach to the media, textbook publishers, etc., can be found in Richmond P. Hobson, "The General Status of Narcotic Drug Education in America," *Narcotic Education 1* : 4–7 (1927).

34 "The Struggle of Mankind against Its Deadliest Foe," broadcast 1 March 1928, printed in *Narcotic Education 1* : 51–54 (1928).

35 "Extract from an Address by Richmond Pearson Hobson, Broadcasted over KMTR, Los Angeles, 28 February 1929," printed in *Narcotic Education 2* : 67–69 (1929).

36 E. George Payne, "Narcotic Addiction as an Educational Problem," *Narcotic Education 5* : 26–30 (1931). Payne was Director of Education for the World Conference on Narcotic Education, and Professor of Educational Sociology in the School of Education, New York University.

37 Hobson to Harry J. Anslinger, Commissioner of Narcotics, 11 Dec. 1936 (AP, box 12).

38 *Exportation of Opium,* Hearings before a Subcommittee of the Committee on Ways and Means on *HR 14,500,* House, 66th Cong., 3rd Sess., 8 and 11 Dec. 1920 and 3 and 4 Jan. 1921 (GPO, 1921), p. 10. The interest of the China Club in narcotics is described by its secretary, William K. McKibben, and the formation of the White Cross from the China Club was described by a Seattle *Times* reporter, J. J. Underwood, in the House Committee on Foreign Affairs hearings (*Limiting Production of Habitforming Drugs and Raw Materials from Which They Are Made, Hearings on HJR 430 and HJR 453,* 67th Cong., 4th Sess., 13–16 Feb. 1923, rev. print. pp. 63–67). By the latter date McKibben was executive secretary. The name the China Club selected, "The White Cross: International Anti-Narcotics Society," may have been original with the founders, or may have had some connection with an earlier reform movement called The White Cross which began in England in 1883 and spread to the U.S. the following year. The latter had chapters scattered across the nation and had as its goal the preservation of the purity of women and especially the prevention of prostitution; although only men could belong, one of its goals was women's suffrage which was seen as an integral part of giving women the power to protect themselves from exploitation (B. F. DeCosta, *The White Cross: Its Origin and Progress* [Chicago: Sanitary Publishing Co., 1887]).

39 McKibben to Butler, 9 July 1925 (BuP); the White Cross also supported

a measure in the Washington State Legislature to permit addiction maintenance in 1940 (see below, ch. 8, n. 41).

40 Hobson stated, "It would be more accurate and psychologically more
useful as a warning to youth to portray narcotic drug addiction in its true
colors, that of an incurable living death" (*Narcotic Education* 2 : 55
[1929]). Interestingly, New York City warned youth in a radio spot
broadcast in spring 1972 against "the living death" of heroin addiction.

41 Harry D. Smith, District Supervisor, Minneapolis, to Commissioner of
Narcotics, 15 Sept. 1939 (FBN file no. 0145-18, "Interstate Narcotic
Association"). A bill to authorize clinics was considered by a committee
of the Washington State House of Representatives and successful opposition to it was mounted by the FBN and other groups. The Chicago-
based Interstate Narcotic Association also favored a clinic system but is
better known for its fight against "marihuana—the weed of madness,"
illustrated by its often-reprinted poster warning parents and children of
the "killer weed." The Association also sold marihuana seals to support
its work. The White Cross of California had attempted to inaugurate a
narcotic clinic in Los Angeles in 1934 but was unsuccessful.

42 Anslinger's lack of respect for the efforts of Hobson, whom he considered
a dilettante who lived off the wealthy financial backers of his antinarcotic
efforts, was revealed in my interview with Anslinger. In his words, organizations like the White Cross, which were once considered supportive of
federal activity, "went sour" and endorsed clinics—"barrooms for addicts"
or "morphine feeding stations"—two terms he favored for the concept.

43 The Knights of Columbus in 1922 "launched upon a ruthless campaign
for the nationwide suppression of opium and other narcotic evils" (*Survey*,
4 Feb. 1922, pp. 718–19). In Rep. Porter's hearings on *HJR 453* (Feb.
1923), numerous service clubs and lodges took official stands in the fight
against drug abuse, including the Loyal Order of the Moose, The Grotto,
Mystic Order of Veiled Prophets of the Enchanted Realm (a Masonic
order); and the Benevolent and Protective Order of Elks, as well as many
local organizations, women's clubs, etc. President Harding was a member
of the Grotto, his Secretary of Labor James J. Davis was Director General
of the Loyal Order of Moose. Davis was planning, when he appeared
before the Porter Committee, to meet soon with officials of the National
Fraternal Congress to coordinate a more extensive campaign by its constituent members against drug abuse.

44 Hobson, "General Status of Narcotic Drug Addiction in America," *Narcotic Education* 1 : 6 (1927); Hobson estimates that in twelve months
prior to July 1927, 2.5 million documents were mailed to educators, clubs,
etc., and 200,000 letters were mailed, one-third typed, the rest mimeo-
graphed. "The very large volume of work is accomplished on a modest
budget," explained Hobson, "because we utilize the services of the public
printer and the congressional frank, and the machinery of education and
of great organizations."

45 *Exportation of Opium*, hearings, pp. 115, 121. Concern was expressed by
Secretary of State William Jennings Bryan when urging passage of the
Harrison Bill and allied proposals in 1913 ("Abolition of the Opium

Evil," House Doc. no. 33, 63rd Cong., 1st Sess., 21 April 1913, p. 5). In 1922 the House report on the *Exportation and Importation of Narcotic Drugs* reemphasized the damage to China's purchasing power by addiction and consequent decrease in trade with the U.S. (House Report no. 852, 67th Cong., 2nd Sess., 27 March 1922, p. 6).

46 See U.S. Treasury Dept., *The Treasury Department's Special Committee of Investigation Appointed March 25, 1918, by the Secretary of the Treasury: Traffic in Narcotic Drugs* (GPO, 1919), p. 7. This report provided statistics on the rapid rise in narcotic exports to Canada after passage of the Harrison Act. See also *Exportation of Opium,* hearings, pp. 132–33.

47 *Exportation of Opium,* hearings, pp. 22, 36, 39–40.

48 *Exportation of Opium,* hearings, pp. 81–82, 49.

49 Dr. J. W. Scherechewsky, Assistant Surgeon General, USPHS, Chief of the Division of Scientific Research explained that the U.S. "probably consumes more narcotic drugs per capita than almost any other country in the world right now" (*Exportation of Opium,* hearings, pp. 133, 105–08).

50 *Limiting Production,* hearings on *HJR 430* and *HJR 453,* p. 1070. In this hearing Terry still maintained that 75% of addicts were made so "through the therapeutic use of drugs in sickness" (p. 109).

51 *Prohibit Importation of Opium: Report to Accompany HR 16,118,* House, Committee on Ways and Means, 66th Cong., 3rd Sess., 21 Feb. 1921, H. Report 1345. Rep. Rainey introduced *HR 16,118* on 17 Feb. 1921.

52 *Public Law no. 227,* 26 May 1922, 67th Cong., 2nd Sess.

53 Andrew Mellon to J. W. Fordney, chairman, Committee on Ways and Means, House of Representatives, 22 June 1921, printed in *Importation and Exportation of Narcotic Drugs: Report to Accompany HR 2193,* House, Committee on Ways and Means, 67th Cong., 2nd Sess., 27 March 1922, H. Rept. 852, pp. 19–20.

54 Porter (1869–1930) studied medicine for two years before entering law school and gaining admission to the bar in 1893; he served in the House from 1911 to his death (*Biographical Directory of American Congressmen, 1774–1961,* pp. 1471–72).

55 Taylor, *Narcotics Traffic,* pp. 232–41.

56 Porter to Secretary of State Charles Evans Hughes, 12 Feb. 1923, printed in *Limiting Production of Habit-forming Narcotic Drugs and the Raw Materials from Which They Are Made: Report to Accompany HJR 453,* House, Committee on Foreign Affairs, 67 Cong., 4th Sess., 21 Feb. 1923, H. Rept. 1678, pp. 5–6. In the report submitted by Rep. Porter he emphatically declared that "no domestic law . . . can control this [narcotic] traffic; [the] only effective and permanent remedy . . . is to be obtained by the concurrence of the producing countries . . . in behalf of the moral and physical welfare of our people," to limit production of plants from which the drugs are made to strictly medicinal and scientific purposes (pp. 4–5).

57 Taylor, *Narcotic Traffic,* pp. 150–59.

58 *Limiting Production,* 21 Feb. 1923, House Rept. 1678 pp. 4–5; condemnation of the Assembly's action was also contained in *Hearings on HJR 430 and HJR 453,* p. 2.

59 *Hearings on HJR 430 and HJR 453,* p. 2. Public Resolution no. 96, 67th Cong., 4th Sess., passed 2 March 1923.

60 Taylor, *Narcotic Traffic,* pp. 146–70.

61 *Prohibiting the Importation of Opium for the Manufacture of Heroin: Hearings on HR 7079,* House, Committee on Ways and Means, 68th Cong., 1st Sess., 3 April 1924, pp. 41–43.

62 Ibid., pp. 2–3, 39. The American Association of Pharmaceutical Chemists had opposed the use of heroin in 1917 (N.Y. *Times,* 8 Aug. 1919). The Public Health Service considered the national prohibition of heroin a wise step also (Surgeon General Rupert Blue to William McAdoo, Chief Magistrate, City of New York, 14 May 1919, PHSR).

63 *Prohibiting Importation,* hearings on *HR 7079,* p. 5. The Commissioner of Health of Chicago, Dr. Herman N. Bundesen, asserted that "the root of the social evil is essentially in our dope, our habit-forming drugs [the] main cause of prostitution and crime" (Hearings on *HJR 430* and *HJR 453,* pp. 72–75). Other examples of growing attribution of crimes to heroin use by responsible officials in the early 1920s are: W. G. Shepherd, "Youth + Drugs = Crime" (*American Legion Weekly,* 30 Nov. 1923, pp. 7–8, 27–30): "Insane daring, utter merciless and vicious cruelty are characteristics of the dope fiend's crimes" (p. 27); "It is estimated that there are 2,000,000 drug fiends in the United States" (p. 28). F. Wallis, (Commissioner of Corrections, City of New York, Former U.S. Commissioner of Immigration), "The Menace of the Drug Addict" (*Current History,* Feb. 1925), pp. 740–43): "Heroin . . . is the most insidious and crime-inspiring of all drugs. When we consider that the United States uses more of these powerful opiates than all the leading nations of Europe combined we begin to understand why there are more murders in a single American city than in all the countries of Western Europe" (p. 741); "In my opinion no measure is too radical or severe that would prohibit the manufacture and sale of habit-forming drugs" (p. 743).

   R. H. Lampman, "Heroin Heroes: An Interview with Capt. Richmond Pearson Hobson" (*Saturday Evening Post,* 20 Sept. 1923, pp. 41–42): "The great expansion of narcotic addiction in America, given impetus by heroin, dates from about 1910, and . . . the great increase in crimes of violence in the United States has a parallel rise . . ." (p. 41).

64 *Prohibiting Importation,* hearings on *HR 7079,* p. 24, statement of Dr. Amos O. Squires, Chief Physician, Sing Sing Prison. Hobson seized on the increase of "900%" in heroin addicts (from 1% to 9%) without explaining that it came after the antimaintenance enforcement of 1919, or that the "peak" was merely 132 addicts in a prisoner total for one year of 1,450 in 1922. He used the simpler statistic to dramatize the peril to the nation. For example, Hobson introduced the figure in a "Sample Lesson for Senior High School":

   Teacher: The actual number of drug addicts has been estimated to be from 250,000 to 2,000,000. Prison authorities at Leavenworth in 1921 reported 15.5 percent of drug addicts and in 1922, 24 percent. The chief physician at Sing Sing says there was an increase in addicts of 900 percent from 1919 to 1922. What do these figures show?

Pupil: That it is becoming a more serious problem all the time.

(*Cong. Rec., House, 66, pt. 4* : 4088–91, 18 Feb. 1925, 68th Cong., 2nd Sess.); see *Prohibiting Importation,* hearings on *HR 7079,* p. 47, for statement of Sidney W. Brewster, Asst. Superintendent and Deputy Warden of the Reformatory Prison at Harts Island, New York City.

For Richardson's disclaimers after making dogmatic and exaggerated statements, see p. 11; for Blue, see pp. 28–29; also Dr. Hobart A. Hare to Rep. H. G. Watson, 1 April 1924, reprinted on pp. 18–19; for discussion see p. 14. Porter (see pp. 51–52) believed also that most crime by addicts was caused by their need to buy more opiates, but he did not press the point against witnesses who gave the impression that heroin had an effect of stimulating a person to crime by its psychological action; see his questioning of Dr. Squires (p. 22).

65 *Prohibiting Importation,* hearings on *HR 7079,* p. 41.

66 *Public Resolution no. 20,* 68th Cong., 1st Sess., 15 May 1924. Porter held hearings on *HJR 195* in February; the resulting publication was something of a handbook on American attitudes toward narcotic control and was consciously directed at foreign governments that would be present at the forthcoming Geneva Conference (*The Traffic in Habit-forming Drugs: Hearings on HJR 195,* House, Committee on Foreign Affairs, 21 Feb. 1924, 68th Cong., 1st Sess.). For Senator Lodges's amendment see *Appropriation for Participation of the United States in Two International Conferences for Control of Narcotic Drugs: Report to Accompany HJR 195,* Senate, Committee on Foreign Affairs, 68th Cong., 1st Sess., S. Report. no. 499, 5 May 1924, p. 1.

67 Taylor, *Narcotic Traffic,* pp. 171–209, esp. pp. 207–08.

68 Porter's attitude can be summarized by an excerpt from a letter to the Secretary of State: "An effective remedy cannot be secured by compromise," Porter to Hughes, 12 Feb. 1923 (*Traffic, Hearings on HJR 195,* p. 35).

69 *Establishment of Two Federal Narcotic Farms,* hearings.

70 Ibid., p. 18; H. E. Mereness, "Some Remarks on the Narcotic Situation as Applying to the Federal Prison System," pp. 133–39. Mereness, Inspector of Prisons, estimated the chance of cure as "a thousand to one against success" (p. 138). Similarly a physician-representative from New York, William I. Sirovich, in a lengthy speech in the House, stated that addicts always relapsed because of their "peculiar psychopathic constitutionally inferior types" (*Cong. Rec., House, 72: pt. 5* : 4975–81, 71st Cong., 2nd Sess., 7 March 1930). Rep. Porter, who spoke at the end of Rep. Sirovich's speech, agreed (p. 4980).

71 Albert S. Gregg, "United States Narcotic Farms," *Narcotic Education* 2 : 9–10 (1928).

72 *Cong. Rec., House, 69, pt. 9* : 9412–13, 70th Cong., 1st Sess., 21 May 1928.

73 *Establishment of Two Federal Narcotic Farms*, p. 42. Porter's arguments
    against the high use of narcotics in the U.S. rested on an analysis made
    by Edwin L. Neville of the State Department, who claimed that the
    rate of per capita opium consumption quoted against the United States,
    36 grains annually, was an error based on total imports and not on con-
    sumption. The year in which this would have been grossly in error was
    1919, when a large proportion of the imported American opium was
    exported to Japan, but it would not have been true of import figures
    prior to 1915. For Neville's argument see Neville to Porter, 13 Feb.
    1924 (in *Prohibiting Importation*, hearings on HR 7079, pp. 42–43).
    When Porter was asked whether he was familiar with the earlier sta-
    tistics he replied, "I have never read the testimony" (p. 43). Porter based
    his rebuttal to foreign charges of massive American narcotic use on the
    official import statistics, which gave an average of 8 grains per capita
    annually, a figure close to that of other Western nations. For a further
    statement of Porter's position see W. W. Willoughby, *Opium as an
    International Problem: The Geneva Opium Conferences* (Baltimore:
    Johns Hopkins Univ. Press, 1925), pp. 1–7, 304–06.
74 *Establishment of Two Federal Narcotic Farms*, p. 42.
75 Porter's argument was that on official statistics the U.S. consumption of
    opiates was similar to other nations; figures on smuggling were difficult
    to estimate for any nation and therefore could not be used to compare
    American and foreign consumption. Porter's aim was apparently to de-
    fend against assigning to the U.S. the cause for America's drug problem,
    which he often said was increasing and a great menace, and to transfer
    the cause to foreign and uncooperative, perhaps even conspiratorial, gov-
    ernments.
76 From my interview with Anslinger it appears that the PHS officers were
    occasionally "brought to heel" as irregularities were detected by FBN
    agents (interview, Hollidaysburg, Pa., 30 May 1970).
77 *Bureau of Narcotics: Hearings on HR 10,561*, House, Committee on
    Ways and Means, 7–8 March 1930, 71st Cong., 2nd Sess., p. 13. Porter
    declared that he was convinced of the "wisdom of separating narcotics
    from Prohibition, for the very simple reason that there is absolutely no
    relationship between the two. The latter is highly controversial and the
    former is not."
78 Newspaper accounts are summarized in Leo Katcher, *The Big Bankroll:
    The Life and Times of Arnold Rothstein* (New York: Harper's, 1959).
    For Rothstein's entry into narcotics and revelations from documents left
    after his death, see pp. 290–99, 337–99.
79 "Presentment and Report by the Grand Jury on the Subject of the Nar-
    cotic Traffic," January, Morning Session, 1930, filed 19 Feb. 1930; re-
    printed in *Bureau of Narcotics: Hearings on HR 10,561*, pp. 73–77.
80 *Bureau of Narcotics, Hearings on HR 10,561*, p. 45.
81 From the Anslinger interview.
82 *Bureau of Narcotics, Hearings on HR 10,561*, p. 57; see testimony of
    Alfred L. Tennyson, legal advisor to the Deputy Commissioner of Pro-
    hibition in charge of narcotic law enforcement; also p. 51.

Chapter 9

1 The following account of Commissioner Anslinger's career and the occasional quotations are based on my interview with him in Hollidaysburg, Pa., on 30 May, 1970; examination of his papers deposited in the Archives of Pennsylvania State University, University Park, Pa.; interviews with his associates and foes; as well as brief published accounts (*Current Biography*, 1948, pp. 20–22; Stanley Meisler, "Federal Narcotics Czar," *The Nation*, 20 Feb. 1960, pp. 159–62). Anslinger was the co-author of two melodramatic books on the narcotics traffic, *The Murderers: The Story of the Narcotic Gangs* (with Will Ousler, New York: Farrar, Straus and Cudahy, 1961), and *The Protectors* (with J. D. Gregory, New York: Farrar, Straus and Co., 1964). A somewhat more detailed study is his *Traffic in Narcotics* (with W. F. Tompkins, New York: Funk and Wagnalls, 1953).

2 Anslinger to Prize Committee on the 18th Amendment, New York City, 19 Nov. 1928 (AP, box 12).

3 Rep. John M. Coffee, "An Investigation of the Narcotic Evil," *Cong. Rec., House, 83, pt. 11* : 2299–3370, 75th Cong., 3rd Sess., 14 June 1938. Coffee demanded an investigation by the PHS of the extent of narcotics use in the U.S. and the FBN's mode of enforcement. No such investigation was authorized.

4 *Public Law 255*, 82nd Cong., 1st Sess., approved 2 Nov. 1951; *Public Law 728*, 84th Cong., 2nd Sess. approved 18 July 1956.

5 *Cong. Rec., House, 61, pt. 3* : 3113–14, 27 June 1921, 67th Cong., 1st Sess. Volk predicted increased drunkenness, insanity, criminality, and narcotic use as a result of Prohibition.

6 "The Referendum on the Use of Alcohol in the Practice of Medicine: Final Report," *JAMA 78* : 210–31 (1922); 37% of American physicians were polled (53,900); of these 58% replied and of the responders 83% were general physicians. To the basic questions, 51% said whiskey was necessary in the practice of medicine, 32% favored also the use of wine, and only 26% said beer was a necessity. To the question, "Should physicians be restricted in their prescription of alcohol?" 58% replied yes. A large number of physicians favored regulations like those under the Harrison law (217–18).

7 Arnold H. Taylor, *American Diplomacy and the Narcotics Traffic, 1900–1939* (Durham, N.C.: Duke Univ. Press, 1969), pp. 3–40.

8 *Pure Food and Drug Act* (1906), ch. 3915, sect. 8, 59th Cong., 1st Sess.

9 *Importation and Use of Opium*, Hearings before the Committee on Ways and Means, House, 61st Cong., 3rd Sess., 11 Jan. 1911, pp. 50, 75–78.

10 Ibid. 80.

11 *Importation and Use of Opium*, Hearings before the Committee on Ways and Means, House, 61st Cong., 3rd Sess., 14 Dec. 1919, p. 7.

12 Letter from H. J. Finger to Dr. Hamilton Wright, 2 July 1911 (WP, entry 39).

13   "International Opium Convention," *Amer. J. Internat. Law* 6 : 177–92 (1912).

14   "The Second Geneva Convention," reprinted in C. E. Terry and M. Pellens, *The Opium Problem* (New York: Bureau of Social Hygiene, 1928, reprint ed. Montclair, N.J.: Patterson Smith, 1970), pp. 945–61.

15   Dr. Oscar Dowling to Gov. John M. Parker, 21 Aug. 1920; and to Surgeon General Hugh S. Cumming, 25 Aug. 1920 (PHSR).

16   *Public Law No. 672,* 70th Cong., 2nd Sess., approved 19 Jan. 1929.

17   J. Samora, *Los Mojados: The Wetback Story* (Notre Dame, Ind.: Univ. of Notre Dame Press, 1969), pp. 38–46.

18   W. E. Safford, Economic Botanist, Bureau of Plant Industry, U.S. Dept. of Agriculture wrote: "There is a very pernicious habit-forming drug used by the lower class of Mexican in certain localities, the use of which the Mexican government is endeavoring to stamp out. This is *Cannabis indica,* the hashish of the Orient, in Mexico called marihuana. It has found its way into prisons and penitentiaries, sometimes mixed with tobacco, and has been the cause of several uprisings." ("Narcotics and Intoxicants Used by American Indians," typed memorandum prepared for the U.S. Indian Service, undated but accompanying letter to PHS dated 10 May 1921 [PHSR]).

19   A. E. Fossier, "The Marihuana Menace," *New Orleans Med. Surg. J.* 84 : 247–51 (1931).

20   P. S. Taylor, "More Bars against the Mexicans?" *Survey,* April 1930, p. 26.

21   N.Y. *Times,* 15 Sept. 1935.

22   W. Bromberg, "Marihuana Intoxication," *Amer. J. Psychiat.* 91 : 303–30 (1934).

23   E. Stanley, "Marihuana as a Developer of Criminals," *Amer. J. Police Sci.* 2 : 252 (1931).

24   "Report by the Government of the United States of America for the Calendar Year Ended December 31, 1931: On the Traffic in Opium and Other Dangerous Drugs," Federal Bureau of Narcotics (GPO, 1932), p. 51.

25   "Uniform State Narcotic Act," reprinted in W. B. Eldridge, *Narcotics and the Law,* 2nd ed. (Chicago: Univ. of Chicago Press, 1967), pp. 161–75.

26   N.Y. *Times,* 3 Jan. 1937.

27   *Sonzinsky v. U.S.,* 57 S. Ct. 554, decided 29 March 1937.

28   "Don't Be a 'Mugglehead'," Worcester (Mass.) *Telegraph,* 11 Oct. 1936.

29   Floyd K. Baskette to FBN, 4 Sept. 1936 (AP, box 6).

30   Confidential memorandum from Harry J. Anslinger to Asst. Secretary of the Treasury Stephen B. Gibbons, 1 Feb. 1936 (AP, box 12).

31   Taylor, *Narcotics Traffic,* p. 292.

32   Marihuana questionnaire filled out by Dr. Walter L. Treadway (AP, box 6).

33   Transcript of the conference on *Cannabis sativa,* held 14 Jan. 1937, in the Treasury Building (AP, box 6).

34 *Taxation of Marihuana,* Hearings before the Committee on Ways and Means, House, 27–30 April and 4 May 1937, 75th Cong., 1st Sess.

35 "Inter-state Narcotic Association," Bureau of Narcotics and Dangerous Drugs, FBN file 0145-18.

36 "Report . . . for 1938: On the Traffic in Opium," p. 49.

37 Mayor's Committee on Marihuana, *The Marihuana Problem in the City of New York* (Lancaster, Pa.: Cattell Press, 1944).

Chapter 10

1 National Commission on Marihuana and Drug Abuse, First Report, *Marihuana: a Signal of Misunderstanding* (GPO, 1972), chapter five, "Marihuana and Social Policy," pp. 127–67.

2 Opium Poppy Control Act of 1942, *Public Law 797,* 77th Cong., approved 11 Dec. 1942.

3 G. Piel, "Narcotics: War Has Brought Illicit Traffic to All-time Low but U.S. Treasury Fears Rising Post-war Addiction," *Life,* 19 July 1943, pp. 82–94. See also H. J. Anslinger and W. F. Tompkins, *Traffic in Narcotics* (New York: Funk and Wagnalls, 1953), p. 166.

4 H. J. Anslinger, "The Federal Narcotic Laws," *Food, Drug, and Cosmetic Law Journal 6* : 743–48 (1951).

5 *Public Law No. 255,* 82nd Cong., approved 2 Nov. 1951, known as the Boggs Act.

6 Anslinger's warnings were accepted by the Daniel's Subcommittee which investigated narcotics traffic in 1955. The Committee's final report, *The Illicit Narcotics Traffic* (Senate Rept. no. 1440, 84th Cong., 2nd Sess., 1956) stated that "subversion through drug addiction is an established aim of Communist China" and that American civilians and military were prime targets. See also H. J. Anslinger and J. D. Gregory, *The Protectors* (New York: Farrar, Straus and Co., 1961), p. 223; H. J. Anslinger and W. F. Tompkins, *Traffic in Narcotics,* pp. 69–116.

7 "Proceedings of the House of Delegates," *Annual Report of the American Bar Association 80* : 408–09 (1955).

8 See above, ch. 10, n. 6 for the subcommittee's report.

9 Narcotic Control Act of 1956, *Public Law 728,* 84th Cong., approved 18 July 1956.

10 "Report of the ABA Commission on Organized Crime," *Annual Report of the ABA 76* : 411–13 (1951).

11 "Report on Drug Addiction by the New York Academy of Medicine," *Bull. of the N.Y. Academy of Medicine 31* : 592–607 (Aug. 1955). An interesting comparison can be made with the Academy's recommendations of 1918 (*Med. Record 73* : 468, 16 March 1918).

12 ABA and AMA Joint Committee on Narcotic Drugs, *Drug Addiction: Crime or Disease* (Bloomington, Ind.: Indiana Univ. Press, 1961), introduction by A. R. Lindesmith, p. 11.

13 Ibid., Appendix B, Rufus King, "An Appraisal of International, British,

and Selected European Narcotic Drug Laws, Regulations, and Policies,"
pp. 121-55.

14   Ibid., Appendix A, Morris Ploscowe, "Some Basic Problems in Drug
     Addiction and Suggestions for Research," pp. 15-119.

15   Federal Bureau of Narcotics, *Narcotic Clinics in the United States* (GPO,
     1955). A similar one-sided report is contained in Anslinger and Tomp-
     kins, *Traffic in Narcotics,* pp. 195-206.

16   U.S. Bureau of the Budget, *The Budget of the U.S. Government, Fiscal
     Year 1969,* Appendix (GPO, 1968), pp. 445, 820.

17   *Message from the President: Mental Illness and Retardation,* House Doc.
     no. 58, 88th Cong., 1st Sess., 5 February 1963. President Kennedy relied
     on "the new knowledge and new drugs acquired in recent years which
     make it possible for most of the mentally ill to be successfully and
     quickly treated in their own communities and returned to a useful place
     in society" (p. 3).

18   For example, this comment by A. R. Lindesmith in 1947: "At first glance
     it might seem that [the British system] would make opiates more avail-
     able than they are now and lead to a spread of the habit. Further con-
     sideration reveals, however, that the opposite would be the case" (*Opiate
     Addiction* [Bloomington, Ind.: Principia Press, 1947], p. 205). By 1965
     the implication that addiction maintenance through physicians would re-
     duce the number of addicts is less clearly stated: "It is characteristic of
     Britain and apparently of virtually all countries with this type of pro-
     gram that the number of addicts is relatively low, that there are very
     few youthful users, and that addiction contributes little to the crime
     problem in proportion to the number of addicts. If a program of this sort
     contributes to creating these effects, it deserves more serious considera-
     tion than it has yet been given" (*The Addict and the Law* [New York:
     Vintage Books, 1965], p. 170).

19   "Drug Addiction" (London: H.M.S.O., 1965).

20   For a recent optimistic review on the rapidly changing British experi-
     ence see Edgar May, "Narcotics Addiction and Control in Great Britain,"
     in Drug Abuse Survey Project, *Dealing with Drug Abuse, A Report to
     the Ford Foundation* (New York: Praeger, 1972), chapter 7, pp. 345-94.

21   J. V. DeLong, "Treatment and Rehabilitation," *Dealing with Drug
     Abuse* . . . , pp. 173-254.

22   "Methadone Maintenance and Its Implication for Theories of Narcotic
     Addiction," in A. Wikler, ed., *The Addictive States* (Baltimore: Williams
     and Wilkins, 1968), p. 359.

23   *Proceedings of the White House Conference on Narcotic and Drug Abuse,
     Final Report,* Washington, D.C. (GPO, 1962).

24   *President's Advisory Commission on Narcotics and Drug Abuse, Final
     Report,* Washington, D.C. (GPO, 1963).

25   Drug Abuse Control Amendments of 1965, *Public Law 89-74,* 89th
     Cong., approved 15 July 1965.

26   Narcotic Addict Rehabilitation Act of 1966, *Public Law 89-273,* 89th
     Cong. approved 8 Nov. 1966.

27   Dennis A. Aronowitz, "Civil Commitment of Narcotic Addicts and Sen-

tencing for Narcotic Drug Offenses," Appendix D of The President's Commission on Law Enforcement and Administration of Justice, *Task Force Report: Narcotics and Drug Abuse, Annotations and Consultants' Papers*, Washington, D.C., (GPO, 1967), pp. 148–58.

28 Comprehensive Drug Abuse Prevention and Control Act of 1970, *Public Law 91–513*, 91st Cong., approved 27 Oct. 1970.

Chapter 12

1 T. Ramsaye, ed., *1947–1948 International Motion Picture Almanac* (New York: Quigley Publications, 1947), pp. 737–44.

2 Interview of 30 May 1970 at Hollidaysburg, Pennsylvania.

3 Bureau of the Census, *Statistical Abstract of the United States, 1981* (GPO, 1981), p. 31.

4 National Commission on Marihuana and Drug Abuse, *Marihuana: A Signal of Misunderstanding* (GPO, 1972), p. 106.

5 Op. cit., pp. 32–33.

6 Domestic Council Drug Abuse Task Force, *White Paper on Drug Abuse* (GPO, 1975), p. 15. Hepatitis has no direct relationship to the number of heroin users, but at the time, the rise in this disease was associated with spread of needle-injected drugs, a common mode of hepatitis transmission.

7 Drug Abuse Council, *The Facts about "Drug Abuse"* (New York: Free Press, 1980), p. 29. Budget figures for drug abuse cannot be precise because of overlap with other federal activities but are a useful guide to changes in emphasis and overall effort.

8 Vincent P. Dole and Marie Nyswander, "Rehabilitation of heroin addicts after blockade with methadone," *N.Y. State J. Med. 66* : 2011–17 (1966).

9 N.Y. *Times*, 9 Apr. 1972.

10 Drug Abuse Council, *Facts*, pp. 37 ff. and 79 ff.

11 Sibyl Cline, *Turkish Opium in Perspective* (Washington, D.C.: Drug Abuse Council, 1974).

12 Drug Abuse Council, *Facts*, p. 29.

13 John F. Holahan, "Economics of Heroin," in Drug Abuse Survey Project, *Dealing with Drug Abuse, A Report to the Ford Foundation* (New York: Praeger, 1972), p. 263.

14 Drug Abuse Council, *Facts*, p. 57.

15 See, for instance, the editorial in the N.Y. *Times*, "Police Terror," 2 July 1973. Also see the important series of articles on ODALE raids by Andrew H. Malcolm in the N.Y. *Times* during 1973.

16 N.Y. *Times*, 30 June 1973.

17 N.Y. *Times*, 22 May 1973.

18 Drug Abuse Council, *Facts*, p. 57.

19 Richard Nixon, "Rremarks on Signing the Drug Abuse Office and Treatment Act of 1972," 21 Mar. 1972, *Public Papers of the Presidents of the United States: Richard Nixon: Containing the Public Messages, Speeches, and Statements of the President, 1972* (GPO, 1974), pp. 451–57.

20   H. Wayne Morgan, *Drugs in America, A Social History, 1800–1980* (Syracuse, N.Y.: Syracuse Univ. Press, 1981), p. 154.

21   Lee N. Robins, *A Follow-up of Vietnam Drug Users*, SAODAP monograph series A, no. 1 (GPO, 1973).

22   Jerome H. Jaffe, "The Pitfalls of Promulgating Policy," *Pharmacologist* 15 : 53–59 (1973).

23   Strategy Council on Drug Abuse, *Federal Strategy for Drug Abuse and Drug Traffic Prevention, 1973* (GPO, 1973), pp. 75–76, 83.

24   See, for example, John N. Chappel, "Methadone and Chemotherapy in Drug Addiction—Genocidal or Lifesaving?" *J. Amer. Med. Assoc.* 228 : 725–28 (1974).

25   For a review of methadone's value and limits, see Joyce H. Lowinson, "Methadone Maintenance in Perspective," ch. 26 in Joyce H. Lowinson and Pedro Ruiz, eds., *Substance Abuse, Clinical Problems and Perspectives* (Baltimore, Md.: Williams & Wilkins, 1981), pp. 344–54.

26   Strategy Council on Drug Abuse, *Federal Strategy*, pp. 60, 62.

27   Virginia Berridge and Griffith Edwards, *Opium and the People, Opium Use in Nineteenth-Century England* (New York: St. Martin's Press, 1981), p. 113 ff.

28   National Commission on Marihuana and Drug Abuse, *Marihuana: Signal of Misunderstanding*, p. 151 ff.

29   N.Y. *Times,* 25 Mar. 1972.

30   National Commission on Marihuana and Drug Abuse, *Drug Use in America: Problem in Perspective* (GPO, 1973), pp. 462–81.

31   Drug Abuse Council, *Facts,* p. 45 ff.

32   Domestic Council Drug Abuse Task Force, *White Paper,* pp. 97–98.

33   Lloyd D. Johnston, Patrick M. O'Malley, and Jerald G. Bachman, *Drug Use Among American High School Students, College Students, and Other Young Adults: National Trends through 1986* (GPO, 1986), pp. 47, 114.

34   National Commission in Marihuana and Drug Abuse, *Drug Use in America,* pp. 218–19.

35   Ch. 1, n. 17, p. 401.

36   Peter G. Bourne, "The Great Cocaine Myth," *Drugs and Drug Abuse Education Newsletter* 5 : 5 (1974).

37   *Taxation of Marihuana,* hearings before the Committee on Ways and Means, House, 27–30 Apr. and 4 May 1937, 75th Cong., 1st Sess. (GPO, 1937), p. 36.

38   United States General Accounting Office, *Report: Gains Made in Control of Illegal Drugs, Yet the Drug Trade Flourishes* (GPO, 1979), p. 17.

39   Richard Nixon, "Remarks at the First National Treatment Alternatives to Street Crime Conference," 11 Sept. 1973, in *Public Papers of the Presidents: Richard Nixon: Containing the Public Messages, Speeches, and Statements of the Presidents, 1973* (GPO, 1975), p. 788.

40   See, for instance, Office of Legislative Research, State of Oregon, *Effects of the Oregon Laws Decriminalizing Possession and Use of Small Quantities of Marijuana,* 31 Dec. 1974.

41   *Decriminalization of Marihuana,* hearings before the Select Committee

on Narcotics Abuse and Control, 14–16 Mar. 1977, House, 95th Cong., 1st Sess. (GPO, 1977) p. 5.

42 "President's Message to the Congress on Drug Abuse," in Strategy Council on Drug Abuse, *Federal Strategy for Drug Abuse and Drug Traffic Prevention, 1979* (GPO, 1979), pp. 66–67.

43 Peter G. Bourne, "Statement before the Fifth Special Session of the United Nations Commission on Narcotic Drugs," press release, White House Press Office, 14 Feb. 1978.

44 Heroin Indicators Task Force, NIDA, *Heroin Indicators Trend Report—An Update* (GPO, 1979), p. 5.

45 Strategy Council on Drug Abuse, *Federal Strategy 1979*, p. 40.

46 Patrick Anderson, *High in America: The True Story behind NORML and the Politics of Marijuana* (New York: Viking Press, 1981), p. 190 ff.

47 Op. cit., p. 274 ff.

48 Ron Shaffer, "The Cocaine Incident," *Washington Post*, 21 July 1978.

49 Later nullified by PL 97–113, sect. 502 (29 Dec. 1981).

50 L. D. Johnston et al. *Drug Use*, p. 114.

51 L. D. Johnston, P. M. O'Malley, and J. G. Bachman, "Drug Use Among American High School Students," press release, University of Michigan, 23 Feb. 1987, p. 8.

52 Peggy Mann, *Marijuana Alert* (New York: McGraw-Hill, 1985), pp. 411–55.

53 Marsha Manatt, *Parents, Peers and Pot*, NIDA (GPO, 1979).

54 *Health Consequences of Marihuana Use*, hearings before the Subcommittee on Criminal Justice of the Committee on the Judiciary, Senate, 16–17 Jan. 1980 (GPO, 1980), p. 199.

55 Domestic Council Drug Abuse Task Force, *White Paper, 1975*, p. 101.

56 R. A. Lindblad, "A Review of the Concerned Parent Movement," *Bulletin on Narcotics* 35 : 41–52, p. 48.

57 Nancy Reagan, "We Must be Intolerant of Drug Use," *USA Today*, 8 Aug. 1986.

58 N.Y. *Times*, 10 Aug. 1986.

59 Lester Grinspoon and James B. Bakalar, "Drug Dependence: Non-Narcotic Agents," in H. I. Kaplan, A. M. Freedman, and B. J. Sadock, eds., *Comprehensive Textbook of Psychiatry*, 3rd ed. (Baltimore, Md.: William & Wilkins, 1980), pp. 1621–22.

60 The fate of the law remains uncertain. In January 1987 the Reagan Administration reduced in its proposed budget the funds requested, and the monies ultimately to be appropriated remain to be decided by Congress and the President.

61 Board on Mental Health and Behavioral Medicine, Institute of Medicine, *Research on Mental Illness and Addictive Disorders: Progress and Prospects* (Washington, D.D.: National Academy Press, 1984), p. 47 ff.

62 Eric J. Simon, "Recent Developments in the Biology of Opiates: Possible Relevance to Addiction," in J. Lowinson and P. Ruiz, *Substance Abuse*, pp. 45–56.

63 Charles P. O'Brien and Robert A. Greenstein, "Treatment Approaches:

Opiate Antagonists," in J. Lowinson and P. Ruiz, *Substance Abuse*, pp. 403–07.

64 Eugene Garfield, "Controversies over Opiate Receptor Research Typify Problems Facing Award Committees," *Current Contents*, no. 20, 14 May 1979, pp. 5–18.

65 M. S. Gold, D. E. Redmond, Jr., and H. D. Kleber, "Clonidine in Opiate Withdrawal," *Lancet* 1 : 929 (1978).

66 R. M. Bray et al., *Worldwide Survey of Alcohol and Non-medical Drug Use Among Military Personnel: 1985* (Research Triangle Park, N.C.: Research Triangle Institute, 1986).

67 "ACLU Denounces Drug Testing Recommendations of President's Commission on Organized Crime," *ACLU News*, 4 Mar. 1986.

68 Hugh J. Hansen, Samuel P. Caudill, and Joe Boone, "Crisis in Drug Testing, Results of CDC Blind Study," *J. Amer. Med. Assoc. 253* : 2382–87 (1985).

Index

Acetanilid, 17, 285n27

Acquired Immune Deficiency Syndrome (AIDS), ix, 274–77

Adams, Samuel Hopkins: attacks patent medicines, 10–11, 285n27

Addiction: increasing fear of, 5, 93–94, 103, 106, 107, 115, 149, 189–93, 232; theories of, 69, 75–79, 82–84, 307n23, 309n24, 309n27, 313n40; new concepts for control of, 230–43; reliability of figures for, 246; categories of, 281n13, 318n3. *See also* Maintenance clinics; Maintenance, institutionalized; Methadone maintenance; Towns-Lambert method

Adee, A. A., 39

Agricultural Appropriation Act of 1918, 327n28

Alamosa (Colo.) *Daily Courier:* asks for marihuana control, 223

Albany clinic, 151, 175, 178–80, 337n6

Albert, José, 27

Alcohol, 1, 7, 15, 245, 250; move for prohibition of, 6; controlled during World War I, 327n28; crime related to, 349n32. *See also* Prohibition

Alcoholism: as vice disease, 75; of World War I draftees, 323n62

Alcohol Tax Unit, 183, 208

Alexandria clinic, 15, 163–64, 167

Allbutt, Clifford: on addiction, 73–74

Allied Patriotic Societies, 220

AMA. *See* American Medical Association

Ambrose, Myles J., 258

American Association for Labor Legislation, 337n8

American Association of Pharmaceutical Chemists: opposes Harrison bill, 55; opposes heroin, 354n62

American Bar Association: opposes mandatory sentencing, 231–34

American China Development Company, 291n29

American Coalition, 220

American Druggist and Pharmaceutical Record, 48, 297n89

American Federation of Labor, 220

American Federation of Physicians, 338n16

American Medical Association, 55–56, 152, 183, 200, 337n8, 340n26; its growth, 13, 56–57; its restrictive policies, 57–58, 144, 184, 186, 213, 227–28, 300n13, 320n39, 348n24, 357n6; Bureau of Legislation, 57; Medicolegal Bureau, 57; its position on narcotic sales, 64; its clinic policy, 148, 167; works with ABA, 232–33; attacks patent medicines, 285n27; Council on Pharmacy and Chemistry, 286n35; Narcotic Committee, 309n27, 313n40, 315n41; *Opium Addiction,* 316n45

American Medical Society for the Study of Alcohol and Narcotics, 307n18

American Medicine, 168–69

American Pharmaceutical Association, 91; opposition to, 14; its restrictive policies, 14–21, 47, 54–55, 281n8, 286n35, 286n43, 300n13; Committee on Acquirement of the Drug Habit, 16, 19; its goal, 56; demands equality in restrictive legislation, 60; makes patent medicine surveys, 94

American Pharmaceutical Manufacturers Association, 285n34

American Psychiatric Association: opposes mandatory sentencing, 237

American Public Health Association, 97, 318n15, 347n12

Amphetamines, 213, 222, 236, 239

Andrews, Lincoln C., 188–89

Anslinger, Harry J., 192, 215, 238, 316n44, 359n6; on harassment, 185, 346n9; heads FBN, 207–10 passim, 212–13; his early career, 210–12; his Prohibition work, 211; his marihuana policies, 221–29 passim; favors mandatory sentencing, 230; his